COMMUNITY AS PARTNER:

Theory and Practice in Nursing

COMMUNITY AS PARTNER:

Theory and Practice in Nursing

Third Edition

Elizabeth T. Anderson, RN, DrPH, FAAN
Professor
Director
World Health Organization Collaborating Center for
  Nursing/Midwifery Development in Primary Health Care
University of Texas Medical Branch
School of Nursing
Galveston, TX

Judith McFarlane, RN, DrPH, FAAN
Parry Chair in Health Promotion and Disease Prevention
Texas Woman's University
College of Nursing
Houston, TX

With 13 Contributors

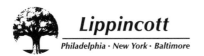

Lippincott
Philadelphia · New York · Baltimore

Sponsoring Editor: Margaret Zuccarini
Editorial Assistant: Hilarie M. Surrena
Project Editor: Debra Schiff
Senior Production Manager: Helen Ewan

Senior Production Coordinator: Nannette Winski
Design Coordinator: Carolyn O'Brien
Indexer: Lynne Mahan
Manufacturing Manager: William Alberti

3rd Edition

9 8 7 6 5 4 3

Library of Congress Cataloging-in-Publication Data
Anderson, Elizabeth T.
   Community as partner : theory and practice in nursing / Elizabeth T. Anderson, Judith McFarlane, with 13 contributors.—3rd ed.
     p. ; cm.
   Includes bibliographical references and index.
   ISBN 0-7817-2125-3
   1. Community health nursing. 2. Community health nursing—Case studies. I. McFarlane, Judith. II. Title.
   [DNLM: 1. Community Health Nursing. WY 106 A546ca 2000]
   RT98 .A533 2000
   610.73'43—dc21
                                                    00-021600

For inspiriting *Community as Partner*, we wish to acknowledge communities everywhere . . .

public health service areas;

rural villages;

shelters for battered women, the homeless, refugees, and migrants;

factories;

urban neighborhoods;

schools . . .

and the nurses who work in partnership with them.

Community as Partner: Theory and Practice in Nursing is dedicated to you.

CONTRIBUTORS

Elizabeth T. Anderson, RN, DrPH, FAAN
Professor
Director
World Health Organization Collaborating Center for
 Nursing/Midwifery Development in Primary Health Care
University of Texas Medical Branch
School of Nursing at Galveston
Galveston, Texas

Susan Scoville Baker, RN, PhD, CS
Associate Professor and Director
Canseco School of Nursing
Texas A&M International University
Laredo, TX

Judith C. Drew, RN, PhD
Associate Professor
University of Texas Medical Branch
School of Nursing and the Sealy Center on Aging
Galveston, TX

Beverly C. Flynn, RN, PhD, FAAN
Emeritus Professor
Emeritus Director of the Institute of Action Research
 for Community Health
Emeritus Head, World Health Organization Collaborating
 Center in Healthy Cities

Indiana University
School of Nursing
Indianapolis, IN

Nina Fredland, RN, MS
Assistant Professor
Texas Woman's University
College of Nursing
Houston, TX

Sally Gadow, PhD
Professor
University of Colorado
School of Nursing
Denver, CO

Janet Gottschalk, RN, DrPH, FAAN
Visiting Professor
Canseco School of Nursing
Texas A&M International University
Laredo, TX

Shirley Hutchinson, RN, DrPH
Associate Professor
Texas Woman's University
College of Nursing
Houston, TX

Charles Kemp, RN, MS, CRNH
Assistant Professor
Baylor University
School of Nursing
Dallas, TX

Bruce Leonard, RN, MSN, APN, NRC, CS
Doctoral Student
University of Texas Medical Branch
School of Nursing
Galveston, TX

Ann T. Malecha, RN, PhD
Assistant Professor of Nursing
Texas Woman's University
College of Nursing
Houston, TX

Judith McFarlane, RN, DrPH, FAAN
Parry Chair in Health Promotion and Disease Prevention
Texas Woman's University
College of Nursing
Houston, TX

Robert W. McFarlane, PhD
Consulting Ecologist
McFarlane & Associates
Houston, TX

Carole Schroeder, RH, PhD
Associate Professor
University of Washington
School of Nursing
Seattle, WA

Pamela Schultz, RN, MSN
Clinical Nurse Specialist, Research Investigator
University of Texas, MD Anderson Cancer Center
Doctoral Student
Texas Woman's University
College of Nursing
Houston, TX

Maija Selby-Harrington, RN, DrPh
Professor and Director of Research (retired)
University of North Carolina at Greensboro
School of Nursing
Greensboro, NC

Anita Tesh, BSN, MSN, EdD
Assistant Professor (formerly)
University of North Carolina at Greensboro
School of Nursing
Greensboro, NC

Mary Wainwright, RN, MSN
East Texas Area Health Education Center
Galveston, TX

Pam Willson, RN, PhD, FNP-C
Postdoctoral Research Associate
Texas Woman's University
Houston, TX

FOREWORD

In the 4 years since the publication of the second edition of *Community as Partner*, the world has been witness to unprecedented social, political, and economic changes. And, while the final balance of these changes is yet to be measured, it is safe to say that the outcomes will be good as well as ill. As we stand on the threshold of a new millennium, the nursing profession must be prepared to accomplish its mission in a world that is radically different than that which existed just a few years ago. Perhaps one of the greatest realizations of the latter part of the 20th century was the transnational nature of health care policy and the need to both understand as well as act on a global level.

As the nursing profession advances into this new world there are certain principles and procedures that must to be maintained while there are new relationships to explore. It is fair to state that *Community as Partner* effectively covers issues from both perspectives. This work continues to provide a sound foundation in the key methodological aspects of the profession as it currently exists. Yet, the third edition also provides important insights into numerous aspects of community health promotion—one of the central issues that will face health care professionals in the years ahead.

The nursing community in the United States and around the world has realized that community health promotion does not take place in a vacuum and if it is to be successful, partnerships within the community need to be promoted. *Community as Partner* offers us a useful discussion of key issues and the most important partnerships that need to be formed in order to promote the health and welfare of our communities. It is important to note that the subject matter covered is applicable to many societies, regardless of geography or economic system. Globally, the importance of primary health care cannot be overstated, and the relationship between this issue and partnerships with key groups within the community is of immense importance. Further, establishing strong partnership relations with the elderly, immigrant communities, schools, those in rural areas, and other vulnerable groups that might otherwise be disenfranchised is the responsibility of nursing practitioners throughout the world and is one of the greatest strengths of this text.

In *Nursing in Action* (Salvage 1993), the practice of nursing has been defined as: ". . . to help individuals, families, and groups to determine and achieve their physical, mental, and social potential, and to do so within the challenging context of the environment in which they live and work." As the issues facing our society and societies around the world become more complex, the role of the nurse will become both more important and more challenging. Nurses involved with health promotion and primary health care will increasingly have to take on many roles. In order to be effective, these nurses must be educators, social workers, managers, advocates, and politicians in addition to handling their traditional responsibilities. *Community as Partner*'s union of traditional nursing skills with the more contemporary concern of establishing strong working relations within the community makes this text appropriate for nurses working in any society. Further, the subject matter covered will remain important for years to come, and thus the relevance of this work will not diminish in the foreseeable future.

Julia R. Plotnick, RN, MPH
Assistant Surgeon General, Retired
United States Public Health Service

(Nursing in action: Strengthening nursing and midwifery for all. [1993]. In J. Salvage [Ed.], *WHO Regional Publications European Series, No. 48*, p 15.)

PREFACE

Building on an earlier edition in which the community was characterized as "client," we expanded our thinking and elaborated the community-as-*partner* concept as the basis for nursing practice in and for the community. This third edition expands this even a bit further as we have included two new chapters in the theoretical foundations section and illustrate the concept as well in the group of chapters that make up Part III. Key theoretical underpinnings of the nurse/community partnership are delineated and illustrated throughout this edition. The nursing process (assessment, analysis, planning, implementation, and evaluation) provides the framework for a real-life, step-by-step, community partnership.

Part I: Theoretical Foundations of Community as Partner

This section describes content areas basic to the practice of community health nursing. The areas encompassed include primary health care; epidemiology and demography; environment and ecology; cultural competence; health policy; empowerment and healing; and ethics, an advocacy approach. Emphasis is on theory-based practice, with those theories critical to community-as-partner described and explicated.

Part II: The Process of Community as Partner

This section begins with a model for practice in the community. The model and one sample community are used to apply each step of the nursing process to the practice of community health nursing. The student is guided through the processes of community assessment; data analysis; formulation of a community nursing diagnosis; and the planning, implementation, and evaluation of a community health promotion program. The emphasis throughout is on understanding the community as a dynamic system that is both more than the sum of its parts and in continual interaction with its environment.

Part III: Strategies for Health Promotion

Beginning with an overview of the diverse areas in which nurses promote health in the community, this section provides a number of examples where nurses played a major role as partners in the promotion of health. Communities/ aggregates included in this section are immigrants, schools, faith communities, homeless, workplace, elderly, rural, and the chronically ill.

Postscript

An editorial describing some of the roots of public health nursing is reproduced here as we enter the new millennium. It is included as both a reminder of our past as well as a beacon for our future.

Elizabeth T. Anderson, RN, DrPH, FAAN
Judith McFarlane, RN, DrPH, FAAN

ACKNOWLEDGMENTS

Our colleagues who contributed to this edition have enriched both the book and our lives. Along with our families they have sustained this process and helped us to feel proud of our profession.

Community as Partner: Theory and Practice in Nursing could not have been written without the thoughts, critiques, and examples provided by our students and colleagues in public health.

The fine folks at Lippincott Williams and Wilkins have facilitated the process of doing this third edition so that it was an enjoyable experience.

We thank each of you.

Elizabeth T. Anderson
Judith McFarlane

CONTENTS

CHAPTER   **22**

Promoting Healthy Partnerships With the
Chronically Ill / **402**

Pamela Schultz

THEORETICAL
FOUNDATIONS

Janet Gottschalk **and** Susan Scoville Baker

PRIMARY HEALTH CARE

OBJECTIVES

This chapter initiates the conceptual underpinning of community as partner. As such, it introduces the concept of primary health care, which is the foundation for work in the community.

After studying this chapter, you should be able to

- Describe primary health care.
- Describe the eight essential elements of primary health care.
- Analyze the impact of globalization on the health of communities.
- Evaluate multisectoral approaches to improve the community's health.
- Analyze the nurse's role in promoting health for all.

INTRODUCTION

Today, community health nurses and most community workers throughout the world base their practice on the concepts of partnership, collaboration, and empowerment. Together with others in their communities, they commit themselves to the attainment of health for all. Their goal is only achieved when the human rights of all, especially women, children, and those most marginalized and vulnerable, are promoted and protected. In other words, community health nurses direct their efforts to the achievement of social justice and equity for all. To achieve this goal, experienced community health nurses have long understood that any health-promotion efforts must be based within the broader socioeconomic contexts of people's local, regional, and even global issues and concerns.

In a time when national borders in their traditional sense continue to disappear and other barriers are being lifted, the interconnected nature of our world and its problems can be seen readily in the multiplicity of international, regional, and local efforts to solve these problems. At the same time, our world is much more politically unstable than it was during the Cold War, when identifying our "friends" and "enemies" was relatively easy. New forms of nationalism, ethnic identity, religious fundamentalism, and even fascism appear to be gaining ground and threatening people's earlier hopes for a "new" world based on peace and justice for all.

GLOBALIZATION

The same forces that are affecting political structures and their functioning around the world are also reshaping health issues, gradually transforming them from national and international concerns to *global* ones (Morgan & Mutalik, 1992). However, the major factor affecting our lives today and in the foreseeable future is the phenomenon known as *globalization*. It has been summarized as the "integration of capital, technology, and information across national borders, in a way that is creating a single global market and, to some degree, a global village" (Friedman, 1999). Most commonly understood in *economic* terms, globalization can seriously affect our daily lives whether we realize it or not. When global financial markets go up or down, when trade agreements are negotiated, when recessions threaten the countries that purchase the products made in our towns and communities, we and our communities can be in danger. When recessions or political instability occur in other countries, foreign companies often lower their prices to make their products more financially tempting. They are able to do this and still make a profit because the levels of local unemployment create conditions in which those competing for jobs are willing to work for less and less. When this happens over a period of time and is widespread, companies and factories, once considered sources of stable employment in our communities, frequently close their US operations and move to countries where salaries are lower and labor laws are weak or nonexistent. Anyone doubting this trend needs only to look at the labels on the clothes, electrical appliances, toys, food, flowers, and other merchandise in our local stores.

A major consequence of economic globalization and its emphasis on free trade, free financial markets, and economic profits is the nearly unbridled power and strength of international capital. Governments, especially those of resource-poor nations, find themselves losing the ability to define and control their own futures. Political scientists and sociologists warn us of the declining strength of the "nation state" and the questionable future of international organizations such as the United Nations (UN) and its related units such as the World Health Organization (WHO). If many of our countries are weakening in relation to powerful international forces, what does this mean for the development of our local communities? How are they affected by the emphasis on *profit*—usually for a few privileged individuals and companies?

Globalization, however, can have many positive consequences in our lives. New technologies bring almost instant communication with other parts of the world. A few years ago, Chinese students with access to fax machines were able to bypass government controls and alert the world about their democratic struggles. More recently, individuals and groups in Serbia and Kosovo with access to e-mail were able to be in constant communication with the rest of the world. Today, mobile phones, many connected to satellites, bring nearly instant access to previously remote areas. Cyberspace with its Internet listserves and chat rooms allows us to learn of other people's realities—their dreams, needs, and challenges. How can these same advances in technology and information be used by communities in their struggles for social justice and equity for all?

COMPETING GLOBAL FACTORS

Powerful positive forces are at work in our world today and should be of assistance to all those working with communities to achieve a more just society. They include a growing environmental consciousness and concern for the destruction of our present and future planet, an increased sensitivity to gender issues and the strength of the worldwide women's movement, a stronger commitment to the promotion and protection of human rights for all peoples, a widespread emphasis on democratic principles, and the nearly global recognition of the positive role civil society can and must play in the building of a more humane and peaceful world. All of these global movements contain forces that reinforce community health nursing's emphasis on working *with* communities—in partnerships, coalitions, and networks.

At the same time, equally strong competing forces are at work and frequently cause disastrous and divisive consequences for communities and nations. They include discrimination in all its forms; ethnic, tribal, and religious hatreds; radical fundamentalism; and violence of all kinds, including militarism. Unfortunately, the 20th century has been the bloodiest in history with two world wars and countless local and regional conflicts. The awful consequences of these hatreds were seen nightly on the world's television screens as genocide was committed in Rwanda, as violent conflicts uprooted millions throughout the world, and as landmines crippled or killed countless innocent civilians merely trying to grow food for themselves and their families. Thousands of refugees were filmed fleeing a *new* genocide in the former Yugoslavia. As more and more stories were told of beatings, forcible rapes, and the wanton destruction of lives and communities, the world watched in horror. Seemingly, all communities and nations contain within themselves the seeds of both good and evil.

How do these global realities affect our understanding of the concept of "health" at all levels locally, nationally, and globally? How should they influence our nursing practice in communities that have within them some of these same seeds?

FACTORS DIRECTLY AFFECTING HEALTH

As recently as 1991, Dr. Hiroshi Nakajima, who was then director general of WHO, identified some of the changes occurring in our understanding of health. He called the new components in the definition of health a "paradigm shift" (WHO, 1991). Up until 20 or 30 years ago, *health* was defined biologically and quantified in negative terms such as the absence of death, disease, and disability. However, during the past three decades, it has become evident that social, economic, and political issues are also essential determinants of a society's health. During this time, a strong link was identified between a society's health and its economic development, especially when the benefits of that development were equitably shared. More recently, a similar strong link has been suggested between a society's respect for human rights and its level of social and economic development depicted in Figure 1–1.

If current trends are any indication, the peoples and nations of the 21st century will continue to face many of the same health-related problems that we struggle with today: poverty, hunger, unemployment, homelessness, illiteracy, racism, sexism, ageism, environmental deterioration, militarism, and human

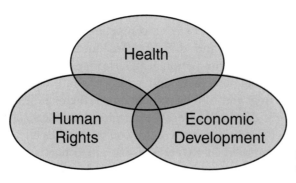

Figure 1–1. Community links to health.

rights violations of all kinds, from torture and death in conflict situations, to the lack of basic necessities such as food, housing, and health care.

Poverty and Growing Inequities

Much of the world, particularly the Western or industrialized parts, has in recent years benefited from economic globalization. However, as indicated above, these benefits have not been evenly distributed in our communities, our nations, or the world as a whole. The number of persons living in absolute poverty is now almost 1.3 billion, and 3 billion people do not have clean water. An estimated 130 million children don't go to school, and at least 40,000 children die daily because of hunger-related diseases (Sen & Wolfensohn, 1999). In addition to struggling with these enormous human needs, people in most resource-poor nations are responsible for huge amounts of debt incurred during the 1980s by previous governments. As a result, these nations spend more in interest payments on these debts than they do to provide the education, social welfare services, and health care so desperately needed by their citizens.

In countries such as the United States, with its emphasis on "privatization" of education and health care and concurrent attempts to move people from "welfare to work," economic globalization has often had similarly negative effects. Although political opinions differ, new data clearly indicate that people's health and well-being suffer the most when they are unable to secure appropriate employment and can no longer access adequate "social safety nets" and supportive services. In a study of results of the United States' emphasis on cutting the welfare rolls during the last years of the 20th century, NETWORK's Welfare Reform Watch Project found that (1) people's poverty was continuing while they received less government assistance, and (2) their suffering continued as their basic needs went unmet. During a time of supposedly unqualified prosperity, 35 million people were living in poverty and one quarter of all US children under the age of 6 lacked life's necessities (Thornton, 1999).

Wherever people live, poverty has been identified as a major cause of undernutrition and illness, thus undermining the efforts of health workers and health services. In cities and peri-urban slums, such as Benton Harbor, Michigan, with its 64.3% poverty rate or East St. Louis, Illinois, and Camden, New Jersey, with nearly similar poverty rates of 42% to approximately 43%, the poor are usually found in unsafe and overcrowded housing (US Department of Housing and Urban Development, 1999). In rural areas such as Mission or San Benito, Texas with poverty rates of nearly 39%, poor people often live in areas labeled "underserved," lacking sufficient health care personnel, facilities, and transportation needed for people to live healthy and productive lives. Whether at home or at work, the poor are often more exposed to pollution and other health risks than others. They frequently eat poorly, whether in quantity or in quality, and are more likely to smoke tobacco and be exposed to other harmful substances. Differences such as these are found not only in the United States but throughout the world. Global social indicators found in the *Human Development Report*, published annually by the United Nations Development Program (UNDP), "point to massive inequalities in income, employment, housing, security and health"(UNDP, 1998).

Demographic and Epidemiologic Changes

World health experts tell us that "increased life expectancy, lower birth rates, and a rise in noncommunicable diseases, combined with exposure to new threats, define the challenges for the future" (Pan American Journal of Public Health, 1998). Both the sheer increase in population in some countries and the high resource consumption in countries such as the United States are sources of grave concern to those struggling to meet the needs of future generations.

Many countries with very large populations have shown great progress in lowering their birth rates. However, the very size of their current populations means that, in absolute terms, their populations will continue to increase for many years. As large numbers of young people become sexually active, they, in turn, will place greater pressures on local health services, schools, and employers. In the United States, certain ethnic and cultural groups with young populations are presenting similar challenges to local education and social service systems.

Many of the poorest countries, those already heavily burdened by communicable diseases like human immunodeficiency virus/acquired immunodeficiency syndrome (HIV/AIDS), cholera, malaria, and tuberculosis, are facing a double challenge known as an *epidemiologic transition*. While these countries continue to struggle with problems caused by poverty and underdevelopment, they must also now cope with the new challenge of treating and controlling diseases such as cancer, heart disease, stroke, and diabetes—diseases formerly regarded as primarily restricted to the industrialized nations (WHO, 1993). Another factor adding to the burden on frequently overstretched health and social support systems is the increased number worldwide of elderly persons, many of whom suffer with disabilities and mental disorders.

Family structures and living arrangements are also changing rapidly in much of the world. Fewer people live in traditional family groups or extended family support networks. The stress that often results from these changes, as well as the growing disruption of traditional cultural patterns, is another factor adding to the erosion of social support systems and people's burden of disease.

Communicable Diseases, Malnutrition, and Maternal Mortality

Although great strides have been made in the control of many communicable and vaccine-preventable diseases, new and reemerging diseases such as HIV/AIDS and tuberculosis are a growing threat to global health. The consequences of living in a *global village*—trade, travel, urbanization, major movements of peoples displaced due to natural or human-made disasters, plus microbial evolution/antibiotic resistance—compound the problem.

Acute respiratory infections, diarrhea, malaria, and measles can be life threatening for malnourished children. Unfortunately, efforts to reduce malnutrition in many countries, especially those in Africa, have stagnated in recent years. Even today, almost a billion people do not have enough food to meet their minimum daily requirements for energy and protein, while more than 2 billion have micronutrient deficiencies (Pan American Journal of Public Health, 1998).

According to a study conducted during 1998 by the US Conference of Mayors, there was a 14% increase in requests for emergency food from families with children and a 6% increase from the elderly. Contrary to public opinion, 37% of the adults asking for assistance were employed, and in 92% of the cities, people relied on emergency food assistance not only in emergencies but over long periods of time. Unfortunately, the study found that an average of 21% of requests for emergency food went unmet. The most frequently cited causes of hunger were "low-paying jobs, high housing costs, unemployment and other employment-related problems, food stamp cuts, poverty or lack of income, low benefit levels in public assistance programs, and substance abuse" (Hartnagel, 1999).

Most women in countries such as the United States have little or no fear of dying in childbirth. However, at the end of the 20th century, only about 55% of the women in developing countries are assisted at delivery by a trained birth attendant, much less a physician. Although maternity should not be considered a disease, an estimated 600,000 women die each year from pregnancy-related causes. Another 50 million women suffer ill health and disabilities as a result of pregnancy (International Planned Parenthood Federation [IPPF], 1998).

The unmet needs of women during their entire life span, but most especially during their childbearing years, were emphasized in the *Programme of Action of the International Conference on Population and Development*, which states:

"All countries, with the support of all sections of the international community, must expand the provision of maternal health services in the context of primary health care"(United Nations, 1994).

Unfortunately, the gaps between the richest and the poorest people in our world—between countries and within countries—have been steadily increasing. According to James Gustave Spaeth, the recent administrator of the UN Development Program, the sad reality is that "expectations have gone global but the affluence has not" (Crossette, 1998).

Diseases of Modern Life

A diverse group of diseases and health conditions is emerging just as some traditional health problems are being brought under control. The vector-borne diseases, such as Lyme and hantavirus, have become widespread as wildlife habitats and suburban sprawl have become intertwined. Technologic advancement in the workplace has been accompanied by orthopedic conditions, such as carpal tunnel syndrome, caused by repeated stress. "Environmental allergies," particularly latex, are placing an increased cost burden on care providers and facilities (Phillips, 1999). As yet unquantified are the consequences of other lifestyle changes, such as long-term exposure to liquid crystal display (LCD) terminals and cellular telephones.

Noncommunicable diseases, many caused by unhealthy lifestyles, contribute significantly to the global burden of disease. If current trends continue, it is likely that tobacco use, high-fat diets, obesity, and related lifestyle risks will become the principal causes of death, disease, and disability by 2020. The solution to these and many other health problems of the 21st century will require broad-based *community health promotion* efforts.

Violence, Injuries, and Social Disintegration

Violence takes many forms and ranges from highly visible armed conflict to the many instances of women's physical and sexual abuse hidden behind closed doors in homes and neighborhoods. Thanks to modern technology, our entertainment media have long been able to produce extremely violent movie scenes and "games" in which the aim is to "kill." In the United States, with its rugged individualism, powerful groups such as the National Rifle Association have made easy access to guns a "right." Although it is very difficult to establish a cause-and-effect relationship between the number of guns available, the violence of the entertainment media, and the number of gun-related crimes committed by younger and younger persons, communities have become increasingly concerned about violence. They are also concerned about the weakening of human relationships—in families, between generations, and in communities—that often result in social disintegration.

PRIMARY HEALTH CARE

In their annual assessment of the world's health, delegates to the 28th World Health Assembly, meeting in Geneva, judged the current global situation to be both unhealthy and unjust (WH0, 1975). Numerous examples from different parts of the world convinced them that the use of an approach called *primary health care (PHC)* could contribute greatly to freeing all people from *avoidable* suffering, pain, disability, and death. They predicted that, if sufficient political will and commitment on the part of the global community could be guaranteed, much of the massive burden of unnecessary illness and death borne by millions throughout the world could be prevented through the use of PHC (Bryant, 1969; Newell, 1975). These predictions led them in a spirit of social justice to set in motion a new global revolution in health care.

Because of the global nature of the problem, a worldwide mobilization of personnel and resources was considered necessary. Two of the UN specialized agencies, WHO and the United Nations Children's Fund (UNICEF), began immediately to coordinate the world's effort to study and implement PHC on a global scale.

As with all UN conferences, initial preparatory meetings were held in many parts of the world to gather additional experiences and further refine the principles and basic elements of PHC. Although most of these meetings were held in what were then called the "developing," or poorer, nations of Asia, Africa, and Latin America, one meeting for the nations of the Western, or "industrialized," world was held in New York. At this conference, efforts were made to counter the belief that PHC was appropriate *only* for poor countries and not for the richer, more industrialized ones. A final preparatory meeting was held in Halifax, Nova Scotia, where nongovernmental organizations (NGOs), ranging from large, internationally active humanitarian organizations to small religious groups active in only one country, were able to review the final draft of the actual conference document.

After such extensive preparation, delegates from 134 nations of the world, plus representatives from those NGOs officially accredited by WHO, met during September 1978 in what was then known as Alma Ata, USSR (now Almaty,

Kazakhstan). In that historic meeting, the nations of the world committed themselves and their resources to the achievement of health for all by the year 2000 through PHC.

From the very beginning, *The Health for All* (HFA) era was based on the defining principles of social justice and equity. In Alma Ata, the original WHO definition of health, "a state of complete physical, mental, and social well-being and not merely the absence of disease" (WHO, 1975), was revised on the basis of the newer understanding of health and its many component parts. According to WHO, health was now to be defined as "a state of enough physical, mental, and social well-being to enable people to work productively and participate actively in the social and economic life of the community in which they live" (WHO, 1978). A major consequence of this new definition is that every nation is now challenged to provide a basic level of health for *all* its citizens so they are able to lead socially and economically productive lives.

As determined at Alma Ata, the principal means by which this level of health can be realized is primary health care, which was defined as follows:

Primary Health Care
- Is essential health care;
- Based on practical, scientifically sound, and socially acceptable methods and technology;
- Universally accessible to all in the community through their full participation;
- At an affordable cost; and
- Geared toward self-reliance and self-determination. (WHO, 1978)

Although PHC was conceived as a global strategy, the issues addressed and the solutions adopted should be country specific. In other words, HFA efforts should be conceptualized and utilized within national and local contexts. As explained in the original *Alma Ata Declaration*,

Primary Health Care
- Forms an integral part of both the health system and . . . the overall social and economic development of the community;
- Is the main focus and central function of the health system;
- Is the first level contact of people with the health system;
- Is health care as close as possible to where people live and work;
- Constitutes the first element of a continuing health process. (WHO, 1978)

Many of the concepts basic to PHC are familiar to community health practitioners: prevention, universal coverage and accessibility, affordability, teamwork, priority setting to address local problems, effective management, community participation, and cultural sensitivity. However, building on the delegates' new knowledge and understanding, four additional concepts were identified in Alma Ata as *essential* to the achievement of health for all:

• Maximum involvement of people in their own health care and the development of their self-reliance;
• Involvement and cooperation of persons and agencies from many sectors (including housing, employment, environment, education, safety and transportation, and communications);
• Use of scientifically sound technologies that are appropriate, acceptable, and affordable; and,
• Availability of essential medicines.

PHC shifts the emphasis of health care to the people themselves and their needs, reinforcing and strengthening their capacity to shape their own lives. Although hospitals and health centers will always be extremely important to people in their search for healthier lives, PHC is based on the principle that health begins where people live and work; that is, in their homes, schools, communities, and places of employment. Understood in its totality, PHC becomes not only a level of care but a philosophy and a strategy as well.

As a philosophy, PHC is based on the tenets of social justice, equity, and self-reliance. As a strategy, PHC focuses on individual community needs; maximizes the involvement of the community; includes all relevant sectors and agencies; and uses only health technologies that are accessible, acceptable, affordable, and appropriate. As a level of care, PHC is the one closest to the people; it relies on the maximum use of both lay and professional workers and includes a minimum of eight essential components, which will be discussed later in this chapter.

This shifting of emphasis away from dependence on health professionals and toward personal involvement, as well as the need for more than improved health and medical services, was echoed again in 1986 at another international conference in Ottawa, Canada. *The Ottawa Charter for Health Promotion* defined health promotion as "enabling people to increase control over and improve their health." Repeating many of the same concepts identified at Alma Ata, the Ottawa Charter stresses that the prerequisites to health promotion include "peace, shelter, education, food, income, a stable ecosystem, social justice, and equity" (WHO, 1986).

Although representatives from 134 nations signed the original Alma Ata document affirming their commitment to the goals of PHC, significant differences continue to arise over how the basic concepts of PHC should be put into practice in specific countries. In the United States, an affluent country, many policymakers believed until recently that they could afford to emphasize optimum functioning and a "high level of wellness." It has become evident that the technologies required for such high-level functioning may be excessively expensive and more than the present system can afford. In addition, many millions of people have no access to health care or health insurance, raising serious ethical questions regarding the maldistribution of health resources in the country. People are beginning to question the appropriateness of US health care priorities and the possible need to revise them.

THE EIGHT ESSENTIAL ELEMENTS OF PRIMARY HEALTH CARE

The eight elements essential to the PHC approach reflect the priorities identified in 1978 at Alma Ata (see display). Although applied differently around the world, they remain valid for all countries, at all levels of socioeconomic development.

1. *Education for the identification and prevention/control of prevailing health problems.*

    In countries like the United States, emphasis should be placed on health-related problems such as violence (homicide, suicide, domestic violence, and sexual exploitation), unhealthy lifestyles, growing numbers of elderly persons with special needs, substance abuse of all kinds, HIV/AIDS, tuberculosis, increasing homelessness, and environmental pollution. It was once

---

The Eight Essential Elements of Primary Health Care

In the globalized 21st century, community health nurses committed to PHC need to focus on:
Education for the identification and prevention/control of prevailing health problems
Proper food supplies and nutrition
Adequate supply of safe water and basic sanitation
Maternal and child care, including family planning
Immunization against the major infectious diseases; prevention and control of locally endemic diseases
Appropriate treatment of common diseases using appropriate technology
Promotion of mental health
Provision of essential drugs

thought that many of these problems were found only in poor communities among ethnic and racial minorities, but it is now clear that they are found at all levels of US society and in all neighborhoods, from the very rich to the very poor. Of course, the poor and those with limited resources suffer the most from the diseases of poverty—malnutrition, diarrhea, acute respiratory infections, and the vaccine-preventable diseases. It is a sad indictment of US social policies that some of the poorer communities in the United States have infant morbidity and mortality rates as high as the poorest, most underdeveloped countries in the world.

HIV/AIDS remains a serious health problem in the United States and throughout the world. In parts of Asia and Africa, HIV/AIDS and other sexually transmitted diseases (STDs) have become the major cause of death for many populations. This epidemic has overwhelmed their already overburdened health care facilities and caused many economic and social problems, especially in those countries without adequate social support systems.

In Nairobi, Kenya, for example, a community health nurse at work in a shanty town of more than 200,000 persons helped develop a community-based hospice and feeding program to meet the immediate needs of AIDS sufferers and their families. However, she soon found another urgent need caused by the large numbers of HIV/AIDS patients in the area. Many children (some as young as 8), finding themselves "heads of household" and unable to cope alone with their enormous physical, economic, and social responsibilities, began coming for help, particularly psychological support.

In all countries, the education required to identify and prevent the prevailing community health problems should extend to health professionals, who may know more about the diseases treated in secondary and tertiary health care facilities than the health-related problems in their communities. Alert and sensitive community health nurses will often uncover major "hidden" health problems and challenges by careful observation and by listening to community members.

2. *Proper food supplies and nutrition.*
   Because of the direct relationship between nutrition and illness, attention to the "food security" of communities is essential. Hunger in the United States is not due to inability to produce sufficient food. People are hungry because they are trapped in low-paying jobs, cannot afford adequate housing or child care, have mental health or addiction problems that make it difficult for them to hold jobs or care for their families, and suffer food stamp cuts and low benefit levels in public assistance programs. People also go hungry because they are recent or "illegal" immigrants to the United States and are trapped in marginal areas and occupations that pay inadequate wages and

rarely provide other benefits. Besides overt malnutrition, these same social and economic problems often cause micronutrient deficiencies and other hidden forms of malnutrition. In more affluent communities, malnutrition may result from unhealthy lifestyles, excessive consumption patterns of food and alcohol, and eating disorders such as anorexia and bulimia.

"Food security" has become a critical issue in many parts of the world where civil disturbances exacerbate existing problems of drought and underdevelopment. In many of the world's war-torn areas, food or the denial of food is used as a weapon specifically directed at civilian populations. One of the ways armies use this weapon is to put land mines in the agricultural fields of local farmers. Community health nurses throughout the world who see the connection between food security and land mines should be active in the international campaign to ban their use.

Few nurses routinely think of trade agreements, such as the North American Free Trade Agreement (NAFTA) between Canada, the United States and Mexico, as having any relationship to their community health practice. However, in the "globalized" world of the 21st century, trade agreements and organizations such as the World Trade Association will have a direct impact on world food production. It is projected that fewer and fewer companies will have control over the world's agriculture. This may endanger the world's environment as well as food security for its population now nearing 7 billion persons. Community health nurses, concerned about adequate food and proper nutrition, should be alert for developments in this area.

3. *Adequate supply of safe water and basic sanitation.*
    A safe water supply and clean disposal of wastes are essential to the health and well-being of any community, and, over the years, there have been many improvements in access to safe water and adequate sanitation. Nearly 2 billion people have gained access to safe water and 400 million people to basic sanitation in recent years. However, during this same decade and a half, many of these gains have bypassed the poor. Nearly 30% of the population of developing countries (1.3 billion people) do not have access to safe water and over 60% (2.5 billion people) lack basic sanitation. Excrement is routinely discharged directly into open ponds, rivers, ditches, and onto open ground, and more than 90% of waste water in the developing world remains untreated (UNDP, 1998).

    Water and sanitation problems are becoming more prominent even in the United States where they were thought to be long resolved. News of the inadequate disposal of toxic waste, nuclear by-products, and medical waste is routinely reported in the media. Unable, safely and locally, to dispose of the mountains of waste generated by our consumer societies, some countries (and individual states) are attempting to dump these wastes in poorer countries (or states) that have less stringent environmental regulations. As a result of this practice, additional health hazards are being added to economic and ecologic systems that are often already overburdened.

Areas such as those found along the 2,000-mile US–Mexican border have major environmental health problems related to industrial development in the region's fragile ecosystem. Rapid urbanization, caused by major movements of people seeking better lives, has placed new strains on already inadequate water treatment and human and toxic waste disposal facilities. Although the poor suffer most from these problems, many environmentally caused diseases respect no borders or social class and affect the whole community. Community health nurses in such areas, aware of the links between industrial development, trade, the environment, and health, see involvement in these and similar issues as an integral part of their practice.

4. *Maternal and child care, including family planning.*
   UNICEF has played a major role in alerting the Western world to the enormous burden of disease and death that is borne by the world's children. However, in spite of decades of concentrated efforts to address this problem, it is estimated that throughout the world 12 million children die each year of disease or malnutrition before their fifth birthday (UNDP, 1998). Ironically, the majority of these deaths could be prevented.

   It is equally tragic that, according to the IPPF (1998), an estimated 600,000 women worldwide die in pregnancy and childbirth each year. Another 50 million women suffer ill health and disabilities as a result of their pregnancies. Dr. M. Fathalla, an Egyptian professor and gynecologist, has written: "It is true that women in the North have almost forgotten what a maternal death is. But, for their sisters in the South, pregnancy and childbirth are still a dangerous journey from which many do not return" (IPPF, 1998).

   In the literature, a number of different terms will be found that refer to the poorer and richer countries of the world. Consider the implications of the contrasting terms listed in the displayed material.

   The voices of women throughout the world are becoming louder and louder as they demand increased respect for their rights as women (including their reproductive rights). In addition to highlighting the needs of their female children, who are often discriminated against from conception, women are also calling attention to the needs of their entire families for PHC. No one doubts improved maternal and child health (MCH) care is essential for healthier families. However, it is important to realize that education, employment opportunities, an end to gender discrimination, and

---

Terms of Reference

In the literature, a number of different terms will be found that refer to the poorer and richer countries of the world. Consider the implications of the following contrasting terms.

Poorer	Richer
Agrarian	Industrialized
Third World	First World
Developing	Developed
Underdeveloped	
East	West
South	North

---

the general empowerment of women may ultimately have more impact on women's and children's health status than specific MCH efforts. Women's groups and networks became a visible and vocal part of important international conferences such as the UN-sponsored Earth Summit held in Rio de Janeiro in 1992, the 1994 International Conference on Population and Development in Egypt, and the 1995 Women's Conference in Beijing. Since then, women continue to demand an end to gender discrimination and violence against women, recognition of their human rights, and access to health care across the life span for themselves and their children. Believing that health is a fundamental human right, women are further demanding that they be ensured access to adequate nutrition, clean water, sanitation, and shelter for all. They make this demand, recognizing that "living conditions to support good health involve far more than simply having access to health care" (Health Caucus Statement, 1999).

5. *Immunization against the major infectious diseases; prevention and control of locally endemic diseases.*

    Great strides have been made in immunizing the world's children against the six major vaccine-preventable diseases. UNICEF and WHO reported in 1993 that their campaign for universal immunization against these killers was reaching more than 80% of the world's children before their first birthday (UNICEF, 1993). However, even with such progress, millions continued to slip through the "safety net." Now that a new generation of vaccines has come on the market—vaccines capable of saving millions more children's lives each year—it should be possible to save many of these children. Unfortunately, though, these new vaccines are relatively costly and the commitment of the world to universal immunization seems to be weakening.

In recent years, brutal regional conflicts have added war trauma and increased exposure to infectious diseases to the health risks of children abandoned in the streets or gathered in refugee camps. We can see the desperate condition of child health worldwide in the faces of suffering children from Somalia, Sudan, and Rwanda or in the eyes of children traumatized by brutal "ethnic cleansing" in Bosnia and Kosovo.

It is a national disgrace that, even with local health departments' and schools' efforts, high immunization levels are rarely found among the poorer populations of the United States. Some sections of US cities have immunization levels similar to or lower than those of many of the poorest countries in the world (UNICEF, 1993). Wherever they live in the world, children have the right to protection from the preventable suffering and death caused by the major childhood diseases. When their lack of immunization is compounded by poverty, malnutrition, abuse, and locally endemic diseases (what UNICEF calls the "silent" emergencies), children have little hope of living "socially and economically productive lives" as adults. For example, poor children in Washington, DC, have little chance to live "productive lives" when child deaths in Washington, DC, rose 81% from 1985 to 1996, and in 1996, 40% of DC children lived in poverty; DC ranked 51st among the states in infant mortality; and DC had the highest percentage of low-birth-weight babies and the highest rates of teen deaths by accident, homicide, and suicide (*The Washington Post*, 1999).

In addressing the main health problems of a community's children, a PHC approach requires the provision of appropriate "promotive, preventive, curative, and rehabilitative services." Where and when this cannot be done locally, referral should be made to "integrated, functional, and mutually-supportive referral systems, leading to the progressive improvement of comprehensive care for all . . . giving priority to those most in need" (WHO, 1978). Hospitals and health professionals who work in tertiary care facilities have, unfortunately, often misunderstood their role in the provision of PHC. Secondary and tertiary care facilities, as well as more complex rehabilitative and long-term care facilities, have a critical role to play in the provision of PHC. Without adequate referral systems to all levels of care, PHC at the local level will ultimately fail (Aga Khan Foundation, 1982). In addition, effective management practices at all levels of the health care system are also critical for successful PHC.

6. *Appropriate treatment of common diseases using appropriate technology.*
Over and over again, community workers of all kinds have found that simple, affordable technologies, often produced locally, can be extremely effec-

tive in easing common health problems. "Technologies" can be as simple, yet scientifically sound, as oral dehydration solutions for diarrhea or orthopedic aids built of local materials to give mobility and independence to a community's disabled members. Other health workers and communities have found the use of herbal medicines and alternative healing methods as effective in the treatment of common illnesses as their more expensive counterparts (Health Action Information Network, 1992). Additional research is desperately needed in alternative healing, including acupuncture/acupressure, Ayurvedic, and "New Age" practices. Although such research is not currently viewed as equal in status to more traditional biomedical studies, it is gradually receiving more support and acceptance.

At all levels, the appropriate treatment of common diseases relies on the appropriate mix of health workers. The PHC health team may include not only physicians, nurses, midwives, and auxiliaries, but also community health workers (agents, promotoras de salud, and so on) and traditional practitioners (herbalists, curanderos, and shamans). When such nontraditional members are added to the health team, care should be exercised in their selection, training, and ongoing supervision. Whatever the makeup of the local health team, the goal should be to concentrate on the expressed needs of the community and to work with it in achieving its health-related goals.

7. *Promotion of mental health.*
   Although not included as an essential element of PHC in all countries, the promotion of mental health is extremely important for the well-being of any community. In the United States, recent developments in mental health and the care of the mentally ill have a profound impact on the overall health of the community. With the development of effective psychotropic medication and the civil rights movement in the 1960s, the philosophy of community mental health care turned from an institutional to community-based system. Heralded as a humanitarian revolution, mainstreaming and community care have placed tremendous burdens on local communities. Deinstitutionalization has led not to inclusion of the mentally ill into all facets of society but to an increased number of persons living marginal lives and requiring substantial public assistance. An estimated 50% of the homeless are mentally ill, many choosing a life on the streets to the restrictions or victimization of shelters or other group living arrangements. In 1999, a federal research agency reported that about 10% of total health care spending ($80 billion) goes to mental health treatment. One third of that amount addresses the severely mentally ill, a population group estimated at about 5 million people, many of them poor and unemployed as a result of their illness (Sharkey, 1999).

There is general consensus on the need to provide care for the seriously, persistently mentally ill. More controversial is the expenditure of two thirds of the $80 billion mental illness dollars on the stress-related conditions of the "worried well." Modern life can be extremely stressful and provoke mental difficulties. Parents struggle to work and care at the same time for aging parents and young children. Gender roles are changing, along with traditional family structures and cultural patterns. Working together with the community from a proactive stance, the PHC team should concentrate on those mental health problems that are of highest priority in and for the community. Assistance from and collaboration with many other disciplines and civic groups active in the broader community are usually crucial in such efforts. In communities where persons and groups have often been treated more like "objects than subjects" (Freire, 1982) and have become dependent on welfare systems, the involvement and mobilization of the community are necessary to lessen the burden of mental illness.

8. *Provision of essential drugs.*
   The WHO has long been convinced that adequate provision of essential drugs at a cost that the community can afford is critical to the success of PHC. Efforts to identify and permit the sale of only those drugs essential for a nation's PHC system have, however, met with great opposition from many in the pharmaceutical industry as well as from many health professionals. Appropriate treatment requires the provision of essential drugs that are safe and effective; of high quality; capable of being adequately supplied, stored, and distributed; and, of course, affordable. In addition to the provision of essential drugs, many countries are studying the use of herbal and other traditional medicines and treatments in PHC (leGrand & Wondergem, n.d.).

   To achieve this goal, the pharmaceutical industry, health professionals, communities, schools, universities, and governments must all collaborate and cooperate. An effective, cost-contained drug marketing and distribution policy has, fortunately, become reality in countries such as Uganda and Bangladesh, but not the United States. Broader attainment of this goal, like other goals of PHC, will require political will and commitment.

HEALTH FOR ALL THROUGH PRIMARY HEALTH CARE

PHC builds on traditional public health practices. However, its emphasis on community participation, a multisectoral approach, and the use of appropriate technologies adds new dimensions to community health efforts and brings additional challenges to all those who are involved.

Ten years after Alma Ata, a meeting of international health experts was held in Riga, Latvia, to evaluate the slow progress being made toward achieving the goal of "health for all by the year 2000." At this meeting, the ethical precepts, political imperatives, and technical directions identified at Alma Ata were reaffirmed, and the nations of the world once again committed themselves to achieving health for all. Since the Riga conference, however, the world has continued to change at a rapid pace. Political and economic realignments, social and demographic changes, and the continuation of armed conflicts with their disastrous health and environmental consequences have added a new urgency to the world's need for justice and equity. Four years later, at the UN's "Earth Summit," delegates realized that humanity was at a defining moment in history. In many parts of the world, they found a worsening of poverty, hunger, ill health and illiteracy and the continuing deterioration of the ecosystems on which the well-being of all depend (United Nations Conference on Environment and Development, 1992).

WHERE ARE WE TODAY?

Twenty years after the original conference in Alma Ata, another group met to look at what had happened to the potentially revolutionary Alma Ata Declaration that so optimistically promoted a multisectoral approach called primary health care, an approach based on equity and social justice, an approach in which people's perspectives are key factors in the global quest for health for all. Looking at some of the realities described above, they found that, for the poor in our world, the goal of health for all is still a distant dream. In fact, millions of people remain marginalized because the economically powerful of the world have chosen a model of development based almost exclusively on economic growth for the few with too little regard for the human and environmental costs of economic development (Werner, 1998). Even today, despite unprecedented economic growth for some, a growing disparity of wealth and power continues to breed joblessness, cutbacks in health and welfare services, anger, despair, and, all too often, violence and social unrest. "Those on the 'bottom' know that health is determined more by the fairness—or unfairness—of social structures than by medical or health services per se" (Werner & Sanders, 1998).

True or comprehensive PHC, especially in the United States, was never really attempted. Instead, "selective" PHC concentrated on a few "vertical, quick-fix technologies" targeted at high-risk groups such as children, teenage mothers, or low-birth-weight babies. The goal was to reduce mortality rates quickly, and programs planned by professionals needed the "community" only for "compliance" with their plans. Because of this "quick-fix" approach, underlying socioeconomic causes of poor health went basically unchallenged, and the health gap between rich and poor continued to widen.

Many years ago, the Institute of Medicine identified four factors considered absolutely necessary for the practice of good *primary care:* accessibility, comprehensiveness, coordination, and continuity. Such care emphasized comprehensive health care, professional attention by accountable providers, and the provision of personal health services at the primary level (Franks, Nutting & Clancy, 1993). This form of *primary* care does include some of the fundamental components of *primary health care*, as defined at Alma Ata. It does not, however, include public health services or environmental and occupational dimensions of health. It also depends on professionals, ignoring the assistance and/or participation of lay health workers. One of the greatest differences between *primary* care and *primary health care* is that a PHC approach considers the involvement of the community—with its multiple sectors and organizations—an essential ingredient in the achievement of health for all. Unfortunately, US nursing programs have been slow to incorporate a true PHC approach in their curricula to prepare nurses able to work as "partners" with community-based groups, networks, and coalitions. Today, however, many are following the strong urgings of the Pew Health Professions Commission to include PHC in nursing curricula at all levels (1993).

NURSES FOR THE 21ST CENTURY

On December 10, 1948, when much of the world was recovering from the horrors of World War II, the UN General Assembly, by unanimous vote, adopted *The Universal Declaration of Human Rights* (United Nations, 1948). In its 30 articles, the declaration outlined the basic conditions necessary for optimal health and well-being. Many articles refer to basic human rights to freedom and equality (Art. 1); life, liberty, and security of person (Art. 3); and the economic, social, and cultural rights indispensable for a person's dignity and the free development of one's personality (Art. 22). It is Article 25, though, that spells out all those human rights of critical importance to people committed to social justice and well-being for all. Article 25 could actually become a checklist to measure progress toward the achievement of health for all.

All people have the right to a standard of living adequate for the health and well-being of a person and of one's family, including food, clothing, housing, and medical care and necessary social services, and the right to security in the event of unemployment, sickness, disability, widowhood, old age, or other lack of livelihood in circumstances beyond one's control.

> Motherhood and childhood are entitled to special care and assistance. All children, whether born in or out of wedlock, shall enjoy the same social protection.
> Article 25, *The Universal Declaration of Human Rights*

To help make these rights a reality, nurses of the 21st century will stretch themselves and go far beyond traditional nursing practice in conventional medical and health services. They will join with "social activists, alternative economists, ecologists, grassroots organizers, progressive educators, and other agents of change, to advance a multisectoral strategy that puts the basic needs of all people—especially the disadvantaged—before the interests of the rich and powerful" (Werner, 1998).

Nurses will be advocates, monitors, catalysts, and enablers. They will be scientifically and technically skilled. They will be knowledgeable about economics, politics, and global issues. But, most of all, they will be *partners* with communities at local, regional, and national levels. The process of "enabling people to increase control over and to improve their health" will be an integral part of all nurses' roles. This new partnership, involving nurses, communities, and their environments, is a common search, based on personal choice and social responsibility, for a healthier future (Maglacas, 1988).

REFERENCES

Aga Khan Foundation. (1982). *The role of hospitals in primary health care*. Report of a conference held in Karachi, Pakistan, November 1981. Geneva, Switzerland: Author.

Bryant, J. (1996). *Health and the developing world*. Ithaca, NY: Cornell University Press.

Crossette, B. (1998, September 13). Most consuming more, and the rich much more. *The New York Times*.

Franks, P., Nutting, P., & Clancy, C. (1993). Health care reform, primary care, and the need for research. *Journal of the American Medical Association, 270*(12), 449–453.

Friedman, T.L. (1999). *The lexus and the olive tree. Understanding globalization*. New York: Farrar Straus Giraux.

Freire, P. (1982). *Pedagogy of the oppressed*. New York: Continuum Press.

Hartnagel, N. (1999, January 8). Reports say hunger still a struggle. *Catholic News Service*.

Health Action Information Network (HAIN). (1992, October). Traditional medical practitioners in the Philippines. *Health Alert #134*. Manila.

Health Caucus Statement. (1999, March 11). *Health is a fundamental right*. Statement to the United Nations Commission on the Status of Women.

International Planned Parenthood Federation (IPPF). (1998, April 7). Important background information [press release]. London.

leGrand, A. & Wondergem, P. (n.d.). *Herbal medicine and health promotion: A comparative study of herbal drugs in primary health care*. Amsterdam: Royal Tropical Institute.

Maglacas, A.M. (1988). Health for all: Nursing's role. *Nursing Outlook, 36*(2), 66–71.

Morgan, R.E. & Mutalik, G. (1992). *Bringing international health back home*. A policy paper for the 19th annual conference of the National Council for International Health, Washington, DC.

Newell, K.W. (Ed.). (1975). *Health by the people*. Geneva, Switzerland: World Health Organization.

Pan American Journal of Public Health. (1998, April 2). *Health for all in the twenty-first century* [condensed from WHO Document A51/5]. Washington, DC.

Pew Health Professions Commission. (1993). *Health professions education for the future: Schools in service to the nation.* San Francisco, CA: UCSF Center for Health Professions.

Phillips, D.F. (1999). New paradigms sought to explain occupational and environmental disease. *Journal of the American Medical Association, 281*(1), 22.

Sen, A. & Wolfensohn, J. (1999, May 16–30). A coin with many faces. *The Earth Times.* New York.

Sharkey, J. (1999, June 6). Mental illness hits the money trail. *The New York Times.*

Thornton, K. (1999, May/June). Poverty amid plenty. The unfinished business of welfare reform. *Network Connection.* Washington, DC.

United Nations. (1948). *The universal declaration of human rights.* New York: Author.

United Nations Children's Fund (UNICEF). (1998). *The state of the world's children 1998.* Oxford: Oxford University Press.

_____. (1993, July–September). Setting the water standard. *First Call for Children, 3.*

United Nations Conference on Environment and Development (UNCED). (1992). *Agenda 21 & Proceedings of "Earth Summit."* Rio de Janeiro, Brazil, 1992. New York: United Nations.

United Nations Development Program (UNDP). (1998). Human development report 1998. New York: Oxford University Press.

US Department of Housing & Urban Development (HUD). (1999). *Now is the time. Places left behind in the new economy.* Washington, DC.

Wealth and health [editorial]. (1999, May 18). *The Washington Post*, p. A22.

Werner, D. (1998). *Health & equity. Need for a people's perspective in the quest for world health.* Paper presented at the conference: PHC 21—Everybody's Business, November 27–28. Almaty, Kazakhstan.

Werner, D. & Sanders, D. (1998). *Questioning the solution: The politics of primary health care and child survival.* Palo Alto, CA: HealthWrights.

World Health Organization. (1998). *World health report.* Geneva, Switzerland: Author.

_____. (1993). *WHO director general calls for a new partnership on health* [press release] WHOA/4. Geneva, Switzerland: Author.

_____. (1986). *Ottawa charter for health promotion.* Developed at an International Conference on Health Promotion. Ottawa, Ontario, Canada: Author.

_____. (1978, September). *Report of the International Conference on Primary Health Care,* held in Alma Ata, USSR. Geneva, Switzerland: Author.

_____. (1975). *Official records, Twenty-Eighth World Health Assembly.* Geneva, Switzerland: Author.

Maija Selby-Harrington **and** Anita S. Tesh

EPIDEMIOLOGY, DEMOGRAPHY, AND COMMUNITY HEALTH

2

OBJECTIVES

To assess community health needs and to plan, implement, and evaluate programs to meet those needs, the community health professional must understand basic concepts in epidemiology and demography.

After studying this chapter, you should be able to

- Interpret and use basic epidemiologic, demographic, and statistical measures of community health.
- Apply principles of epidemiology and demography to your practice in community health.

INTRODUCTION

Epidemiology and demography are sciences for studying population health. To restore, maintain, and promote the health of populations, the community health professional integrates and applies concepts from these fields. In this chapter, we explore the meaning and usefulness of these concepts.

DEMOGRAPHY

Demography (literally, "writing about the people," from the Greek *demos* [people] and *graphos* [writing]) is the science of human populations and is concerned with population size, characteristics, and change. Examples of demographic studies (ie, demographic research) are descriptions and comparisons of populations according to such characteristics as age; race; sex; socioeconomic status; geographic distribution; and birth, death, marriage, and divorce patterns. Demographic studies often have health implications that may or may not be addressed by the investigators. The census of the US population is an example of a comprehensive descriptive demographic study that is conducted every 10 years.

Epidemiology ("the study of what is upon the people," from the Greek *logos* [study], *demos* [people], and *epi* [upon]) is the science of population health. Epidemiology investigates the characteristics, distribution, and determinants of health conditions. Epidemiology overlaps with demography. Epidemiologic studies sometimes take on the intrigue of detective stories as the investigators track the factors associated with illness and death. In fact, a number of novels concerning epidemiologic studies have become popular classics. (Try *The Black Death* [Cravens & Mair, 1977], *The Andromeda Strain* [Crichton, 1969], and *The Scourge* [Dunne, 1978].)

Early epidemiologic studies were concerned chiefly with the control of epidemics. (An epidemic is an outbreak of an illness beyond the levels expected in a population.) John Snow's study of a cholera epidemic in London in 1853 is a classic in epidemiologic history. At that time, the mode of transmission of cholera was unknown. Snow suspected it was spread by contaminated water. Applying epidemiologic principles, Snow determined that death rates from cholera were highest in areas served by two specific water pumping systems. He learned that the water from these systems came from portions of the Thames River in which London sewage was discharged. Thus, this early epidemiologist was able to identify a waterborne mode of transmission of cholera and determine measures to control its spread (Snow, 1936).

CONTEMPORARY COMMUNITY HEALTH AND PRACTICE

Today, advanced epidemiologic and demographic measures and research methods are used not only to study disorders such as food poisoning and acquired immunodeficiency syndrome (AIDS) but also to investigate environmental conditions, lifestyles, health-promotion strategies, and other factors that influence health. This chapter provides an introduction to epidemiologic and demographic concepts that are useful for the practice of community health. If you need more in-depth study, numerous textbooks are available (eg, Lilienfeld & Stolley, 1994; Mausner & Kramer, 1985).

LEVELS OF PREVENTION IN COMMUNITY HEALTH PRACTICE

The concept of prevention is a key component of modern community health practice. In popular terminology, prevention means warding off an event before it occurs. In community health practice, we consider three levels of prevention: primary, secondary, and tertiary.

Primary prevention involves true avoidance of an illness or adverse health condition through health-promotion activities and protective actions. Primary prevention encompasses a vast array of areas, including nutrition, hygiene, sanitation, immunization, environmental protection, and general health education, to name but a few. Research into the causes of health problems provides the basis for primary prevention. For example, just as Snow's 1853 investigation of cholera paved the way for provision of pure water to the residents of London, modern research into motor vehicle accidents has led to seat belts and air bags.

Secondary prevention is the early detection and treatment of adverse health conditions. Secondary prevention may result in the cure of illnesses that would be incurable at later stages, the prevention of complications and disability, and confinement of the spread of communicable diseases. An important component of secondary prevention is screening, the examination of asymptomatic people for disorders such as tuberculosis, diabetes, and hypertension.

Tertiary prevention is employed after diseases or events have already resulted in damage to individuals. The purpose of tertiary prevention is to limit disability and to rehabilitate or restore the affected people to their maximum possible capacities. Examples of tertiary prevention include provision of "meals on wheels" for the homebound, physical therapy services for stroke victims, and mental health counseling for rape victims.

To plan appropriate methods of primary, secondary, and tertiary prevention, the community health professional must first assess the health of the community. The following section covers some basic measures used in community health assessment.

DESCRIPTIVE MEASURES OF HEALTH

Demographic Measures

Certain human characteristics, or demographics, may be associated with wellness or illness. Age, race, sex, ethnicity, income, and educational level are important demographics that may affect health outcomes. For example, men are more likely than women to develop certain heart diseases, and blacks are more likely than whites to have low-birth-weight infants. To plan for the health of a community, a health professional must be familiar with the demographic characteristics of the community and with the health problems associated with those characteristics.

Morbidity and Mortality

Although epidemiology encompasses wellness as well as illness, wellness is difficult to measure. Therefore, many measures of "health" are expressed in terms of morbidity (illness) and mortality (death). An excellent source of morbidity and mortality data, by state and for select cities, is the Centers for Disease Control and Prevention, *Morbidity and Mortality Weekly Report* (Internet site www.cdc.gov/mmwr).

Incidence

The incidence of a disease or health condition refers to the number of persons in a population who develop the condition during a specified period of time. The calculation of incidence, therefore, generally requires that a population be followed over a period of time in what is called a prospective (forward-looking) study.

Prevalence

The prevalence of a disease or condition refers to the total number of persons in the population who have the condition at a particular time. Thus, prevalence may be calculated in a "one-shot" cross-sectional ("slice of time") or retrospective (backward-looking) study.

Interpretation of Incidence and Prevalence

Measures of incidence and prevalence provide different information and have different implications. For example, an increase in the prevalence of cancer means that there are more persons with cancer in the population. This may be because there are more new cases (in other words, increased incidence) or because persons with cancer are living longer. In either case, the community may need to direct resources toward cancer. However, if knowledge of incidence is lacking, it will be difficult to decide whether to target the resources toward primary prevention or toward secondary and tertiary treatment services.

Rates

Incidence and prevalence usually are expressed as mathematical measures called rates. Because epidemiology is the study of population health, these measures must relate the occurrence of a health condition to the population base. Rates do exactly this. They express a mathematical relationship in which the *numerator* is the number of persons experiencing the condition and the *denominator* is the *population at risk*, or the total number of persons who have the possibility of experiencing the condition.

Rates must not be confused with other proportions that do not use the population at risk as the denominator. For example, the death rate from cancer is not the same as the proportion of deaths from cancer. In each, the numerator is the number of deaths from cancer. However, the denominators differ. In the death rate, the denominator is all persons at risk of dying from cancer. Therefore, the cancer death rate is an expression of the risk of dying from cancer. In the proportion of deaths, also called *proportionate mortality*, the denominator is the total number of deaths from all causes. Therefore, the proportionate cancer mortality simply describes the proportion of deaths attributable to cancer.

Calculation of Rates

Rates are calculated in this general format:

$$\text{Rate} = \frac{\text{number of persons experiencing condition}}{\text{population at risk for experiencing condition}} \times K$$

K is a constant (usually 1,000 or 100,000) that allows the ratio, which may be a very small number, to be expressed in a meaningful way. Let us apply this formula to the calculation of the infant mortality rate, which estimates an infant's risk of dying during the first year of life.

Example of a Rate: The Infant Mortality Rate

The infant mortality rate (IMR) usually is calculated on a calendar-year basis. The number of infant deaths (deaths before the age of 1 year) during the year is divided by the number of live births (infants born alive) during the year. The numerator represents the number of infants experiencing the "condition" of dying in the first year of life, and the denominator represents the population of infants at risk for dying in the year.

If 4,084,000 live births and 34,400 infant deaths were reported for the United States for a given year, then we can calculate a rate. Applying the formula for a rate, we divide 34,400 by 4,084,000 and find that 0.0084 of the infants died during the first year of life. Because it is difficult to relate to 0.0084 of an infant, we multiply by a constant, in this case 1,000, and find that 8.4 infants per 1,000 live births died during the first year of life; that is, the infant mortality rate was 8.4 infant deaths per 1,000 live births.

Interpretation of Rates

Rates enable researchers to compare different populations in terms of health problems or conditions. To assess whether the population in a specific community is at greater or lesser risk for the problems or conditions, the rates for the community should be compared with rates from similar communities, from the state, or from the United States as a whole.

Some cautions must be taken in interpreting rates. Like most statistical measures, rates are less reliable when based on small numbers. This must be kept in mind when assessing relatively infrequent events or conditions, or communities with small populations.

Many rates are based on data from a calendar year, which may also present some difficulties. When calculating an infant mortality rate, be aware that some of the infants who die during a given calendar year, such as 2001, were actually born in 2000 and thus were not part of the 2001 population at risk, and some of the infants who were born in 2001 might die in 2002 and not be reflected in the 2001 infant mortality rate. Also, populations may increase or decrease during a calendar year. In such cases, the midyear population estimate is generally used because the population at risk cannot be determined exactly. A study that follows a *cohort*, or specified group, forward into time can help overcome the limitations of the conventionally calculated calendar-year rate.

Commonly Used Rates

Table 2–1 summarizes a number of important rates. Note that the measures of natality and mortality are, in essence, measures of incidence of the conditions of "being born" and "dying." Note also the various ways in which the denominator, or population at risk, is determined in different rates.

TABLE 2–1 ■ Commonly Used Rates

Measures of Natality

$$\text{Crude birth rate} = \frac{\text{Number of live births during time interval}}{\text{Estimated midinterval population}} \times 1000$$

$$\text{Fertility rate} = \frac{\text{Number of live births during time interval}}{\text{Number of women aged 15–44 at midinterval}} \times 1000$$

Measures of Morbidity and Mortality

$$\text{Incidence rate} = \frac{\text{Number of new cases of specified health conditions during time interval}}{\text{Estimated midinterval population at risk}} \times 1000$$

$$\text{Prevalence rate} = \frac{\text{Number of current cases of specified health condition at a given point in time}}{\text{Estimated population at risk at same point in time}} \times 1000$$

$$\text{Crude death rate} = \frac{\text{Number of deaths during time interval}}{\text{Estimated midinterval population}} \times 1000$$

$$\text{Specific death rate} = \frac{\text{Number of deaths in subgroup during time interval}}{\text{Estimated midinterval population of subgroup}} \times 1000$$

$$\text{Cause-specific death rate} = \frac{\text{Number of deaths from specified cause during time interval}}{\text{Estimated midinterval population}} \times 1000$$

$$\text{Infant mortality rate} = \frac{\text{Number of deaths of infants aged} < 1 \text{ year during time interval}}{\text{Total live births during time interval}} \times 1000$$

$$\text{Neonatal mortality rate} = \frac{\text{Number of deaths of infants aged} < 28 \text{ days during time interval}}{\text{Total live births during time interval}} \times 1000$$

$$\text{Postneonatal mortality rate} = \frac{\text{Number of deaths of infants aged} \geq 28 \text{ days but} < 1 \text{ year during time interval}}{\text{Total live births during time interval}} \times 1000$$

Crude, Specific, and Adjusted Rates

Rates that are computed for a population as a whole are called *crude rates*. Subgroups of a population may have differences that are not revealed by the crude rates. Rates that are calculated for subgroups are referred to as *specific rates*. Specific rates help identify groups at increased risk within the population and also facilitate comparisons between populations that have different demographic compositions. Most frequently, specific rates are computed according to demographic factors such as age, race, or sex.

In comparing populations with different distributions of a factor that is known to affect the health condition being studied, the use of *adjusted rates* may be advisable. An adjusted rate is a summary measure that statistically removes the effect of the difference in the distributions of that characteristic. In essence, adjustment produces an estimate of what the crude rate would be if the populations were identical in respect to the factor for which adjustment is made. A rate can be adjusted for age, race, sex, or any factor or combination of factors suspected of affecting the rate. Adjusted rates are helpful in making community comparisons, but they are imaginary rates and so must be interpreted with care.

ANALYTIC MEASURES OF HEALTH

As you have learned, rates are used to describe and compare the risks of dying, becoming ill, or developing other health conditions. It is also desirable to determine if health conditions are associated with, or related to, other factors. The related factors may point the way to preventive actions (eg, the linking of air pollution to health problems has led to environmental controls). To investigate potential relationships between health conditions and other factors, analytic measures of community health are required. In this section, three analytic measures will be discussed: *relative risk, odds ratio,* and *attributable risk.*

Relative Risk

To determine if a relationship or association exists between a health condition and a suspected factor, it is necessary to compare the risk of developing the health condition for the population exposed to the factor with the risk for the population not exposed to the factor. The relative risk (RR) does exactly this by expressing the ratio of the incidence rate of those exposed and those not exposed to the suspected factor:

$$RR = \frac{\text{incidence rate among those exposed}}{\text{incidence rate among those not exposed}}$$

The relative risk tells us whether the rate in the exposed population is higher than the rate in the nonexposed population and, if so, how many times higher it is. A high relative risk in the exposed population suggests that the factor is a *risk factor* in the development of the health condition.

Internal and External Risk Factors

The concept of relative risk is understood readily when one group of people clearly is exposed and another is not exposed to an external agent such as a virus, cigarette smoke, or an industrial pollutant. However, it may be confusing to see relative risks applied to internal factors such as age, race, or sex. Nevertheless, as can be seen in the next example, persons are also "exposed" to intrinsic factors that may carry as much risk as extrinsic ones.

Example of Relative Risk: Homicide

Sinauer, Bowling, Moracco, Runyan & Butts (1999) studied female homicide (termed *femicide*) over a 5-year period in North Carolina and found the overall homicide rate was 6.2 per 100,000. However, among young (age 15 to 33 years) black females (women exposed to the two intrinsic factors of age and race), the rate was 19.5 per 100,000 compared to 5.4 homicides per 100,000 for white women of the same age. With this information, we can calculate a relative risk. Among young black women (those "exposed" to the intrinsic condition of being black), the rate was 19.5 per 100,000, and among young white women (those "not exposed" to the condition of being black), the rate was 5.4 per 100,000. Thus, the relative risk of homicide for young black women compared to young white women can be calculated as follows:

$$RR = \frac{19.5 \text{ per } 100,000}{5.4 \text{ per } 100,000} = 3.61$$

In other words, the risk of dying from homicide was three and one half times greater for blacks than for whites. Clearly, race is a risk factor. The risk factor itself cannot be altered, but the information provided by this analysis can be used to plan protective services for the population at greatest risk.

Odds Ratio

Calculation of the relative risk is straightforward when incidence rates are available. Unfortunately, not all studies can be carried out prospectively as is required for the computation of incidence rates. In a retrospective study, the relative risk must be approximated by the *odds ratio*.

As shown in Table 2–2, the odds ratio is a simple mathematical ratio of the odds in favor of having a specific health condition when the suspected factor is present and the odds in favor of having the condition when the factor is absent. The odds of having the condition when the suspected factor is present is rep-

TABLE 2–2 ■ Crosstabulation for Calculation of Odds Ratio			
	Health Condition		
	Present	**Absent**	**Total**
Exposed to factor	a	b	$a + b$
Not exposed to factor	c	d	$c + d$
Total	$a + c$	$b + d$	$a + b + c + d$

resented by a/b in the table. The odds of having the condition when the factor is absent is c/d. The odds ratio is thus:

$$\frac{a/b}{c/d} = \frac{ad}{bc}$$

An example may help. When toxic shock syndrome (TSS), a severe illness involving high fever, vomiting, diarrhea, rash, and hypotension or shock, was first reported, it was neither practical nor ethical to consider cases only on a prospective basis. Therefore, existing cases were compared retrospectively with noncases, or controls. Early studies noted an association between TSS and tampon use and suggested that users of a specific brand of superabsorbent tampon might be at especially high risk. To clarify the issue, researchers analyzed data from TSS cases and controls, all of whom used tampons. Let's use the TSS data in Table 2–3 to calculate the odds ratio for users of the specific brand of tampon.

$$\text{odds ratio} = \frac{ad = 30\,(84)}{bc = 30\,(12)} = 7$$

Users of the specific brand were seven times more likely to develop TSS than were users of other brands. Based on this and other studies, the brand was voluntarily withdrawn from the market.

TABLE 2–3 ■ Toxic Shock Syndrome Cases Among 156 Tampon Users			
	Toxic Shock Syndrome		
Brand of Tampon Used	**Present**	**Absent**	**Total**
Suspected brand	30	30	60
Other brands	12	84	96
Total	42	114	156

(Data from Centers for Disease Control, 1980.)

Relative Risk and Odds Ratio: Caution in Interpretation

A word of caution: Regard a high odds ratio or relative risk with appropriate concern, but do not allow the finding to obscure the potential involvement of other factors. Refer to Table 2–3 again and note that 12 persons in the sample had TSS although they did not use the specific brand of tampon. In other words, this product was not the sole cause of TSS. Subsequent research showed that certain superabsorbent materials in tampons or certain aspects of tampon use foster growth of *Staphylococcus aureus*, the probable causal organism in TSS (Centers for Disease Control [CDC], 1983, 1981; Davis, Chesney, Ward, LaVenture, & the Investigation and Laboratory Team, 1980).

Attributable Risk and Attributable Risk Percent

Another measure of risk is *attributable risk* (AR), or the difference between the incidence rates for those exposed and those not exposed to the risk factor. This measure estimates the excess risk attributable to the factor being studied. It shows the potential reduction in the overall incidence rate if the factor could be eliminated:

$$AR = \frac{\text{incidence rate in exposed group } minus \text{ incidence}}{\text{rate in nonexposed group}}$$

AR usually is further quantified into attributable risk percent:

$$\frac{\text{attributable risk}}{\text{incidence rate in exposed group}} \times 100$$

This provides an estimate of the percentage of occurrences of the health condition that could be prevented if the risk factor were eliminated. For example, studies of the relation between physical inactivity and mortality from coronary heart disease (CHD) showed that the attributable risk associated with physical inactivity was 35% (CDC, 1993). Thus, improved physical activity has the potential to greatly reduce CHD mortality.

Cause and Association

Ultimately, community health professionals hope to determine causes of health conditions so steps can be taken to improve health. In view of the complexity of the human body and human behavior, establishing causality is very difficult.

Therefore, investigations of population health generally examine relationships or *associations* between variables. The *variables* are the characteristics or phenomena (such as age, occupation, or physical exercise) and the health conditions (such as heart disease) being studied.

Variables and Constants

An important requirement in any study is that the factors studied must have the potential to vary from person to person. If a factor cannot vary, it is not a variable but a *constant*. It is impossible to establish an association between a constant and a variable because the constant, by definition, cannot change when the variable changes. Thus, a study that looks only at men cannot establish an association between gender and, for example, heart disease; the study has made gender a constant. A study that looks only at persons with heart disease cannot establish an association between heart disease and any other variable; heart disease has become a constant in the study.

Control or Comparison Groups

To ensure that associations between variables can be examined, *control groups* or *comparison groups* may be needed. A study of heart disease might compare persons with the disease with a control group of persons without the disease. An investigation of a new treatment would study persons who receive the treatment and a control group of persons who do not receive the treatment.

Independent and Dependent Variables

Frequently variables are referred to as *dependent* or *independent*. The dependent variable is the outcome or result that the investigator is studying. It is a characteristic that conceivably could be altered (eg, health status, knowledge, or behavior). The independent variable is the presumed "cause" of or contributor to variation in the dependent variable. For example, in the heart disease study cited earlier (CDC, 1993), physical inactivity, the independent variable, is seen to contribute to heart disease, the dependent variable. An independent variable may be a naturally occurring event or phenomenon such as level of usual physical activity, exposure to ultraviolet radiation, or type of employment, or it might be a planned intervention such as an exercise regimen, a medical treatment, or an educational program. An independent variable might also be an intrinsic quality such as age, race, or sex. (Note that these intrinsic qualities, although they cannot vary within an individual, can vary from person to person; thus, they can be studied as independent variables.)

Confounding Variables

When an association is identified between variables, it is tempting—but incorrect—to assume that one variable causes the other. If, for example, a study found that communities with lower salaries for public health workers had higher crime rates, we could not conclude that low public health salaries lead to high crime rates. Common sense suggests that economic conditions might influence both salaries and crime; that is, economic conditions intervene in the study and confound the results. Any factor that may influence a study's results is referred to as an extraneous, intervening, or confounding variable.

Criteria for Determining Causation

If an association is found between variables, it means the variables tend to occur or change together, but it does not prove that one variable causes the other. Because of the possibility of confounded results, very strict criteria for determining causation have been established. An association must be evaluated against all of these criteria; the more criteria that are met, the more likely it is that the association is causal. However, an association may meet all the criteria for causation and later be shown to be spurious because of factors that were not known at the time the study was done. For this reason, investigators must interpret their results with great caution; they rarely consider a cause "proven." Six widely used criteria for evaluating causation are listed below.

1. *The association is strong.*
   The strength of the relationship may be evaluated statistically by a variety of measures. For example, the higher the relative risk or odds ratio, the stronger the association.

2. *The association is consistent.*
   The same association must be found repeatedly in other studies, in other settings, and with other methods.

3. *The association is temporally correct.*
   The hypothesized cause of the health condition must occur before the onset of the condition.

4. *The association is specific.*
   The hypothesized cause should be associated with relatively few health conditions. For example, speaking English may be associated with many health conditions, but it is a cause for none. This criterion must be tempered

by the knowledge that certain factors, such as cigarette smoking, have been shown to have multiple effects.

5. *The association cannot be explained as being the result of a confounding variable.* Not all potential intervening variables can be explored, of course, but alternate explanations for the association must be examined carefully before considering an association to be causal.

6. *The association is plausible and consistent with current knowledge.* An association that contradicts current scientific views must be evaluated very carefully. However, associations may be inconsistent with current knowledge simply because current knowledge is not as advanced as a new discovery.

SOURCES OF COMMUNITY HEALTH DATA

To be an effective community health professional, you will also need to interpret and use data from various sources. In this section, we review the use of several important sources of data.

Census

The census is probably the most comprehensive source of health-related data for the United States. Every 10 years, the Bureau of the Census enumerates the US population and surveys it for basic demographics such as age, race, and sex as well as numerous other factors such as employment, income, migration, and education. Only a limited number of questions are asked of the entire population. More detailed surveys are taken of selected samples of the population.

Census data are available in many public libraries. The Census of the Population addresses the entire census. Special *Subject Reports* (eg, on Hispanic populations) also are published. In noncensus years, segments of the population are surveyed to monitor ongoing demographic trends. These are published as *Current Population Reports*.

Although census data are comprehensive, bias does occur. For example, people may answer personal questions dishonestly. Perhaps more significantly, the census is believed to underrepresent low-income residents, minorities, and transients. These people are more difficult to locate and enumerate and tend to be less likely to respond to census surveys.

Vital Statistics

Vital statistics are the data on legally registered events (such as births, deaths, marriages, and divorces) collected on an ongoing basis by government agencies. State health departments usually publish vital statistics annually. The US Public Health Service also gathers data from the states and publishes annual volumes as well as periodic reports on specific topics.

Beginning researchers tend to consider vital statistics "hallowed" because they are, after all, legal data. However, legality does not guarantee validity. For example, a person's race sometimes differs on birth and death certificates, and the manner in which cause of death is recorded on death certificates is inconsistent. The numbers of unmarried but cohabitating couples—and the occasional news reports of newly discovered bigamists—also demonstrate that marriage and divorce records are also not completely valid measures of reality. Despite their limitations, vital statistics are often the best available data and much useful information can be gained from them.

Notifiable Disease Reports

The Centers for Disease Control and Prevention of the US Public Health Service reports data collected by state and local health departments on legally reportable diseases and also periodically requests voluntary reporting of non-notifiable health conditions of special interest. The CDC weekly publication, *Morbidity and Mortality Weekly Report (MMWR)*, is valuable for community health practice.

Even legally mandated disease reports may not be representative of all cases of the disease. Thus, they may not provide valid descriptions of the disease as it exists in the community. In practice, health care providers may fail to report diseases that should be reported.

Medical and Hospital Records

Medical and hospital records are used extensively in community health research. These records, however, do not provide a completely representative or valid picture of community health. In the first place, not all clients with health problems receive medical attention, so medical records are obviously biased. Second, medical documentation is not always complete. Finally, hospitalized patients are also more likely to have another illness along with the one being studied. This phenomenon, called *Berkson's bias*, creates the likelihood of finding a false association between the two illnesses.

Autopsy Records

Autopsy records have a very severe inherent bias: The patients were so sick that they died. Autopsies are not performed for all deaths. Autopsy records include a disproportionate number of cases of violent death and persons for whom the cause of death was unknown until after autopsy (eg, the manifestation of the illness was unusual). Religious groups that do not sanction autopsy are underrepresented. These factors influence the validity and representativeness of the findings of any study using autopsy records.

SCREENING FOR HEALTH CONDITIONS

Thus far, we have focused on methods for studying community health problems and assessing health risks for populations. In this section, we discuss *screening*, a method of secondary prevention. Screening is an effort to detect unrecognized or preclinical illness among individuals. Screening tests are not intended to be diagnostic. Their purpose is to rapidly and economically identify persons who have a high probability of having (or developing) a particular illness so they can be referred for definitive diagnosis and treatment.

Considerations in Deciding to Screen

Screening goes further than identifying groups at risk for illness; it identifies *individuals* who may actually have an illness. Screening carries an ethical commitment to continue working with these individuals and provide them access to diagnostic and treatment services. In general, screening should be conducted only if

- Early diagnosis and treatment can favorably alter the course of the illness
- Definitive diagnosis and treatment facilities are available, either through the screening agency or through referral
- The group being screened is at risk for the illness (in other words, the group is likely to have a high prevalence of the illness)
- The screening procedures are reliable and valid

Screening Test Reliability and Validity

Reliability refers to the consistency or repeatability of test results; *validity* refers to the ability of the test to measure what it is supposed to measure. A few considerations specific to screening tests are discussed below.

Screening Test Reliability

A reliable screening test yields the same result even when administered by different screeners. Training for all screening personnel in use of the test is essential. Lack of reliability may suggest that the screeners are administering the test in an inconsistent manner.

Screening Test Validity: Sensitivity and Specificity

To be valid, a screening test must distinguish correctly between those individuals who have the condition and those who do not. This is measured by the test's sensitivity and specificity, as shown in Table 2–4.

Sensitivity is the ability to correctly identify individuals who have the disease; that is, to call a true positive "positive." A test with high sensitivity will have few false negatives.

TABLE 2–4 ■ Sensitivity and Specificity of a Screening Test

	Reality	
Screening Test Results	**Diseased**	**Not Diseased**
Positive	True positive	False positive
Negative	False negative	True negative
Total	Total diseased	Total not diseased

$$\text{Sensitivity (true positive rate)} = \frac{\text{True positives}}{\text{Total diseased}}$$

$$\text{Specificity (true negative rate)} = \frac{\text{True negatives}}{\text{Total not diseased}}$$

$$\text{False negative rate} = \frac{\text{False negatives}}{\text{Total diseased}} \quad or \quad 1 - \text{Sensitivity}$$

$$\text{False positive rate} = \frac{\text{False positives}}{\text{Total not diseased}} \quad or \quad 1 - \text{Sensitivity}$$

Specificity is the ability to correctly identify individuals who do not have the disease, or to call a *true negative* "negative." A test with high specificity has few *false positives*.

Relationship Between Sensitivity and Specificity

Ideally, a screening test's sensitivity and specificity should be 100%; in practice, however, screening tests vary in this regard. As shown in Table 2–4, *sensitivity*, or the *true positive rate*, is the complement of the *false negative rate*, and *specificity*, or the *true negative rate*, is the complement of the *false positive rate*. Thus, as sensitivity increases, specificity decreases. Therefore, decisions regarding screening test validity may require uncomfortable compromises, as you will see from the following examples.

Decision Making in Screening: Practical and Ethical Considerations

Suppose you are screening for a deadly disease that is curable only if detected early and you have a choice between a test with high sensitivity and low specificity or one with high specificity and low sensitivity. To save the most lives, you need high sensitivity; that is, a low rate of false negatives (people who have the disease but are not detected by the screening test). However, if you select the test with high sensitivity, its low specificity means that you will have a high rate of false positives (people who do not have the disease but whom the test identifies as having it). That is, you will alarm many people needlessly and will cause unnecessary expenses by overreferring them for nonexistent disease. Which test would you choose?

Now, suppose you are screening for the same disease, but the diagnostic and treatment facilities in the community are already overloaded, and further budget cuts are projected. To minimize unnecessary referrals of false positives, you would want the test with high specificity. However, because of the low sensitivity of this test, you will have to weigh the benefits of a low false positive rate against the ethics of a high false negative rate. Is it justifiable to lull the undetected diseased persons into a false—and potentially fatal—sense of security? Which test would you choose now?

Decisions regarding screening involve seeking the most favorable balance of sensitivity and specificity. Sometimes, sensitivity and specificity can be improved by adjusting the screening process (eg, adding another test or changing the level at which the test is considered positive). At other times, evaluating sensitivity and specificity may result in a decision not to conduct a screening program because the economic costs of overreferral or the ethical considerations of underreferral outweigh the usefulness of screening. An understanding of the principles discussed in this section will help you make informed decisions regarding community screening. You also are encouraged to pursue further study regarding screening.

EPIDEMIOLOGIC APPROACHES TO COMMUNITY HEALTH RESEARCH

In studying the determinants of population health, investigators may be guided by epidemiologic models. This section describes three models and explains how each might guide the approach to the same problem.

The problem to be considered is an increase in the infant mortality rate in a hypothetical community. The infant mortality rate is a particularly important health index that should be understood even by health professionals whose main concern is not maternal or child health. Because infant mortality is influenced by a variety of biologic and environmental factors affecting the infant and mother, the infant mortality rate is both a direct measure of infant health and an indirect measure of community health as a whole.

The Epidemiologic Triangle

The *epidemiologic triangle* or *agent–host–environment model* is a traditional view of health and disease, developed when epidemiology was concerned chiefly with communicable disease. As you will see, however, the model is applicable to other health conditions as well. In the model, the *agent* is an organism capable of causing disease. The *host* is the population at risk for developing the disease. The *environment* is a combination of physical, biologic, and social factors that surround and influence both the agent and the host. According to this model, health and illness can be understood by examining characteristics of, changes in, and interactions among the agent, host, and environment.

Figure 2–1 shows the triangle in its normal state of equilibrium. Equilibrium does not signify optimum health but simply the usual pattern of illness and health in a population. Any change in one of the sides (agent, host, or environment) will result in disequilibrium, in other words, a change in the usual pattern.

How would this model guide the investigation of increased infant mortality? To understand this, let us consider the three facets of the model.

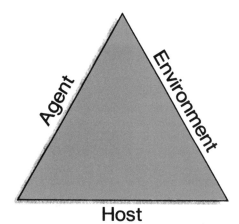

Figure 2–1. The epidemiologic triangle is the traditional view, showing health and disease as a composite state of three variables.

Agent

At first glance, it might be concluded that the investigation should focus on types of infections as agents that cause infant deaths. However, major causes of infant mortality in the United States include prematurity and low birth weight, birth injuries, congenital malformations, sudden infant death syndrome (SIDS), accidents, and homicides. Therefore, the investigation will try to determine whether there has been a change in any of these other agents.

Host

The investigators also will want to know the characteristics of the host; that is, the infant population. This involves examining infant birth and death patterns in terms of age, ethnicity, sex, and birth weight. These characteristics have been shown to be important risk factors for infant mortality. By studying these factors, it may be possible to identify groups of infants who are at particularly increased risk of dying.

Environment

Finally, the environment must be assessed. The mother is a significant part of the infant's prenatal and postnatal environment. Therefore, the investigators will analyze birth and infant mortality patterns according to factors such as maternal age, ethnicity, parity (number of previous live births), prenatal care, and education or socioeconomic status. Analysis of these factors, which have also been shown to be related to infant mortality, will help provide further identification of at-risk groups. Other conditions in the environment also need to be considered. For instance, has migration into the community from other areas increased? Has adult morbidity or mortality, particularly among pregnant women, increased? Have there been changes in health services, policies, personnel, funding, or other factors that could affect infant health?

Practical Application

The analysis of these three areas—the agent, host, and environment—should provide information regarding groups at risk for increased infant mortality and may point the way toward a program aimed at reducing that risk. Thus, the epidemiologic triangle, although it was designed with a communicable disease orientation, can provide a useful guide for studying the multifaceted problem of infant mortality, as well as other health problems.

The Person–Place–Time Model

An approach similar to the epidemiologic triangle is one that guides the investigators to consider the health problem in terms of person, place, and time (Mausner & Kramer, 1985). The investigators examine characteristics of the persons affected (the host in the triangle model), the place (environment) or location, and the time period involved (which could relate to the agent, host, or environment). In studying infant mortality according to the person–place–time model, infant and maternal factors are considered traits of "person." Aspects of "place" are such factors as whether the community is rural or urban, affluent or poor. Aspects of "time" include seasonal or age-specific patterns or trends in mortality.

The Web of Causation

The *web of causation* (MacMahon & Pugh, 1970) views a health condition not as the result of individual factors but of complex interactions among multiple factors. One factor may lead to others, which, in turn, lead to others, all of which may interact with one another to produce the health condition.

Central to this model is the concept of *synergism*, wherein the whole is more than the sum of its separate parts. For example, the effects of a *Shigella* infection of the infant, combined with the effects of poverty, youth, and low educational level of the mother, are more deleterious to infant health than the sum of the effects of the individual risk factors.

Use of the web of causation may result in a more expansive study of infant mortality than one guided by other models. Ideally, investigators using this model first identify all factors related to infant mortality. Next, they identify factors that are related to each of these factors. These two comprehensive steps provide the outline for the web of causation for infant mortality. Finally, the investigators examine the relationships among all the identified components of the web and attempt to determine the most feasible point of intervention to improve infant mortality in the community. Figure 2–2 depicts a web of causation for infant mortality.

Practical Application

This multifaceted approach addresses the concept of causation in a manner consistent with current knowledge of human health. However, it may be overwhelming to carry out in everyday practice. In fact, it is more usual to examine only a portion of the web, acknowledging that other relationships exist. Thorough examination of one portion of the web may provide sufficient information for initiation of useful actions to improve community health.

Models: Guides to Investigation and Practice

In this section, we showed how three models each provide a slightly different approach to a community health problem. As you continue to study community health, you will find other models that can guide your practice and investigation. There is no one "correct" model; as you gain experience, you will be able to choose or adapt those that are most appropriate for your work.

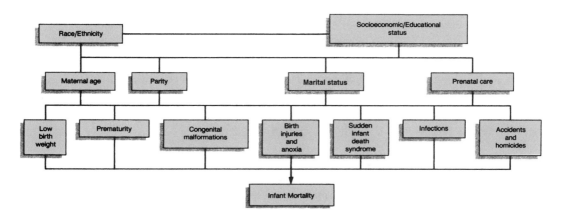

Figure 2–2. A web of causation for infant mortality, based on information available from birth and death certificates.

SUMMARY

In this chapter, you have been introduced to demography, the broad science of populations, and epidemiology, the specific science of population health. Examples have been offered as to how these two sciences can be used to guide community health nursing practice. Now, you should be able to apply epidemiologic and demographic principles to your community health practice. For more detailed information on epidemiology and demography, you may wish to consult the reference list.

REFERENCES

Centers for Disease Control and Prevention. (1993, September 10). Public health focus: Physical activity and the prevention of coronary heart disease. *Morbidity and Mortality Weekly Report, 42*, 398–400.

_____. (1983, August 5). Update: Toxic shock syndrome—United States. *Morbidity and Mortality Weekly Report, 32*, 398–400.

_____. (1981, June 30). Toxic shock syndrome—United States, 1970–1980. *Morbidity and Mortality Weekly Report, 30*, 25–33.

_____. (1980, September 19). Follow up on toxic shock syndrome. *Morbidity and Mortality Weekly Report, 29*(37), 441–445.

Cravens, G. & Mair, J.L. (1977). *The black death.* New York, NY: Dutton.

Crichton, M. (1969). *The Andromeda strain.* New York, NY: Alfred A. Knopf.

Davis, J.P., Chesney, P.J., Ward, P.J., LaVenture, M., & the Investigation and Laboratory Team. (1980). Toxic shock syndrome: Epidemiologic features, recurrence, risk factors, and prevention. *New England Journal of Medicine, 303*, 1429–1435.

Dunne, T. L. (1978). *The scourge.* New York, NY: Coward, McCann, & Geohegan.

Lilienfeld, D.E. & Stolley, P.D. (1994). *Foundations of epidemiology* (3rd ed.). New York, NY: Oxford University Press.

MacMahon, B. & Pugh, T.F. (1970). *Epidemiology: Principles and methods.* Boston, MA: Little, Brown & Co.

Mausner, J.S. & Kramer, S. (1985). *Epidemiology: An introductory text.* Philadelphia, PA: W.B. Saunders.

Sinauer, N., Bowling, J.M., Moracco, K.E., Runyan, C.W., & Butts, J.D. (1999). Comparisons among female homicides occurring in rural, intermediate, and urban counties in North Carolina. *Homicide Studies, 3*(2), 107–128.

Snow, J. (1936). *Snow on cholera, being a reprint of two papers by John Snow, M.D., together with a biographical memoir by B.W. Richardson, M.D., and an introduction by Wade Hampton Frost, M.D.* New York, NY: The Commonwealth Fund.

INTERNET RESOURCES

www.cdc.gov/mmwr
The Centers for Disease Control and Prevention has morbidity and mortality weekly reports by state and select cities as well as reportable disease trends. This is an excellent site for information on measures and determinants of community health.

Robert W. McFarlane **and** Judith McFarlane   CHAPTER

ECOLOGIC CONNECTIONS   3

O BJECTIVES

The community health nurse needs to have an understanding of the principles and applications of human ecology as they affect human health.

After studying this chapter, you should be able to

- Understand the ecologic mechanisms that facilitate the migration of
  pollutants from their sources to human populations.
- Apply this ecologic knowledge to the promotion of health and the
  identification of human health problems of environmental origin.

INTRODUCTION

No person or community is an independent entity. Each is intimately linked to
the environment, frequently in ways we have never imagined. Thus, the environment influences health, directly and indirectly, through subtle, indirect
pathways. Conversely, human activities affect the health of the environmental
system. One aspect of human ecology is the study of these linkages. This chapter explores the ways in which interconnections, transport mechanisms, and
constant change combine to affect health.

Political action in the United States during the 1970s produced new legislation and strengthened a number of existing laws protecting human populations and the environment. Pollution-control efforts concentrated on reducing
the quantities of pollutants emitted by major point sources, such as smokestacks or water-discharge pipes. These pollutants affected large numbers of

people over broad areas of the nation. The success of these efforts can be gauged by the measurable reduction of the major air and water pollutants that has been achieved in our environment.

The current challenge is to control pollutants from nonpoint sources—pollutants that are released in smaller quantities from innumerable locations. These arise from agricultural activity, urban development, motor vehicle operation, and the disposal of solid wastes, among other sources. They are present in our homes and workplaces as well as at industrial sites. These pollutants may be released in smaller quantities and may affect fewer people than the point-source contaminants, but many are potentially more toxic. Many exhibit carcinogenic, mutagenic, or teratogenic effects.

The carcinogenic potential of hazardous pollutants in air, water, and solid waste is perceived by the public as a major health problem. An effective public policy must be developed to define and reduce any significant risks to public health that may arise from exposure to hazardous substances. Determining if and when and how human exposure to potentially hazardous substances should be regulated will be an essential, yet difficult, governmental task. Risk management decisions are always complex and almost always involve some degree of uncertainty that cannot be resolved with the available scientific facts.

The difficulties of creating a public policy are further compounded by the observation that everyone does not respond in the same way to the same exposure to the same chemical substance. The effects of a given substance may be magnified in some people by a concurrent exposure to other chemicals or minimized in other people because of genetic characteristics. The cost of providing complete protection to everyone may not be justified if the benefits would apply to only a small fraction of the exposed population. Further, the existence of health problems unrelated to pollution can complicate evaluation. For instance, in a milieu in which voluntary substance abuse and obesity are major community health problems, it is difficult to determine the limits of regulated exposure to an environmental risk.

In recent history, the interdependency of the human species and the natural world has been too frequently overlooked or ignored. As we seek ways to alleviate problems associated with health, it is imperative to be cognizant of nature's operating principles. The "laws of nature" have not been repealed, and knowledge of these laws is vital to understanding the origin of health problems and in successfully designing strategies to reduce them. The law of gravity is particularly important to the ecologic system. Everything that goes up, including pollutants, must come down, and everything dumped on the surface of the earth must ultimately flow downhill. Water and even land masses, such as mountains, move slowly to the sea. It is imperative that we learn to design with nature, exploiting these principles to advantage, rather than expending resources in a useless struggle, because nature always wins.

It is important to remember three commonsense observations that are frequently overlooked because of their inherent simplicity.

Everything is connected to everything else, but some things are connected more tightly than others. This observation is the least obvious, and it will be the objective of this chapter to demonstrate its validity. As we go from a climatically controlled workplace to a correspondingly pleasant home, insulated from the vagaries of the weather even while en route, it is easy to forget that working in a climate-controlled environment is a very recent phenomenon, restricted to a minority of the world population. As we select foodstuffs from the bounty of 24-hour supermarkets, we seldom stop to wonder where a particular item came from; what chemical abuses it may have suffered during its growth, harvest, or transportation; or what unsuspected surprises may lurk beneath the protective cellophane.

Everything has to go someplace. Although this observation is readily acknowledged, "someplace" is generally considered synonomous with "away" and is not considered to be a problem until the "away" becomes your living space. This may produce the now familiar "NIMBY" reaction (not in my back yard!). As human populations and industrial development grow, pollutants are produced in greater quantities and dispersed over longer distances. At the same time, unpopulated areas are diminishing. Some pollutants are conspicuous and readily detected. Others, perhaps more insidious, are detected only when sought; the search frequently requires elaborate instrumentation and methodology.

Everything is constantly changing. Although constant change is universally recognized, the nature and rate of change are generally unappreciated. The natural environment undergoes continual change. Some changes seem irreversible, permanent, or barely detectable from our perspective in time (eg, geologic transformations and continental drift). Other changes are cyclic (such as the seasonal climate) or transient (floods or droughts). However, changes produced by the actions of human beings have become more prominent. Significant human-induced changes began with the domestication of animals and the development of agriculture. These led to the growth of large human settlements, soon followed by deforestation and the depletion of local resources. The rate of change increased greatly as muscle power was replaced by mechanical power and renewable energy resources (wood, wind, and water) were replaced by energy derived from fossil fuels.

During the last few decades, human impacts have reached an unprecedented intensity and now affect the entire world, owing to a vastly increased population and higher per capita consumption. The nature of change has also been altered as development projects redirect rivers, create lakes, alter sedimentation patterns, and introduce new crops, in addition to producing agricultural-industrial air, water, and soil pollution. The desire to control the environment often creates conflicts between our goals and natural environmental patterns. In the quest to increase production, people often deflect natural flows of energy, bypass natural processes, sever food chains, simplify natural systems, and consume large energy subsidies to maintain the equilibrium in artificial systems. The pursuit of short-term gains often results in irreversible environmental degradation. Humanity has become a geologic agent and is rapidly altering both the face of the earth and the planet's capacity to support human populations.

When exploring these interconnections, it may be useful to remember that only one rule has no exceptions: *There are exceptions to every rule.*

ENERGY AND NUTRIENTS

All living organisms require both nutrients with which to build and maintain their bodies and energy to drive the chemical reactions that permit them to function. The nutrients are continuously recycled by way of natural processes and are used over and over again. The energy literally arrives from outer space and cannot be recycled. The sun is the only significant source of energy in our solar system.

Living organisms exist by capturing the physical energy of sunlight and transforming it into the energy of chemical bonds in organic molecules. This process, photosynthesis, is unique to green plants. Therefore, humans and all other animals are totally dependent on the productivity of the plant world for survival. When animals eat green plants, they release the energy stored in the chemical bonds and use it to power their own activity. Both plants and animals are capable of respiration, which releases the energy stored in organic molecules.

The laws of thermodynamics apply to these biologic energy processes. The first law states that energy may be transformed from one type of energy to another, as from light to chemical bonds to heat, but it is never created or destroyed. The second law specifies that no process involving an energy transformation will occur spontaneously unless there is a degradation from a concentrated form into a dispersed form; that is to say, no energy transformation is 100% efficient. Thus, although living organisms are successful in channeling the energy of sunlight into a series of chemical reactions that store and release energy in small, manageable amounts, the end result is always the same: the release of heat to the environment and eventually to outer space. This process is at work constantly, as when the metabolic heat of our bodies is released in expired air, urine, and feces or radiated from our body surfaces. The time delay in these biologic processes may be considerable, as the amount of energy bound up in organic fuel (such as wood) and fossil fuel (coal, petroleum, and natural gas) attests. Today's primary fuel sources were produced by biologic activity under environmental conditions that no longer exist on earth. It is important to note that biologic energy transformation is a flow-through process. Energy enters the earth's environment, is stored and used, and departs in a transformed state. Energy is never cycled.

Nutrients behave in a very different manner. The chemical elements of living organisms circulate from the environment to the organisms and, following death of an organism, back to the environment. These paths, known as biogeochemical cycles, exhibit varying degrees of complexity and time scales. Most elements cycle from a sedimentary reservoir in the earth's crust, and a given molecule may have a limited geographic range. A molecule absorbed from the earth may enter plant tissue and persist until the death and decomposition of the plant. If the plant is eaten, the molecule may move a short distance as part of the animal before returning to the earth when the animal decomposes. Other substances cycle as gases from an atmospheric or hydrospheric reservoir, and these may be distributed globally, particular examples being nitrogen, oxygen, carbon dioxide, and water.

At this point, you may ask what all this has to do with health. The essential point is that human beings have complex and elaborate chemical and homeostatic mechanisms that function to acquire and retain nutrient- and energy-containing molecules from the environment. Any toxic or undesirable chemicals that mimic required nutrients or are otherwise incorporated into these natural cycles and pathways will also be transported into our bodies. Frequently, it is not a question of whether a given chemical will find its way into our bodies but rather how long will it take, how much will be acquired, and how long will it persist in both our bodies and the environment. Two decades after the pesticide dichlorodiphenyltrichloroethane (DDT) was banned from use in the United States, it was still present in measurable quantities in all people examined.

THE ORGANIZATION OF LIFE

The capture and use of energy by living organisms is accomplished by the high degree of organization characteristic of all levels of the biologic world. Within free-living organisms, the hierarchy includes subatomic particles, atoms, molecules, macromolecules, organelles, cells, tissues, organs, and organ systems. Beyond individuals, we find populations of similar organisms, communities of different species of plants and animals (note an essential difference here: health professionals consider only people when describing a community, whereas ecologists include all organisms), and ecosystems including both biotic communities (organisms) and the abiotic environment, each influencing the properties of the other and both necessary for maintenance of life. Within an ecosystem, the flow of energy and materials follows distinct pathways. Green plants capture the energy of sunlight and manufacture energy-rich organic compounds. Animals eat the plants or eat other animals that have fed on plants. This transfer of energy from plant to animal to another animal is known as a food chain. Humans and other animals typically consume many different kinds of food. Food chains are rarely simple; they are generally extensively interconnected with one another in a "food web."

In complex natural communities, organisms whose food is obtained from plants through the same number of steps are considered to belong to the same trophic level. At each trophic level, energy is lost due to metabolism, and nutrients are lost in waste products. A given species may function at more than one trophic level according to the source of energy actually eaten. For example, humans function at the second level when eating plant material, the third level when consuming beef, and the fifth level when dining on carnivorous fishes such as tuna or salmon. Understanding the trophic concept and energy loss between trophic levels is important when problems of human nutrition are considered. As food becomes scarce, food chains must be shortened to avoid energy loss. Staple foods are commonly highly productive grasses—cereals, rice, corn, and so forth. It is inefficient to use such plant foods to produce meat for human consumption. Cattle are efficient converters of nonedible grasses (nonedible, that is, for humans, who lack the necessary digestive enzymes) to meat and have evolved a complex four-chambered stomach (which incorporates bacteria that help break down the food) for this purpose. Affluent societies circumvent nature's energy-efficient food chains by feeding corn to cattle to increase the fat content of beef intended for human consumption. Although more delectable, this marbled beef subsequently creates new health problems.

Food webs and trophic levels are phenomena associated with ecosystems. The physical boundary of a given ecosystem is often indistinct. Even such a discrete habitat as a pond is used by species that alternate between aquatic and terrestrial environments. Minerals can reach the pond from anywhere within its watershed, an area typically much larger than the pond itself. Other chemicals can reach the pond from hundreds of miles away, as the spread of pollutants that create acid rain has taught us. Many food webs overlap several ecosystems. A cursory survey of a pantry shelf or supermarket will easily demonstrate the widespread food-transportation system that has been developed to ship staples, fruits, and delicacies across continents and oceans. Pollutants and toxins readily accompany these foodstuffs.

Primitive humans were aware of humanity's niche in the biologic community and exploited numerous plants and animals in pursuing the hunter–gatherer mode of existence. Agricultural humans focused on a few domesticated species and began to regard other plants and animals as weeds and pests. The increased productivity of cultigens permitted larger human populations but also led to dependence on a less diverse nutrient base. Technologic humans, particularly urbanites, have forgotten their dependence on natural ecosystems and agro-ecosystems. The quest to further increase agricultural production and control pest organisms by chemical means has added new threats to health in the name of feeding human populations.

ECOLOGIC INTERACTIONS AND HEALTH

Interactions between organisms are particularly important in the cause, transmission, and persistence of disease. Infectious diseases fall into several broad categories, depending on the number of organisms involved. The simplest consists of only two members, a pathogen and its host. Smallpox is such a system; the virus is the pathogen and a human is the host. Infected individuals who recover are no longer susceptible to reinfection. The immune mechanisms can be stimulated with a vaccine, and, through this action, the host becomes immune to the pathogen. As the potential host population is reduced (by way of vaccination), the pathogen is unable to persist and will eventually become extinct.

Many diseases include a third party, a vector that transmits the pathogen from host to host without becoming infected itself. For example, the pathogen that causes the bubonic plague is a bacterium that is transmitted to humans (and other animals) through the bite of a flea. The bacterium is maintained in populations of rodents of various kinds. The rodents provide the reservoir wherein the bacillus persists; the fleas are merely vectors of transmission from an infected rodent to an uninfected rodent or to a human being. Humans are secondary hosts, but when the bacillus is introduced into a crowded human population, the results can be devastating, as has been demonstrated by the epidemics that occur every few centuries. These epidemics have disappeared on their own, not as the result of human countermeasures.

Pollution

Pollutants are the residues of things humans make, use, and throw away. Nondegradable pollutants either do not degrade or degrade very slowly in the natural environment. Biodegradable pollutants can be rapidly decomposed by natural processes unless input exceeds decomposition or dispersal capacity. Degradable pollutants that provide energy or nutrients may increase the productivity of an ecosystem by providing a subsidy when the rate of input is moderate. However, high rates of input can cause productivity to oscillate, whereas additional input may poison the system completely.

When any pollutant is introduced into the environment, we must be concerned about both the fate of the pollutant (where it goes and how it gets there) and its effect on humans or any of the ecosystems on which we depend. We must always keep in mind that any effects that pollutants have on other species are early warning symptoms that something is amiss in the ecosystem and that humans may well be the next to be affected. There are five mechanisms of particular concern.

Major Pollutant Mechanisms

Transport

Transport of the pollutant, once it is introduced into the environment, is generally accomplished by way of wind patterns or aquatic systems. Pollutants can be dispersed aerially as particulates or in a gaseous state; they can travel long distances before falling to earth as dust or being carried in rainwater. Ironically, the construction of taller smokestacks to relieve local pollution generally results in greater dispersal, thus enlarging the area affected without diminishing the amount of pollutant released. Once air pollutants have settled to earth, they frequently continue their movement by traveling along waterways. Following a single heavy rainfall, stormwater runoff can mobilize more suspended particulates than may be transported during the rest of the year. Dissolved pollutants may be transported long distances before settling onto the bottom sediments through some precipitatory mechanism.

Pollutants generally exert greater influence on aquatic ecosystems than on terrestrial environments. Air pollutants may enter a person's lungs or settle on vegetation and then be eaten with the plants. Water, though, is nature's best solvent, and many pollutants go into solution in aquatic ecosystems, with the result that aquatic animals and plants live in a weakly polluted "soup." Many chemicals enter the biota directly through the skin or across gill surfaces, because there is no escape from a dissolved pollutant. The effects of a given one-time polluting event, such as an accidental spill, are therefore exerted for a longer time in aquatic ecosystems. Not only is a greater portion of the pollution incorporated into and cycled within the biotic nutrient pool, but material that settles into the sediment can also be resuspended and redistributed with every major storm event. The dispersion of pollutants is also more restricted in aquatic systems than in terrestrial ones because movement is always downstream, until the pollutants reach the ocean. The efficacy of ocean transport has been demonstrated by the ubiquitous spread of several insecticides throughout the world; their area of distribution even includes the Antarctic continent.

Transformation

Transformation of a pollutant within an ecosystem takes place in many ways. Harmful substances can be rendered innocuous or even helpful during the biodegradation process. But, occasionally, a relatively harmless substance is transformed into a noxious form. A classic example is the transformation of metallic or inorganic mercury, which is relatively immobile, into methylmercury by microorganisms living in aquatic sediments. Methylmercury is readily incorporated into detrital food chains, which may terminate with human consumption of contaminated fish and shellfish, producing the neurologic disorder known as Minamata disease. Nonbiogenic chemical transformations are more common in the environment (eg, one such transformation is the conversion of sulfur dioxide and nitrous oxides in the atmosphere to form sulfuric and nitric acids and create acid rain).

Bioaccumulation

Bioaccumulation refers to the introduction of substances into ecologic food webs. Chemicals that behave in a manner similar to essential elements are most susceptible to rapid uptake and retention. Chiefly because of human beings and their activities, the ecologist must now be concerned with the cycling of nonessential elements. For example, the radionuclides of strontium and cesium, whose chemical behavior is analogous to calcium and potassium, respectively, are introduced into the environment by nuclear reactors and represent a potential health hazard.

Biomagnification

Biomagnification results when the accumulation of a pollutant greatly exceeds the rate at which an organism eliminates it. The pollutant is concentrated in organisms at a low trophic level, where it is further concentrated and passed to the third level, and so forth. For example, polychlorinated biphenyls (PCBs) are a large class of 209 separate chemical compounds that held many industrial applications before 1976, when they were banned in the United States. Each of these compounds has a different type and degree of toxicity, bioaccumulates at different rates, and behaves differently when free in the environment. In the 1970s, these PCB compounds were associated with adverse health effects in people eating fish from the Great Lakes. The PCBs were acquired by phytoplankton that innocuously acted as tiny scavengers of the pollutant, reaching levels of only 2.5 parts of PCB per billion parts of phytoplankton. These were then eaten by zooplankton, which, in turn, were eaten by larger zooplankton, in which PCB concentrations increased nearly 50-fold, reaching 123 parts per billion. The zooplankton were eaten by small fish, rainbow smelt, with PCBs increasing ninefold to 1 part per million (ppm). Next, the smelt were eaten by lake trout, which reached 5 ppm PCB, and finally consumed by humans (or other end-chain carnivores). At each step, the PCBs were sequestered in the fatty tissue of the carrier and stored. The final concentration of PCBs in herring gull eggs, which are rich in stored fat and sometimes consumed by humans, was 124 ppm, or 50,000 times greater than the original concentration in the phytoplankton.

Synergism

Synergism is the simultaneous action of separate substances or agencies that together produce a greater total effect than the sum of their individual effects. It is common to discover that a given substance behaves in one fashion in a controlled laboratory environment and quite another when introduced into a natural ecosystem, where it interacts with a number of physical and chemical properties of the environment.

Toxic Substances

In recent years, toxic substances have received a great deal of attention in governmental regulations and the news media. Any chemical can be toxic, including table salt, sugar, and the chlorine in drinking water. Toxic substances are generally considered to be any chemicals or mixtures of chemicals, either synthetic or natural, that are poisonous to humans or plants or animals under expected conditions of use and exposure. There are four major categories of toxic substances. Pesticides are lethal chemicals specifically designed to kill weeds, fungi, insects, mites, rodents, and other pests. Four pesticides have been banned from further use in the United States: DDT, aldrin, dieldrin, and chlordane. Industrial chemicals are particularly numerous and a few have proven especially dangerous (eg, asbestos, benzene, vinyl chloride, and PCB). A number of metals, such as arsenic, lead, cadmium, and mercury, have also proven to be very toxic in the environment. The fourth category includes those substances with isotopes that emit various types of radiation, such as strontium, cesium, iodine, and so forth.

There are approximately 60,000 different chemical substances in commercial use in the United States today, and 98% of these chemicals are safe. In 1988, the baseline year for the US Environmental Protection Agency (EPA) Toxics Release Inventory, 20,458 manufacturing facilities released 2.18 billion pounds of toxic wastes directly into the air and 164 million pounds were discharged to surface waters. By 1997, these releases had been reduced to 982 million pounds into the air and 61 million pounds to surface waters from 19,597 facilities.

Chemical toxicity occurs when a chemical agent produces detrimental effects in living organisms. The effects of a toxic substance can be immediate or long term and can harm selected tissues or the entire organism. Both the toxicity of the substance and the expected exposure to the organism must be considered to define the anticipated risk. Neurotoxins are likely the most significant toxic substances in both prevalence and severity that pose a risk to human health. Epidemiologically, a relatively small fraction of major neurologic disorders are inherited; most neurologic diseases appear to be associated with environmental factors. Many commercial chemicals used in very large amounts and known to persist in the environment have neurotoxic properties. In fact, insecticides, designed to have neurotoxic properties, are manufactured for deliberate release into the environment.

Pollutants and Human Population Size

All of the environmental processes described so far can influence human health. Any pollutant or toxic substance introduced into the environment is subjected to these processes, many of which lead directly to human beings. Pollution of the environment occurs when these pollutants overwhelm the capacity of the environment to assimilate them without being thrown out of balance. Thus, pollution is a rate function involving a quantity of pollutant introduced over a period of time. This rate is directly correlated to population size.

It can be said that all pollution is the result of population growth. A single family, living on a subsistence level in the wild, burning wood as their fuel and discarding rubbish and human wastes on the landscape, would seldom be a polluting factor in their environment. The population of a small village would denude the landscape of wood fuel, pollute the air with smoke from numerous wood fires, and litter the ground with rubbish and human wastes randomly dispersed. Cities, with more numerous inhabitants, totally overwhelm the environment with rubbish and human wastes, fostering the development of sewage and garbage disposal systems. Industrial development increases the number of pollutants and environmental insults. Our past practice for handling pollutants has been to just dump them, taking further action only when the natural systems have been overwhelmed. We need to reverse this practice and remove the bulk of pollutants before inflicting them on nature. Then the natural ecosystem can work for us by removing the final bit of pollution that always proves so difficult and expensive to neutralize.

Demographic changes can rapidly alter the stress inflicted on the environment. As population grows, the stress increases. If the population moves, both the nature and the intensity of an environmental problem can shift. For example, the recent decline of industrial productivity in the northeastern United States has resulted in a shift in the population caused by the exodus of workers (particularly younger families) and an improvement in the surface water quality. The growth of population in the south, especially the arid southwest, is both increasing water pollution and straining overall water supply.

The solution to one environmental problem may be the creation of another. Pollutants do not disappear. Sulfur that is scrubbed out of power plant smokestack gases ends up as a sludge stored on the ground, where it may threaten water quality. Pollutants removed from wastewaters by precipitation end up in the bottom sludge, which also requires disposal. Unfortunately, if the sludge is burned, the pollutants may be released into the air, to settle and become incorporated into the water or land once again. If the sludge is buried in a landfill, it may threaten surface water or groundwater supplies. Sewage treatment plants that aerate water as part of the process may discharge substantial amounts of volatile toxic substances to the air. Everything has to go someplace.

In summary, virtually any pollutant that is introduced into the environment will subsequently be transported away from its point of entry. It may be transformed into another chemical form, either less or more hazardous. It will probably be accumulated by biologic organisms, possibly becoming magnified in its concentration. It is likely to react with other chemicals or physical processes and to produce unanticipated effects. Distinct and efficient chemical cycles and pathways that have evolved over millions of years ensure that toxicants will enter biologic systems and eventually reach humans or other organisms on which they depend. Everything is connected to everything else, and everything has to go someplace. There is nowhere to hide. The only solution is to stop the pollution.

INTERCONNECTIONS

Humanity's attempts to intervene in natural processes seldom go smoothly and frequently produce effects far removed from the immediate intervention site. Some of the most profound effects have been experienced in attempts to control or eradicate diseases. The following example reveals some unexpected connections.

Malaria is caused by four species of Plasmodium, a single-celled sporozoan parasite. During the first stage of the disease, elongate sporozoites in the blood penetrate cells within the liver. The sporozoites multiply asexually to produce numerous merozoites. During the second stage of the disease, the merozoites leave the liver and enter red blood cells. The merozoites reproduce, again asexually, within the red blood cells and erupt, with the progeny invading new red blood cells and continuing the cycle. These eruptions eventually synchronize to 48-hour or 72-hour cycles, depending on the Plasmodium species involved. The shock of the simultaneous release of the merozoites can produce chills in the victim, followed by a high fever caused by toxins released with the merozoites. Some merozoites become gametocytes, capable of sexual reproduction.

The human immune system functions by being able to recognize the chemical antigens of an infectious agent and producing specific antibodies to combat it. The malarial pathogen presents three different stages (sporozoite, merozoite, and gametocyte) with three different antigens. Antibodies that counter one antigen are not effective against the other two stages. Also, the antibodies will be effective only when the various parasite cells are free in the bloodstream. Once they have entered either liver cells or red blood cells, they cannot be attacked by the antibodies. Thus, an effective vaccine would have to work against all three stages.

Mosquitoes are found in abundance virtually everywhere in the world. More than 1500 species are known, and a few tropical and subtropical species are involved in the transmission of human diseases. Larval mosquitoes develop in water, and many species are quite adaptable in their choice of breeding sites, using water that collects in abandoned tin cans, rubber tires, and so forth. Adult male mosquitoes suck plant juices for their nourishment and do not bite animals. Adult females require a blood meal to provide nutrients for their eggs. Various species bite reptiles, birds, and mammals (including humans) to obtain the blood. When a female anopheles mosquito bites a human who is infected with malaria, the malarial gametocytes may be drawn up into the digestive system of the insect. The gametocytes are transformed into gametes within the stomach of the mosquito, where they unite to form a zygote and then burrow into the cells in the wall of the stomach. The resulting oocyte produces numerous new sporozoites, which migrate to the salivary glands of the mosquito. When the female mosquito next bites a human, some sporozoites may be injected into the wound by way of saliva. Mosquito saliva contains an anticoagulant to keep the blood flowing until the mosquito has drunk her fill.

This complicated procedure is the only mechanism by which the malaria parasite is transmitted indirectly from one human host to another. It cannot be transmitted by direct human contact (although it has been transmitted by means of blood transfusion and intravenous drug abuse), nor is it passed from one mosquito to another. It persists only by using the mosquito vector to complete its complex lifecycle. Malaria is a widespread and debilitating disease. It has been estimated that each year, worldwide, 250 million people fall ill with this disease, and more than 1 million die. It causes anemia, fever, spleen enlargement, and miscarriage; contributes to high infant mortality; and causes in its victims a greater susceptibility to many kinds of infection. The eradication of malaria has been a top priority goal of the World Health Organization (WHO) for many years.

As the primary hosts of the malarial parasite, humans represent three distinct populations according to their susceptibility to the disease. Some people are susceptible to being infected with the disease, some are already infected, and some are immune to infection. Newborn infants may acquire some antibodies from their mothers, but these do not persist. Children from 1 to 4 years of age are highly susceptible to malaria and constitute most of the deaths from the disease. Older children and adults can develop partial immunity to small numbers of the malarial parasites, but when large numbers are present, the parasites tend to overrun this limited immunity.

Temporary artificial immunity to malaria can be created with the continuous intake of drugs. The South American Indians discovered that the bark of the cinchona tree yielded quinine, which was effective in preventing and treating malaria. The famous gin and tonic, made with quinine water, is reputed to have been developed by the British to ameliorate their daily intake of quinine in malarial regions. Quinine was replaced by quinacrine hydrochloride, which had the side effect of coloring the eyes yellow. The drug in present use is chloroquine, which prevents DNA replication and RNA synthesis in the parasitized red blood cells. For prevention and suppression of malaria, chloroquine must be taken on a weekly basis.

Mosquitoes have no immune system to counteract invasion by malaria parasites. Uninfected females become infected by biting an infected human. Infected mosquitoes never recover from the infection and continue to transmit the parasite to subsequent victims. Malaria can be maintained in areas of low human population density if the mosquito population density is high. However, mosquitoes do have high rates of reproduction. Efforts to eradicate malaria have focused on eradicating the mosquito or at least lowering mosquito populations to the point where they were no longer effective vectors of the disease.

The weapons of choice for this worldwide campaign were insecticides. A favorite was DDT, a chlorinated hydrocarbon that attacks the central nervous system. Although synthesized in 1874, it was not used as an insecticide until 1939. It is a broad-spectrum pesticide, affecting many organisms in addition to the target species. DDT was used widely during World War II to protect US troops from malaria, typhus, and other insect-borne diseases. DDT was inexpensive to manufacture and easy to handle. Its long-lasting residual effect was hailed as one of its chief advantages.

Within a dozen years, unwelcome side effects began to appear. Eggshell thinning in birds began as early as 1947. Fish, crabs, shrimps, and oysters accumulated lethal concentrations of DDT even at very low levels of exposure. Citizen opposition to widespread use, particularly aerial spraying, began in 1957. Domestic production of DDT peaked at 188 million pounds annually in 1963 but declined to 60 million pounds in the 1970s. Domestic consumption peaked at 79 million pounds in 1959 and declined to 20 million pounds by 1971. In 1972, the EPA suspended virtually all uses of DDT in the United States on the grounds that continual use would pose an unacceptable risk to humans and the environment.

DDT was more persistent in some environmental systems than others. Residues in soil degrade slowly. In arid areas, the time required for one half of the DDT to wash out or break down exceeds 20 years. Eventually, DDT breaks down in the environment to DDD or DDE, which are even more potent. DDT applied to soils can evaporate into the air and move long distances (it has even been recorded in antarctic snow). Rainfall and surface runoff transport DDT to streams, rivers, estuaries, and oceans.

The US Food and Drug Administration established a maximum allowable concentration of DDT in foodstuffs at 5 ppm. By the 1960s, several species of fish from the Great Lakes as well as the Atlantic and Pacific Oceans exceeded this level. The National Human Monitoring System tracked selected chlorinated hydrocarbons in human adipose tissue from 1970 to 1983. DDT has been found in more than 99% of all human tissues sampled. Total DDT (including DDD and DDE) in human fatty tissues peaked at 8 ppm in 1971. DDT is concentrated in fatty tissues of the body and frequently contaminates milk and dairy products. At one point, the DDT content of human milk exceeded the 5-ppm level, rendering breast milk unfit for human consumption.

Since DDT was banned in the United States, the level of DDT in food organisms and wildlife has slowly, but steadily, declined. DDT residues in human fat slowly declined to 1.7 ppm in 1983, the final year of the survey.

DDT provides vivid evidence of worldwide environmental transport mechanisms. DDT has spread throughout the world and has been found in both arctic fishes and antarctic penguins, far from any site of direct DDT application. In addition, DDT has been directly implicated in the precipitous decline of brown pelican and peregrine falcon populations. Both species occupy positions at the end of long food chains in which DDT is concentrated at each transfer level. DDT interferes with calcium metabolism, causing the birds to produce eggs with abnormally thin shells that frequently crack during incubation, thus failing to hatch. Consequently, both bird species were classified as endangered. Both of these cases reveal only the tip of the iceberg, because DDT contamination is widespread throughout their food web.

Through the use of these pesticides, the war against malaria appeared to be succeeding for a number of years, with spectacular reductions being made in the prevalence of the disease. Many agencies and governments felt that the benefits gained far outweighed the environmental costs. However, in recent years, the prevalence of malaria has soared to precontrol levels in the very areas that enjoyed the greatest success. The mosquitoes are no longer affected by the insecticides, and, in some regions, the malarial organisms within their human hosts no longer respond to chemotherapy. Human endeavors have encountered the reality of biologic adaptation.

One explanation for this biologic adaption is variability, which is exhibited by all organisms. This is recognized readily in humans, because we not only look different as individuals, but our chemical makeup, reaction to drugs, and even taste sensors also respond differently to a given stimulus. In a parallel fashion, not all targeted organisms will succumb to a given pesticide. In any large population, there always seem to be a few organisms that survive various stressors. Thus, when an area is treated with an insecticide, the majority of the mosquito population, perhaps more than 99%, will die. But the resources that originally supported that mosquito population may be unaffected, and some of the natural enemies and predators of mosquitoes may also have been killed by a broad-spectrum pesticide. So, the few mosquitoes that survive find themselves in an advantageous situation: Their resources are intact, their enemies are gone, and they can reproduce and grow in number as they please. But one significant change has occurred. Assuming that the characteristic that permitted them to survive the pesticide is inheritable, all of their progeny will also possess this characteristic. This means that the new generation will be stronger than the previous one and will not be susceptible to that pesticide.

This description of adaptation is an oversimplification, but the principle is valid. It is applicable equally to the development of drug- or antibiotic-resistant strains of microorganisms. In fact, this has occurred with malaria organisms in some parts of the world, where chloroquine-resistant strains have arisen. Just as the overuse of antibiotics leads to antibiotic-resistant pathogens, the overuse of insecticides leads to insecticide-resistant insects. When the strength and frequency of insecticide applications are increased, insecticide-resistant insects develop all the more quickly.

Widespread insecticide application can have even broader effects. Malaria was a serious, prevalent disease in Borneo, where in some areas, over 90% of the population suffered from enlarged spleens. In 1955, WHO began a successful program of malaria control. Two insecticides, DDT and dieldrin, were sprayed inside the thatched-roof houses to eradicate two species of mosquitoes that were transmitting the malaria. The insecticides also reduced the populations of small parasites of a moth species. The parasites avoided thatch that had been sprayed with DDE and were killed outright by dieldrin. Freed from their parasites, the population of moth larvae expanded rapidly and consumed large quantities of thatch in the housetops. The insecticides were also picked up by cockroaches and geckos (small lizards that lived in the houses and fed on insects). Both cockroaches and geckos were captured and eaten by the domestic cats kept by the villagers. The cats proved to be particularly susceptible to the insecticides and many of them died.

With the cat population drastically reduced, two species of rats, native to the forests and plantations, then invaded the villages. These rats were potential carriers of plague, typhus, and leptospirosis. Thus, although the villagers had gained protection from malaria, they were subsequently exposed to much more virulent pathogens. To redress this imbalance, surplus cats were transported from urban areas to the villages, some even being packed into special containers and parachuted into remote villages.

These examples demonstrate the reality of extensive ecologic interconnections. Environmental transport mechanisms have distributed DDT all over the globe. DDT has been transformed into its breakdown products, DDD and DDE, which are even more dangerous than their precursor. All three forms are accumulated by biologic organisms and concentrated as they progress upward in ecologic food webs. The concentration of DDT in higher food organisms is commonly 30,000 times greater than the concentration dissolved in water at a given site. Biologic populations are both variable in their response to given toxicants and quick to produce toxicant-resistant populations that negate the temporary inroads gained by human actions. Once introduced into the environment, DDT and other pesticides may persist for decades, contaminating and killing numerous nontarget organisms. Humans are not exempt from these processes, and toxic chemicals that are released for very commendable reasons may return to haunt us for years to come. The pathways and interconnections are frequently unpredictable, even when the road is paved with good intentions.

THE COMPLEX HUMAN ENVIRONMENT

The preceding section has described humans interacting with the physical world and other species in a simplistic fashion. The complete human environment is difficult to comprehend because of the multiplicity of interrelated elements. The delivery of health care sometimes goes awry because the influence of certain elements is underestimated or unappreciated. A conceptual model of the human environment from an ecologic viewpoint can often illuminate the problem and guide efficient intervention.

An ecologic model (Figure 3–1), like most models, proposes a framework from which to study and understand a phenomenon. A complete enumeration of all salient components of human health would be too complex to illustrate; therefore, this model is limited to environmental variables. The environment is the world that surrounds people wherever they go, whatever they do. An ecologic approach to the study of human health relates the biologic, physical, sociocultural, and politicoeconomic components of a person's environment to any deviation in him or her from a state of health. The model can be applied to

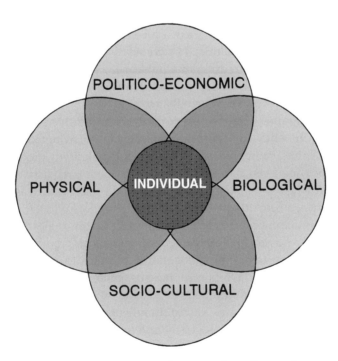

Figure 3–1. The environmental systems that affect each individual.

study the health of any defined subpopulation (eg, infants, children, adolescents, and the elderly) as well.

Environmental systems not only act on the individual person but also interact with one another, and a change occurring in one system will frequently affect others. Each system consists of components that act with and on other systems to bring about equilibrium or disequilibrium within the system.

Change occurs within a system when one variable acts on a second variable to force alteration. Climate and topography are variables within the physical system that can act separately or in unison to cause change within the other systems. For example, food distribution (determined by a set of politicoeconomic variables) depends on the production ability of the land (determined by physical variables such as climate and topography), which, in turn, influence the selection and consumption of food (determined by sociocultural variables); all of these affect human growth (a biologic variable).

The environmental systems show both inter- and intradependence in function and effect. The systems (depicted as circles in Figure 3–1) interface with each other and overlap to form a network that encases the individual (the inner circle of Figure 3–1). At any time, all systems may impinge on the individual simultaneously.

Layered within the systems is a hierarchy of four subsystems: the individual, the family unit, the community (ecologically speaking, the human population), and the nation (Figure 3–2). Each subsystem is conditioned for the occurrence of illness by the environmental systems. When acted on, the subsystems interact both intradynamically and interdynamically to mitigate or reinforce the conditioning influences of the systems' variables; in this way, the subsystems modify the systems. Each subsystem is also influenced by its developmental stage. For instance, an individual may react to an external perturbation differently as an infant, child, adolescent, adult, or elder. A family may be small or extended, with young or school-age children, semi-independent adolescents, or elderly parents to accommodate. A community may be small, homogeneous, and cohesive or large, diverse, and divisive. A nation may be agrarian, industrial, and poor or rich in human and natural resources.

To explain, a family with inadequate access to the basic needs of food and shelter (conditioned by politicoeconomic production and accompanying distribution policies) may act to change these impediments by migrating to an area of improved access to basic needs. Migration, in turn, can force change in the intrafamily physical, biologic, sociocultural, and politicoeconomic composition of the community and nation.

Conceptually, both the subsystems and environmental systems are in a constant state of interaction (everything is connected to everything else and is constantly changing). Enumerating the variables within the systems and mea-

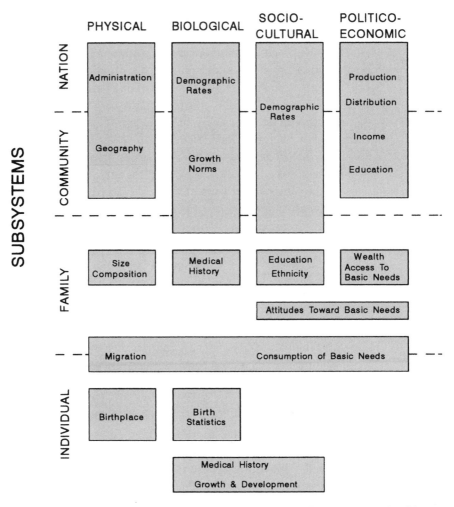

Figure 3–2. The environmental systems and subsystems affecting human health.

suring the interaction among them is the key to operating the model. In Figure 3–2, the environmental systems and subsystems are displayed in a tabular arrangement, with variables boxed according to the systems most acutely affected by their interaction. Certain variables, such as migration and consumption of basic needs, equally interact with all systems as they affect the family and individual's functioning. Other variables, such as birth statistics (age at birth, sex, birth order, and condition), are primarily within one system, affecting one developmental stage (the child) of one subsystem (the individual). Lines encasing variables are not set boundaries; rather, they serve as a guide to identify the system and subsystem most affected by variable manipulation.

The purpose of the conceptual model is to offer a framework from which to select significant variables related to the health status of a chosen individual. The variables that appear in Figure 3–2 are a synthesis of the epidemiologic, demographic, and social health indicators consistently proposed, tested, and recommended as valid and reliable indices of child health. Application of this model is described in the regional case history that follows.

APPLICATION: A REGIONAL CASE STUDY

The Problem

The following study concerned children with infection and the environmental variables they shared. Much is known about the effects of infection; the morbidity and mortality statistics are salient testimony to its impact on child growth, development, and survival. Surprisingly little is known, however, about the ecologic milieu that shrouds infected youngsters or the causal paths by which the environmental variables interact to determine child health.

Epidemiologic studies of infection are plentiful, but their focus is usually on the incidence and seriousness of the problem, with little attention to the associated social or cultural forces. Similarly, sociologic analyses of infection focus on behaviors and attitudes, usually skirting the biologic as well as the economic and political factors. The objective of explaining this study was to demonstrate the usefulness of an ecologic model to identify and quantify the physical, biologic, sociocultural, and politicoeconomic variables related to infection among children.

Health statistics for children in rural communities, especially youngsters of indigenous heritage, reveal that they have more problems than urban children. For example, in Chile, infant mortality rates in rural communities are more than twice those of urban communities. When risk is matched for ethnicity, indigenous children have a far higher risk, which is reduced somewhat if they live in urban areas but still remains substantially higher than that of nonindigenous children living in rural areas. The chance for indigenous children to attain the same mortality rate as nonindigenous children is directly correlated to years of maternal schooling.

In developing countries, income determines food consumption. With inadequate income, nutrient intake suffers. Malnutrition, defined as a deficiency of the essential nutrients required to support normal physiologic functions, has startling effects on health. The Pan American Health Organization found that a preexisting nutritional deficiency or immaturity (defined as a severe growth deficit) was the underlying or associated cause of death in 57% of deceased preschool children in the Americas. Infection was the leading (58%) cause of death, and 61% of those children who died of infection also had a nutritional deficiency (McFarlane, 1985). Malnutrition and infection demonstrate a synergistic and compounding relationship. Infection, a state in which microorganisms reproduce and cause damage to the host, is a radically different and more lethal process in a child than in an adult. Malnutrition and infection affect the vast majority of children in developing countries.

When a community seeks to maximize its resources of health personnel and capital goods to service the greatest number of children, it requires a tool that will (1) appraise the impingement of biopsychosocial variables that surround the child and (2) establish the relationships that link these variables to health status indicators, such as the presence or absence of infection. Because infection is usually a short-term problem, whereas malnutrition is a chronic state of ill health, age-specific prevalence rates of infection are considered crucial indicators of health status and were used to measure health condition in this study.

Population and Methods

The Multinational Andean Genetic and Health Survey assessed the health status of the indigenous population living in Chile's northern province of Tarapacá. Northern Chile is geographically divided into three ecologic zones—the lowland coast, mountainous sierra, and highland altiplano—which differ radically in topography and climate. Associated with the differences are biotic changes that determine the types of agroeconomics, and thus lifestyles, that can be practiced. The health status of 988 children and 1108 adults in 12 communities was determined; these people represented 70% to 90% of the people in any given village.

The International Classification of Diseases codes were used. Children with one or more diagnoses of infection were considered "infected"; children with one or more noninfectious disorders were categorized as "noninfected"; and children without coded diseases were considered "well" and "free of disease." Additionally, family health variables were abstracted from census data collected concurrently. Family wealth was scored according to the number of animals and amount of acreage owned. Four anthropometric measurements—weight, height, arm circumference, and subscapular skinfold—were used to study the relationship between growth and present health status. From known surnames, ethnicity was determined: non-Aymara (Spanish), Mestizo (mixed Spanish and indigenous), or Aymara (indigenous).

The people studied were primarily agriculturists who derived their livelihood from the land. Inhabitants of the highlands had little arable land, but large expanses of grazing pasture were available. They used their livestock (goats, llamas, and alpacas) to convert the inedible (to humans) natural vegetation into animal products (meat, milk, cheese, and fibers) suitable for human use. Conversely, residents of the sierra had more arable land, more irrigated fields, more diverse livestock (adding sheep and cattle) and agricultural crops, and thus more available foodstuffs. Coastal residents had the least arable land (desert stream floodplains) but benefited from a favorable climate and subsidized irrigation. Plant production was high and diverse on the coast, but animal products were restricted.

Population Characteristics

The physical examinations of children of all three ecologic zones revealed that 40% of them had one or more infections, 18% exhibited one or more noninfectious disorders, and 42% were well and free of disease. Infection did not decrease appreciably with age. Non-Aymara children living on the coast were most likely to be well and free of disease, whereas highland children had the highest rates of infection. The prevalence of noninfectious disorders showed little ethnic variability and no appreciable difference between coast and altiplano regions.

A complex clustering of interacting variables prevailed at the family level. Some, such as the number of persons in the household, influenced child health directly (the larger the family, the more potential reservoirs for the incubation and transmission of infection). Other variables exerted their influence indirectly, acting through a web of interrelationships. A primary problem in understanding the ecologic determinants of child health is deciding how to assess the extent to which a given variable acts within the family's environment, directly or indirectly, to affect health status. Analysis of socioeconomic variables (maternal age, education, and health; paternal occupation and health; and family wealth) revealed that well children were likely to have a mother with secondary education and that infected children were likely to have a mother with no education.

Additionally, children with one or more infections were more likely to be cared for by a mother who was also infected, who was younger than 35, and who had minimal or no education. A large number of infected youngsters in the altiplano resided in homes below the median wealth index, but neither wealth nor the father's occupation differentiated the health status of coastal or sierra children. Only among sierra children did the father's health correlate significantly to the child's health. Most early child and maternal health factors varied as a function of region but not of ethnicity.

When compared to well youngsters, infected children consumed fewer foods and, regionally, altiplano children consumed the fewest foods. Region of residence with associated access to food, shelter, education, and health care proved more connected to child health than culture and associated lifestyle behaviors. Child health was determined by environmental factors operant at the individual, family, and community level.

MODEL APPLICATION

Most children in developing nations (and some children in developed nations) reside in abject poverty, resulting in inadequate dietary intakes and significant prevalence of infectious disease. The dilemma facing health workers and planners in all countries is how to use existing resources to the greatest benefit of the largest number of children. To promote child health, causal determinants of infection and malnutrition as well as cost-effective interventions must be identified. The problem is how to define and measure the crucial variables of child morbidity.

Most assessment models are linear, unidirectional, and not designed to look beyond the child or immediate family for health indicators. The ecologic determinants responsible for the prevalence, severity, and duration of the infection–malnutrition cycle are practically unknown. In developing countries, almost all pediatric morbidity data are obtained from hospital records; consequently, they offer uncertain direction for regional or community health planning, especially in rural areas where people have limited or no routine access to medical care.

The Chilean study used an ecologic model to sort physical, biologic, sociocultural, and politicoeconomic variables that impinged on child health. Descriptive and multivariate analyses were used to delineate the variables that exerted an appreciable effect on child health. Using ecologic concepts and the variables found to be important links to child health, a model of the ecologic chain of events has been constructed (Figure 3–3). This "ecologic map" begins with the geographic region of residence—the community.

The region, or community, surrounds the child with a given set of physical forces, including climate, water supply, and topography. These forces interact with demographic structure and political and economic organization to determine the nutrient productivity of the land. Food production in any region is

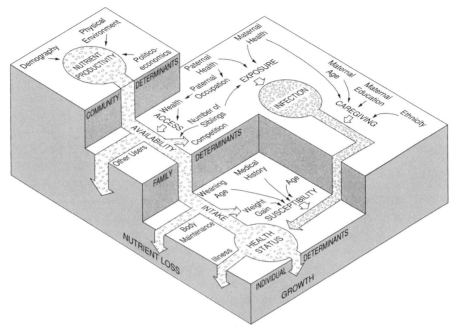

Figure 3–3. The ecologic determinants of child health.

conditioned by economic forces (resources allocated to food production and food distribution), social forces (land tenure), and political edicts (policy and legal implication of land ownership and use). These forces unite and determine the quantity and quality of land used for food production; the persons and technology applied to the land to maximize production; and the diversity, nutritive value, and distribution of the produce. The physical, biologic, sociocultural, and politicoeconomic forces within each region determine the quantity and quality of nutrients available to the family for consumption.

The family consists of a clustering of interacting variables, many of which serve as gates, acting to impede or facilitate members' access to available nutrients. Simultaneously, infection-risk factors abide within the household, variables that mitigate or accentuate the child's risk of illness. Both nutrient intake and infection risk concurrently determine health status, which is reflected in growth patterns.

The web of interconnection continues even further. Paternal health influences paternal occupation, which determines family wealth and, in turn, defines purchasing power and access to available nutrients. The number and age of siblings influence both access to food (through competition) and infection risk (through exposure). In addition, poor maternal health not only exposes the child to illness but also acts as a deterrent to adequate care giving. Care giving is also affected by maternal ethnicity, age, and education. Each factor determines the mother's knowledge and experience regarding basic health-promoting acts, such as hygiene practices, appropriate weaning foods, and needed nutrients and physical care during illness. Obviously, when the care giver is impaired by lack of knowledge or poor health, the child's risk of infection increases.

The child is a composite of risk factors that interact with familial and regional variables to set his or her health status and subsequent growth. The quantity and quality of nutrients consumed by the child determine weight gain and nutritional status. Weight gain is a product of both nutrient intake and a risk variable for infection. The malnourished child has impaired immunocompetence and is prey to infection. Also influencing a child's weight gain are weaning age and weaning foods; both affect the child's nutritive status and susceptibility to infection. Finally, the child's age and past medical history decrease or accentuate susceptibility to infection. In this study, it was the young, preschool children, ill within the last 2 weeks, who experienced the bulk of morbidity.

For most children, the interaction of nutritive intake and infection determines growth. Infection is wasteful and has a negative effect on nutrient absorption, metabolism, and use. As a result, the child loses weight, and growth is halted or retarded. Low nutrient intake equally retards growth. Children have greater nutritional needs relative to body mass; the younger the child, the more kilocalories per kilogram of body weight are needed for normal metabolism and growth. The risk of infection is high for all children, especially for infants and preschool-age youngsters, regardless of their nutritional status; however, when adverse infection-risk factors combine with marginal nutrient intake, the result is morbidity and delayed growth.

POLICY IMPLICATION

Current assessment of world health indicates that lack of basic needs is the primary barrier to wellness. To provide basic needs and improve access to and availability of human services (eg, education, health, sanitation), most countries have focused on providing selected basic needs to designated groups, such as school feeding programs or prenatal care. Unfortunately, regard for the environment, from which the needs arose, is usually omitted. To focus on selected needs without assessing the environment from which the needs arose ignores the complex interrelationships of the biopsychosocial system and negates the structure that created the health problems. Basic-needs intervention programs that do not address ecologic dynamics can create an illusion of success and allow continuation of social and political inequalities that are themselves major contributors of poor health.

Child health is ecologic and relates to the total environment that surrounds children, the physical ecosystem, as well as social, political, and economic organizations. Each system determines the production, availability, and distribution of resources and the eventual access of children to basic needs, which, in turn, dictates both health and growth. Children's health and nutrition problems will not be improved substantially until measures are instituted to eradicate poverty.

Using an ecologic model to identify and sort the determinants of infection among children in northern Chile, researchers found that the region of residence consistently emerged as a significant correlate of health. Region embraces politicoeconomic factors as well as a set climate and demographic state that determine nutrient productivity and access. Once the child acquires food, whether the nutrients are used to maintain and promote growth or are degraded by infection that retards growth and development depends on the family milieu, especially the mother's health, age, and education. Additional risk factors include family wealth, ethnicity, and paternal health. No one risk factor can be addressed independently of the others. Infection is promoted or hindered by a maze of intercorrelated variables, and to address only one or two does little more than vibrate the web of causation.

The root determinants of child health lie deep in the social, economic, and political fiber of the people. Child health cannot be improved independently of changes in the environment surrounding the child. To focus on selected prevention programs (such as improved nutrition or adequate housing) without simultaneously attending to the environment from which the deficits arise (such as existing political and economic policies) negates the determinant values of health and is an inappropriate use of time, money, and personnel.

REFLECTIONS

Where does this knowledge of ecologic processes leave us? As practitioners of community health, how does this information aid us?

First, we must be aware that the health of any population can be affected by its surrounding environment. Next, be skeptical of any claims of perfect disposal schemes for pollutants; they do not exist. Remember that pollutants can travel long distances undetected. Water treatment systems usually precipitate pollutants to a bottom sludge. Eventually, the sludge must be cleaned out. If it is burned, will the pollutants go back up the smokestack, only to settle into another watershed? If it is buried in a landfill, will they remain in place or seep into a groundwater reservoir, only to surface at your kitchen faucet? Everything—including pollutants—has to go someplace, and it may be difficult to keep them in any one place.

Finally, as a consumer or a public advocate, do not demand perfect disposal schemes. Demand honest and realistic estimates of the risk that invariably accompanies any plan, no matter how appealing. Beware of flowcharts that indicate perfect control of pollutants at all stages of the cycle. Remember that it is people who handle pollutants, and the people factor can overwhelm every other part of any plan. It is people who load, transport, and dispose of pollutants. It is people who operate and maintain pollution control systems. It is people who give illegal orders for "midnight dumping and roadside disposal." In some instances, particularly involving the ultimate disposal of nuclear wastes, we may be planning caretaking operations that exceed the realm of past human experience. Our oldest civilizations generally have not persisted for more than 5,000 years, and individual nations typically survive for far shorter periods. Can we honestly listen to glib talk of storing radioactive materials that will require maintenance for 10,000 years or longer—and take such plans seriously?

FURTHER READINGS

Council on Environmental Quality. (Issued annually since 1970). *The annual report of the Council on Environmental Quality, Executive Office of the President*. Washington, DC: US Government Printing Office.

_____. (1981). *Environmental trends*. Washington, DC: US Government Printing Office.

Hardin, G. (1999). *The ostrich factor: Our population myopia*. New York: Oxford University Press.

McFarlane, J. (1985). Use of an ecologic model to identify children at risk for infection and to quantify the expected impact of the risk factors. *Public Health Nursing, 2*, 12–22.

Odum, E.P. (1997). *Ecology: A bridge between science and society*. Sunderland, MA: Sinauer Associates, Inc.

US Environmental Protection Agency. (1987). *The toxics release inventory: A national perspective*. Washington, DC: Office of Toxic Substances.

_____. (1976). *Quality criteria for water*. Washington, DC: US Government Printing Office.

US General Services Administration. (continually updated). Code of Federal Regulations. Title 40—Protection of the environment, part 50. National primary and secondary ambient air quality standards, part 129. Toxic pollutant effluent standards, part 141. National primary drinking water regulations, part 143. National secondary drinking water regulations. Washington, DC: US Government Printing Office.

INTERNET RESOURCES

American Museum of Natural History
www.amnh.org/exhibitions/epidemic/epidemic_index.html
Epidemic! The world of infectious disease.

Committee for the National Institute for the Environment
cnie.org
Congressional Research Service reports.

Program for Monitoring Emerging Diseases
www.Healthnet.org/programs/promed.html

US Environmental Protection Agency
www.epa.gov
Environmental facts, profiles, watershed information, maps of regulated sites by zip
code or county.

Carole Schroeder **and** Sally Gadow

AN ADVOCACY APPROACH TO ETHICS AND COMMUNITY HEALTH

4

OBJECTIVES

After reading this chapter, you should be able to

- Describe the universalist tradition in primary health care.
- Describe advocacy as an alternative ethical model for health care.
- Begin to apply an advocacy approach to your practice with the community as partner.

INTRODUCTION

Traditional health care ethics have tended to emphasize issues involving the individual client rather than the community. To broaden that narrow focus, current discussions of health care ethics include attention to issues of public policy. The conclusion that a health professional might draw from this dichotomy is that nothing of ethical interest happens in the region of health care that falls between the care of individuals, at one extreme, and the formulation of policy, at the other.

Most people, however, live their lives at neither extreme. Their primary experience happens elsewhere. People have, in other words, a lifeworld, a primary situation consisting of places, projects, relationships: they live in communities. Community health care as a distinct ethical domain is largely unexplored, yet it may be more important ethically than either individual clients' care or public policy. Primary health care engages people where they live, in communities. Thus, it is an intimate practice, and intimacy entails the potential for significant harm as well as benefit. Health care at the primary level has the power to affect people's lives in radical, pervasive, and often unseen ways.

One approach to community health ethics would be to define the community as client, but this has two limitations. The first is that this approach ignores significant differences between an individual and a community. The second limitation is that defining communities as clients creates the potential for a traditional client–professional relationship, characterized by client dependence, passivity, and neediness in conjunction with professional authority, expertise, and invulnerability. In that model, "clients are constructed as deviant, and service provision has the character of normalization" (Fraser, 1989). A community as client is subject to the same repressive forces as an individual client is, for example, a gendered or racialized definition of community or a professionalized definition of health. Functioning as official interpreters of community health, primary health professions could become "therapeutocracies," removing clients' powers to interpret their own needs (Fraser, 1987). However, defining the community as partner rather than client of the professional offers a different ethical approach, that of advocacy.

An ethic of advocacy calls for formation of partnerships between professionals and community members in order to enhance community self-determination. In these partnerships, professionals and communities form relationships to help a community discern its values and needs and to develop an encompassing health narrative that includes all views. Unique and nongeneralizable, the narrative is specific to the community that develops it, because it expresses the particular health values of the people involved. Unlike other ethical models, the aim of the partnership is improved community health *as defined by the members of the community* rather than as defined by the professional. By interpreting community as partner and primary health care as intrinsic to the life of a community, advocacy mandates that everyone in the community be represented, not just those with political or professional authority.

Although many professionals value the inclusion of diverse views in health care decisions, enacting that value is limited in practice by a universalist ethical tradition that frames service delivery in the United States.

IMPLICATIONS OF UNIVERSALISM FOR COMMUNITY HEALTH CARE

The universalist tradition that frames service delivery in the United States effectively prohibits community self-determination in health. That tradition views people as identical, equal, and autonomous, thereby excluding people whose autonomy is different or diminished. Significantly, these are usually the people most affected by decisions regarding community health: the poor and uninsured, single women with children, people lacking transportation, alienated teenagers and gang members, homebound elderly people, and homeless people. Yet, the inability of these groups to participate in the public arena and to influence decisions affecting their health must be challenged in a system so committed to abstract equality that actual inequalities are invisible.

Historically, universalism emerged from the search for a single set of principles to ground a system of justice. The effect of basing justice on principles of rationality, equality, and neutrality has been to privilege the autonomous and disembodied self and to create the notion of a "generalized other" (Benhabib, 1992). This tradition has three important implications for health professionals: (1) authorization of a single definition of the good (in this case, health), (2) exclusion of the private domain from the service arena, and (3) professional self-identification as expert authority and needs interpreter.

Single Definition of Health

Universalism assumes that a single morality or view of the good is valid, rather than validating many moralities based on different conceptions of the good. Operating out of the universalist tradition, professionals assume a stance of authority and certainty, believing that the general professional definition of health is valid for all. This belief renders professionals incapable of recognizing the particularity of communities and the various meanings of health within a single community. By ignoring contextual, personal, and cultural meanings of health, professionals generalize an abstract model of health across communities. Generalized models often fail to meet the diverse needs within communities and thus fail to be used. Rather than reexamining abstract assumptions about health, many professionals label groups of people as "noncompliant," assuming that failure to use services represents lack of interest in (the professional meaning of) health.

Exclusion of the Private Domain

The separation of public and private domains, which is inherent in universalism, allows subtle exclusion of people who do not fit current definitions of public needs. For example, in the United States, spheres of family/intimacy historically have been deemed outside the public realm. Privatization of family/intimate relationships has excluded them from attention. Because the lives of women and children are conducted primarily through those spheres, domestic violence, child abuse, child care, and most reproductive concerns traditionally have been relegated to the private realm. Until the women's movement brought these issues to public awareness, they were considered too intimate for public attention. Renegotiating the traditional boundaries between public and private domains is one way to begin addressing the health care needs of an entire community.

The Professional as Normalizer

A further implication of universalism is the professional's self-identification as expert authority and thus as community normalizer. The notion that the professional is the bearer of expert and authoritative knowledge that the community lacks is rarely questioned in modern health care; as a result, little recognition is given to communities as experts regarding their own health needs. Instead, individuals, families, and communities are viewed as deviant, passive, and in need of normalization. The resulting hierarchy privileges the professional interpretation while disempowering communities' interpretations of their own needs. Moreover, the professional's self-identification as expert authority fosters a sense of invulnerability that distances professionals from the people they serve and destroys the possibility for mutuality in relationship.

Because professional knowledge can lag behind social changes, health care delivery is often based on invalid assumptions. For example, despite the fact that the traditional ideal of the two-parent family (husband working, wife providing child care and homemaker services) is no longer the norm in many communities, the model continues to express for many professionals the "normal" family. Consequently, health professionals may view single mothers as failed families, needing psychological intervention instead of affordable child care, housing, health care, and well-paying jobs. Thus, due in part to an outdated ideal of family, professional attitudes can effectively silence the community of families headed by single mothers before they even attempt to speak.

Another example of the failure of universalism is the current obstetric approach to childbirth in which professional goals override personal meanings. The medicalization of pregnancy and birth emphasizes (and sometimes legislates) production of a normal fetus as having priority over the rights or experience of the mother. Emerging from universalism and the entrenched view of professional as expert authority, this view does violence to women's personal meanings of pregnancy and birth and results in underutilization of prenatal and birthing services.

An analysis of obstetric literature suggests that medicine defines childbirth in terms of a manufacturing metaphor in which the fetus is a product (Martin, 1992). In that definition, the pregnant woman is marginal, an obstacle to be removed from the center of the situation and replaced by an expert who externally narrates and technologically produces the desired outcome (a healthy fetus). No longer is the woman central to the birthing experience: "The control over knowledge about the pregnancy and birth process that the physician has through instruments . . . devalues the privileged relation she has to the fetus and her pregnant body" (Young, 1984, p 46).

The medical narration of childbirth is particularly evident in services offered to women receiving public assistance and those experiencing complicated (high-risk) pregnancies. Despite the fact that the efficacy of some obstetric practices, such as childbirth position, enemas during labor, and shaving the mother's pubic area, has not been demonstrated, other choices rarely exist for these women regarding their care. In addition, the medical narrative of pregnancy fosters a woman's feelings of failure: having failed to obtain private medical care and to maintain a healthy pregnancy, she has failed to be a "normal" woman, has become a "problem," and so has abrogated any right to assert herself over the management of the pregnancy and delivery.

Not surprisingly, many of these women also "fail" to obtain or comply with prenatal care regimens offered through public assistance programs and high-risk clinics. Particularly alarming is the fact that the US infant mortality rate is significantly higher than the rates in most developed countries. Buried in that statistic is the fact that the number of infant deaths in African-American families is nearly three times the number in white families. This fact further attests to the failure of a health care system based on universalism to meet the needs of particular women and infants.

By critically reevaluating universalism in light of these implications for health care, professionals can redefine themselves and their values in order to relate to communities in other ways. An ethical framework of advocacy offers an alternative to universalism.

ADVOCACY: AN ETHICAL FRAMEWORK

The term *advocacy* has many uses in the literature of health care ethics (Bernal, 1992; Winslow, 1984). Its meaning here is a professional's commitment to enhance client autonomy and to assist clients in voicing their values (Gadow, 1990).

Advocacy as a moral position is derived from the nature of ethics itself; namely, the possibility of choice. Ethics is reflective inquiry motivated by the question, What is the right decision in this situation? If that question is allowed no more than one answer, dictated by a force claiming greater legitimacy than the questioner (a force such as religious, legal, or scientific authority), choice is impossible and ethical inquiry futile. In answering questions about value, ethical inquiry is the alternative to force. Any form of force that preempts free reflection silences ethical inquiry.

Health questions, like all questions about the direction of human life, involve decisions about value. The very concept of health is based on decisions (often at a level neither client nor professional recognizes) to value some functions, abilities, experiences, and outcomes over others. Certain outcomes—life rather than death, for example—may represent such a crucial value for a culture that they become institutionalized as an element of health and take on the appearance of fact instead of value, necessity rather than choice. But a single person refusing the "fact" and insisting on a different outcome is sufficient to illustrate the value basis of health.

To summarize the two points that are the basis for advocacy

- Health decisions are based on values.
- Value questions can be addressed only when choice exists.

Advocacy in minimal terms means that a client's freedom of choice should not be infringed on. The professional, although obligated to act in the client's best interest, is not permitted to interpret that interest contrary to the client's definition. In positive terms, advocacy has broader implications that extend beyond respect for self-determination. Enhancing client autonomy involves not only respect for but engagement with clients in expressing their values as unique persons.

An individual can express her uniqueness only if her values are clearly in her mind, having been reexamined in the context of her health concern. Yet that clarification is the most difficult just when it is most important, when a health situation threatens to overturn existing values. In those circumstances, the person has the alternatives of (1) revising her values to incorporate the new situation, or (2) recreating the situation to conform to her values. In either case, her decisions will be based on her values. Paradoxically, the situation—if serious enough—may call for a decision affecting the very center of a person's world at the same time that the personal world has tilted disturbingly.

Paternalism makes too much out of this tilt; consumerism, too little. Paternalism is the commitment to professional decision making *for* clients, based on the belief that need renders a person incapable of rational judgment. Client autonomy is by definition impaired; hence, professionals are obligated to impose their expertise. Consumerism, on the other hand, is the commitment to professional *non*involvement in client decisions, based on the belief that rationality transcends a tilted personal world. Autonomy is undiminished by illness or injury; therefore, the professional's obligation is to respect the right of self-determination by not intruding in a client's decision making.

Advocacy differs from both of these positions in that it emphasizes the ambiguity intrinsic to health concerns. Client decisions about values are neither the insuperable tasks that the paternalist assumes they are, nor as facile as the consumerist believes. Advocacy accepts the likelihood that, for most people, significant health alterations require reorientation and a new version of personal autonomy. The professional's role is to participate with clients in developing autonomy in the new situation by helping them to discern their values. On the basis of that reflection, clients can reach decisions that express their own reaffirmed or revised values. Only in this way, when the self is engaged and expressed, can a client make decisions that are *self*-determined rather than merely not determined by others.

A client is an embodied self, and part of self-determination involves the relation between self and body. Disruptions in health often create a sense of the body as an objectlike other, alien to the self. Clinical categories and interventions further objectify the experience of embodiment. As a result of objectification, the body seems to become the property of institutions like science, medicine, or law, without a felt connection to the person. At the same time that objectification overwhelms experience, the subjectivity of humiliation, fear, or pain can further isolate persons from their familiar world; in the subjectivity of extreme pain, the world can disappear altogether (Scarry, 1985).

In advocacy, the health professional involves the client in establishing a self-body relation that reconciles the extremes of subjectivity and objectness. The body may retain the meaning of "other" to the client, but advocacy assists a client in freely deciding how to interpret the otherness of the body—perhaps as crony, sage, or intimate adversary. The specific character of the body-as-other is not crucial, as long as its meaning includes more than objectness (that is, includes the body as self or subject)(Gadow, 1980). This interpretation makes the new self-body relation analogous to the intersubjective relation between persons.

The meaning of the body-as-subject offers enhanced client autonomy, because new complexity has emerged in the individual, making new choices possible. Besides the body, other aspects of the person—emotional, intellectual, spiritual, interpersonal—can also enrich the individual if given voice. In this view, the person is a *community* of interests and subjectivities, each offering a different perspective.

As in any community, however, a hierarchy often exists, so that only a few voices are heard on most issues. Whether in the individual or in the community, hierarchy entails the suppression of views and constriction of choices. Because the primary discourse excludes them, excluded views find expression only in dissident forms, such as protest or revolt. Advocacy is the participation with individuals in recognizing seemingly alien views as their own (and, furthermore, legitimate) voices in decision making. In this way, advocacy assists in amplifying clients' perspectives and, thus, available choices.

Ultimately, self-determination is the freedom to interpret experience and determine meaning for oneself. Advocacy is participation with clients in reaching practical decisions, but, at a more fundamental level, advocacy involves participation with a client in deciding the *meaning* of an experience. The greater the diversity of views available, the more choices open to an individual in deciding how to interpret an experience. Engagement with clients at the level of existential choice is the primary means whereby advocacy can enhance autonomy.

It is this existential engagement that distinguishes advocacy from consumerism and paternalism and suggests a client–professional partnership that is foreign to both of those positions. Advocacy is a partnership in which professional and client compose a mutually satisfactory interpretation of their situation. In the partnership, both persons are moral agents, freely accepting or declining the interpretation that each offers, until they reach a meaning that both affirm. The meaning they compose can be considered a narrative, an interpretation that—to their satisfaction—coherently connects all of the elements of the situation. Ultimately, advocacy becomes participation with clients in coauthorship of a health narrative.

The connection between advocacy and authorship is based on the view that every situation represents a narrative or story, a humanly constructed set of meanings that make sense out of phenomena (Carr, 1986). Because no situation has predetermined, unalterable meanings, none has a literal or correct meaning. Other interpretations are always possible. That ambiguity, the absence of final meanings, makes freedom possible. Ambiguity is the space where choice exists, imagination operates, and new narratives can be created.

However, paternalism imposes on clients its own interpretation of their experience, whereas consumerism is indifferent to the narrative clients adopt. Only advocacy as partnership is based on a mutuality without either imposition or indifference. Both persons have a stake in the narrative they compose, and both are present as particular persons, not as abstract categories that assign expertise to the professional and vulnerability to the client. Each has a different expertise, equally essential to the narrative. And each is vulnerable. In fact, the professional is often more vulnerable than the client, who, lacking recourse to the certainty and authority that professionals claim, may already excel at accommodating ambiguity.

The meaning that persons create through advocacy can be termed a *relational narrative*. This relational narrative is different from narratives derived from impersonal sources like science or policy. Advocacy as coauthoring a relational narrative is an example of communicative or discourse ethics. In contrast to ethics based on abstract principles, communicative ethics is a dialogic model involving concrete, contextual deliberations among particular persons. The narrative a client and professional compose claims no universal validity: "Discourse ethics is not one more thorough experiment in universalizability but an ethics of practical transformation through participation" (Benhabib, 1986).

In summary, advocacy aims to enhance and express client autonomy through client–professional creation of a relational health narrative. What are the implications of this ethical model for primary health care, for a practice in which the community is the *partner* of the professional?

IMPLICATIONS OF ADVOCACY FOR COMMUNITY HEALTH

In an ethic of advocacy, no longer does a single authoritative point of view dominate. Instead, morality becomes contextual, the product of mutual interaction and a willingness to reason from the other's point of view (Benhabib, 1992). That willingness is the basis for a community health ethic in which service recipients have an equal voice in the development and delivery of care. When community is defined as partner, univocal decisions are not valid, for all views become legitimate influences in decision making. In an advocacy approach, practitioners become free to engage with a community as a particular partner rather than as an abstract aggregate and to act on the belief that true expertise regarding health resides in the community itself.

The aim of advocacy is to enhance community self-determination through construction of a unique health narrative that guides delivery of services. Fundamental to construction of a health narrative is knowledge about the community's needs and values. Therefore, research methods congruent with advocacy become as important as care delivery models. Participatory research methods, expanded public health nursing, school-based neighborhood clinics, and nurse-managed care centers are but a few examples of a community health ethic in which the professional and the community are partners.

Participatory Research

Using principles of participatory research is a means of increasing community self-determination and control. Participatory research calls for the involvement of local people to collectively investigate problems, analyze information, and act as a community. Basic to participatory research is the concept of collective or community knowledge and the building of relationships as the basis of collective problem solving. To use participatory principles, professionals are obligated to relate to community research subjects as equals. In this way, both professionals and community members begin to see that each group possesses an area of expertise that can benefit the other (Lather, 1986).

Ethnographic assessment of problems and solutions is one means of approaching communities as equal participants in health care. Traditional needs assessments are typically conducted from the perspective of researchers living outside the community, using secondary data such as epidemiologic, historic, registry, and census data. In contrast, in ethnographic analyses of communities, professionals may live in communities for weeks and months at a time, interviewing diverse community members and participating in community life. Information from community members is considered primary data; by living and participating in the community, professionals are less likely to apply disembodied, abstract knowledge to a generalized other.

Focus groups are another means of ensuring community participation in decisions affecting community health. Focus group techniques are a naturalistic method of qualitative research designed to elicit views from the participant's perspective rather than from the researcher's framework (DesRosier & Zellers, 1989). The groups provide a forum for generating innovative solutions to chronic problems. Gathered in a group to discuss health values and needs, community members are considered the primary informants of the research process. Most importantly, this method mandates inclusion of representatives of all persons affected by the analysis. Open-ended questions are used to elicit information, such as

> What is it like living in your community?
> What are your community's strengths? Weaknesses?
> What is health for your community?
> What does health mean for you?

Members of different focus groups bring their results back to the community for analysis in neighborhood meetings. That information is then used to assist in construction of the health narrative that will guide the development and delivery of services in the community.

Public Health Nursing

The reinterpretation of community health using a model of advocacy involves construction of a health narrative that encompasses all views. But how are views to be expressed by those who historically have been excluded from participation (such as mothers lacking child care and transportation, adolescents, gang members, or the working poor)? The disenfranchised often have little trust in professionals and little belief that their own participation can make a difference in their lives. More effective involvement of public health nurses could build on nurses' already established ability to reach marginalized individuals and families. Public health nurses have a long tradition of empowering those outside the public arena. They are closer to families and their problems than professionals who deliver services out of clinics and hospitals. Because they visit people in their homes, they are experienced in approaching clients from a position of shared power. One nurse characterized her practice as mutual disclosure:

> You don't have all your professional hoopla as a shield. . . . You have no uniform, no stethoscope around your neck, no little gadgets to assert your authority. It's you and that person listening to each other. (Zerwekh, 1992)

Public health nurses' expertise in locating "disappearing" families is well documented (Zerwekh, 1992). Ideally situated as advocates for individual and family health and skilled in building trusting relationships, nurses have a sound understanding of local needs and services. Already experienced as advocates for individual and family health, nurses in a community advocacy model could translate their special knowledge from family services into the larger context of community partnerships.

School-Based Clinics

Expansion of existing school-based clinics into comprehensive neighborhood health and social service centers is another means of delivering care to people in their own locale. Most families are already associated with schools, and by integrating social, health, and educational services into neighborhood centers, school-based clinics could increase underserved families' access to public services (Uphold & Graham, 1993). Because schools are based in neighborhoods, underrepresented people's access to health care services can be increased; people lacking time and transportation can more easily participate when decision making and service delivery occur close to their homes.

Nurse-Managed Centers

Community nurse-managed centers are an especially promising means of actualizing an advocacy ethic in community health practice. They are unique in providing clients with direct access to nurses without first requiring a referral fee. Because their focus is maintenance of health rather than diagnosis and treatment of disease, they deliver a wide range of primary services such as wellness maintenance, assessment and screening, education and counseling, symptom management, medical services, and support of home care rather than hospital care. Guided by a health narrative developed by professionals and community members together, these centers could become models for comprehensive delivery of primary health care based on advocacy.

One example of such a center is the Denver Nursing Project in Human Caring, a nurse-managed outpatient center for people with HIV/AIDS. The center was conceived in 1988 by nurses concerned that the health and social needs of people with HIV/AIDS were not being met in the acute care system. The advisory board includes people affected by the disease and local health professionals. Three local hospitals and the University of Colorado School of Nursing contributed to the center's initial operations. In 1990 and 1993, federal funding was obtained from the US Department of Health and Human Services, Division of Nursing, to increase community access to nurses and expanded services at the Denver center. Services include assessment and referral, education for self-care, maintenance of home care rather than hospital care, prevention and management of symptoms, support and counseling, and alternative health treatments (less than one fourth of services are traditional medical services such as blood, fluid, and medication administration, laboratory tests, and so forth). Due to the chronic nature of HIV/AIDS, assistance in negotiating the health and social service system is emphasized as a means of client empowerment.

Collective decision making operates at the center, and a rotating, elected board of clients meets frequently to provide input into all programs offered by the center. Unilateral power relationships of professional privilege and authority are not tolerated; instead, people utilizing the center are considered experts in interpreting their own needs. In initial interviews, clients are asked to "Tell the story of living with HIV." In this way, aspects of the situation that *the client* deems meaningful become the starting point for care planning.

Mutual engagement between nurses and clients for the purpose of client empowerment is a focus of the center, using a partnership model of nursing care. Based on the results of focus groups conducted at the center in 1990, the partnership model evolved out of expressed client and staff needs, rather than unilateral professional interpretation of needs (Schroeder & Maeve, 1992). Clients have been involved in all phases of planning, implementing, and evaluating the care partnerships.

Despite affiliation with institutions that endorse the medical model of disease intervention, the center endorses no single medical narrative of HIV/AIDS as authoritative. Instead, health is individually defined and actualized by clients and nurses through their personal partnerships. This model of community nurse-managed care has proven to be a well-utilized (as well as cost-effective) method of delivering meaningful service at the community level (Schroeder, 1993).

CONCLUSION

Although the public demand for health care reform is no longer ignored by legislators or health professionals, little will actually change unless the traditional values of universalism and authority underlying community health care are renegotiated by the very professionals who have been mandated to change. Rather than new external structures, a new internal ethic is necessary to guide the efforts of health care reform. An advocacy model of community health returns power to communities through partnerships of professionals and representatives of *all* members of a community. Through partnership, professionals and communities develop a health narrative that expresses the diverse values of the community regarding health. Unique and nongeneralizable, the narrative guides service delivery and reform within the community that participated in its development as partner.

REFERENCES

Benhabib, S. (1986). *Critique, norm, and utopia: A study of the foundations of critical theory.* New York, NY: Columbia University Press.

_____. (1992). *Situating the self: Gender, community and postmodernism in contemporary ethics.* New York, NY: Routledge.

Bernal, E.W. (1992). The nurse as patient advocate. *Hastings Center Report, 22*(4), 18–23.

Carr, D. (1986). *Time, narrative, and history.* Indianapolis, IN: Indiana University Press.

DesRosier, M. & Zellers, K. (1989). Focus groups: A program planning technique. *Journal of Nursing Administration, 19*(3), 20–25.

Fraser, N. (1989). *Unruly practices: Power, discourse and gender in contemporary social theory.* Minneapolis, MN: University of Minnesota Press.

_____. (1987). What's critical about critical theory? The case of Habermas and gender. In S. Benhabib & D. Cornell (Eds.), *Feminism as critique* (pp 31–56). Minneapolis, MN: University of Minnesota Press.

Gadow, S. (1990). Existential advocacy: Philosophical foundations of nursing. In S. Spicker & S. Gadow (Eds.), *Nursing images and ideals: Opening dialogue with the humanities* (pp 79–101). New York, NY: Springer Publishing Company.

_____. (1980). Body and self: A dialectic. *Journal of Medicine and Philosophy, 5*(3), 172–185.

Lather, P. (1986). Research as praxis. *Harvard Educational Review, 56*(3), 257–277.

Martin, E. (1992). *The woman in the body: A cultural analysis of reproduction.* Boston, MA: Beacon Press.

Scarry, E. (1985). *The body in pain: The making and unmaking of the world.* New York, NY: Oxford University Press.

Schroeder, C. (1993). Nursing's response to the crisis of access, costs and quality in health care. *Advances in Nursing Science, 16*(1), 1–20.

Schroeder, C. & Maeve, K. (1992). Nursing care partnerships at the Denver Nursing Project in Human Caring: An application and extension of caring theory in practice. *Advances in Nursing Science, 15*(2), 25–38.

Uphold, C. & Graham, M. (1993). Schools as centers for collaborative services for families: Visions for change. *Nursing Outlook, 41*, 204–211.

Winslow, G.R. (1984). From loyalty to advocacy: A new metaphor for nursing. *Hastings Center Report, 14*(6), 32–40.

Young, I.M. (1984). Pregnant embodiment: Subjectivity and alienation. *Journal of Medicine and Philosophy, 9*, 45–62.

Zerwekh, J. (1992). Laying the groundwork for family self-help: Locating families, building trust, and building strength. *Public Health Nursing, 9*(1), 15–21.

Bruce Leonard

CHAPTER

COMMUNITY EMPOWERMENT AND HEALING

5

OBJECTIVES

Community empowerment and healing are theoretical underpinnings to the concept, community as partner. This chapter is designed to assist community nurses to see how healing and empowerment may be applied in practice.

After studying this chapter, you should be able to

- Understand a framework for empowering communities.
- Expand on the concept of healing as a way to transform communities to develop humanistic relationships and resolve community disharmony.
- Apply participatory research as a method to address inequities and injustices in health and society.

INTRODUCTION

As we begin a journey into the next millennium, nurses have the potential to reframe community partnerships through the integration of healing and empowerment in their practice. Partnerships between community members and health care professionals are critical for collaborative decision making in order to improve health. Nurses form partnerships with clients, families, and communities to promote healing and health. The processes by which nurses develop healing or caring relationships in the community mirror interactions among the four major constructs of the nursing paradigm: health, environment, client, and the nurse. The power community nurses have is reflective of their capacity to influence and reshape the environment.

In developing community partnerships through healing and empowerment, we must first understand what a community is. Behringer & Richards (1996) describe communities not as abstract "ideal states" but as complex webs of people shaped by relationships, interdependence, mutual interests, and patterns of interaction. The community encompasses people in a particular time and place. A shared history and language are identifying characteristics of a community. Community health nursing focuses on health, caring, and relationship building among community members. A few key concepts identified by Drevdahl (1995) that are essential to community organization and intervention by nurses are empowerment, participation, goal selection, and critical consciousness. We will examine how nurses might use these concepts to expand the social consciousness of communities.

Community involvement is one of the critical elements of successful problem solving with communities. Community partnership programs in the 1960s and 1970s frequently embraced the concepts of community empowerment and development but were often under the control of academic experts. Experts introduced many programs to communities, but the projects failed because they lacked true community commitment and involvement. In the 1990s, a new emphasis was placed on having communities solve their own problems with guidance from experts. Partnership alliances were formed. Rather than allow self-interests of experts to guide a community, partnership approaches were formulated. Community partnerships work by integrating ideas, people, and resources, in both the development and implementation processes, from the community perspective. A community's level of commitment and involvement may be increased by giving people the needed information and rationale for participation (Behringer & Richards, 1996). Partnership is a complex process of bringing together academics, community leaders, and health care providers to accomplish change.

Not only are partnerships important in implementing community-based programs, but they must be culturally sensitive to ensure success. When implementing a program, we must find ways of caring for communities that match their perception of health problems. Partnership programs often fail if there is conflict between the health provider's and the community's belief systems. Spector (1996, p 63) notes in her book, *Cultural Diversity in Health and Illness*, that "we are living in a pluralistic society, and it is becoming more and more evident that cultural differences are increasingly serving to isolate and alienate us from the other." We define our own health or illness based on our cultural and ethnic backgrounds and on how to be healthy and to recognize illness (Spector, 1996). Community partnership programs designed to promote health should be aware of the complex issues that surround the delivery of health care from the community's or client's point of view.

Historically, nurses have had a rich practice in the community transforming both individual and public health for the poor and disenfranchised through political advocacy. Lillian Wald (1915), who coined the term *public health nurse* in 1893, provides probably our prime example of working with the community to improve health. During the latter half of the 20th century, however, nurses have been thwarted in their activities to promote community health. The focus of health care has emphasized individualized medical care and has been centralized around the biomedical model of primary care. Assumptions of the medical model identified by DeJong (1979) include:

- The physician is considered the medical expert.
- The physician is the primary decision maker who has ultimate authority in decision making.
- The client is expected to cooperate with the physician and assume the "sick role."
- The primary role of medicine is to cure or restore health through the use of procedures such as drug therapy or surgery.
- Diseases may be identified, diagnosed, and treated only by certified practitioners.

The present "system" of health care has not served our profession well, and this has resulted in fragmented programs and limited return on improving the overall health in communities. "The system had developed a well-defined hierarchy in which nurses have great responsibility but little independence and patients are passive recipients of care" (Roberts, 1998, p 184).

In embracing the biomedical model, nurses have lost their unique voice, innovation, and drive to be proactive in community affairs. We may remain silent or blind to what is going on around us while working for technologically advanced institutions whose focus of care has been on the individual. Through integration of the concepts of empowerment and healing, nurses may learn to transform our present sick–cure medical system of primary care into a model of primary health care. Primary health care, as defined in Chapter 1, embraces the ideals of the World Health Organization's Alma Ata declaration (WHO, 1978) of providing essential health care based on the needs of the community emphasizing health and well-being as a fundamental right for all. Our challenge is to transform our fragmented health care system into one that reflects the values and needs of our communities.

COMMUNITY PARTICIPATION AND HEALING

Community nurses may transform our fragmented system of disease-oriented health care by reformulating a vision for the future. We must look beyond our past and explore new avenues aimed at improvement of health for all. Rather than focusing on disease-specific problems, we should explore developing new programs with a community focus on providing primary health care. People in communities deserve comprehensive nursing care aimed toward improvement of health and quality of life for all. "Health for all through primary health care means that the nurses first ask the people what they want to improve their health and then take the responsibility to work as partners with them to achieve it (empowerment)" (Anderson, 1991, p 1). It is evident that health in this country cannot be improved just by the mere provision of health services, but needs to be based on principles of equity, participation, and involvement of communities in making decisions about health care. Successful community participation implies negotiation without manipulation and equity in relationships between community members and health care workers who embrace common goals in providing health care with accessible programs and services for all.

Community participation is a social process involving people from specific geographic localities who share common values in identifying their needs (Rifkin, 1986). Participation in formulating the framework for primary health care in a community may lead not only to better services but also to services based on existing socioeconomic conditions. Rifkin (1986) described three approaches to community participation in health programs commonly used by different countries (Figure 5–1). One is the medical approach, which is focused on curing diseases and is controlled by the medical profession. The second is a health services approach, which mobilizes people to take an active role in the delivery of services based on modifying unhealthy behaviors. The third is a community development approach in which people are involved in the decision-making process to improve health. The first two approaches to health care are top-down approaches similar to primary care where experts in health care prescribe their values of health care for the public. The third approach is a grassroots approach in which members within a community determine what

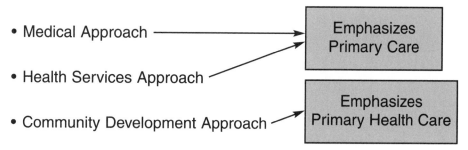

Figure 5–1. Three approaches to community participation in health care (Rifkin, 1986).

health care services should be provided, and it is more consistent with the principles of primary health care.

Our present model of health care in this country is rooted in specialized services for the individual because health care is controlled by the medical profession and the insurance industry, which are designed for capitalistic profit. The current primary care system sometimes dehumanizes our health care and ignores principles of participation as a human right.

Several components are essential for community participation; these include (1) a framework to define the community, (2) the members of the community must share a common awareness of their health concerns, and (3) mechanisms to mobilize the community to recognize their needs and work in partnership with health care professionals to develop a culture of participation (Meleis, 1992). Community nurses have the skills to enable people to make decisions and act on issues communities believe are essential for their health or well-being through empowerment participation.

Empowerment through participation has three essential components to which nurses must be sensitive for community transformations to occur (see displayed material). First, participation is an active process, not a process where one group or organization imposes its values on the community, but a process of mutuality where all have voice. Second, participation involves choice, implying people have the right and the power to make decisions that affect their lives. Third, the decisions made through participation must have the possibility of being effective and there are social systems to allow decisions to be implemented. Community participation, according to Rifkin, Muller, & Bichmann (1988, p 933), "is a social process whereby specific groups with shared needs living in a defined geographic area actively pursue identification of their needs, make decisions and establish mechanisms to meet these needs."

Essential Elements of Community Empowerment

Active process
Nonjudgmental
Mutuality
Choice
Right to make decisions
Effective participation
Decisions are implemented

The role of the nurse in community empowerment is building effective partnerships through community participation. Nurses offer a rich source of skill and knowledge to empower community members while drawing on several paradigms. Only our imagination, vision, and moral or ethical values limit the climate of empowerment we create. Nurses are very familiar with the curative model of health care based on the biomedical model. This model has not served our profession well because it has made health care a commodity and not a lifestyle choice that includes health promotion, disease prevention, and caring beyond curing. Nurses working within this traditional framework have allowed the biomedical sciences to determine the boundaries of moral and ethical concerns based on empirical scientific knowledge rather than honoring the human sacredness of caring or healing (Watson, 1995). An alternate vision comes from the holistic model of nursing based on principles of healing that integrate all human potentials in formulating client-based partnerships. Nursing is about building moral healing relationships, not curing relationships.

HEALING IN THE COMMUNITY

Holism is fundamental to the mind–body–spirit connection necessary for true healing to occur. Healing is a dynamic process involving interplay of human energies that transforms people toward wholeness in understanding their connectedness among themselves, others, and the environment. Healing may be both a process and an outcome with multidimensional possibilities limited only by the human imagination.

The process of being healed is more than just the physical biologic healing of a wound. Although the physical wound may heal completely without leaving a scar, the mental wound of how it occurred may not.

> Nurses recognize that healing is not the same as curing, that casting a broken leg for nine weeks ensures little for the person who has to live out a complex, unique, personal life with that cast for nine weeks. We all want the cast when we have a broken leg, though that is merely the beginning of healing and often the least complex facet of the process. (Kritek, 1995, p 226)

The process of healing involves both the physical and the mental to allow persons or communities to resolve emotional wounds and enjoy our full potential as human beings. Healing is more than curing. Curing as it relates to the biomedical model implies resolution of illness. In situations of community violence, social injustice, poverty, terminal illness, chronic pain, physical disability, for instance, a cure may not be possible beyond the physical relief of symptoms. The biomedical model of health care doesn't get to the "real" causes of community problems. Although this model has brought us wonderful technologies for curing communities, such as in preventing infectious diseases and epidemics, this model is insufficient to use in creating an environment for maximizing our life-sustaining energies to heal.

DEVELOPING RIGHT-RELATIONSHIPS

Nurses relate to clients, communities, and families on many psychosocial levels. Although the concept of healing is applied frequently to an individual, the same concept may be applied to communities or aggregates of people who make up our social systems. In the development of a nurse–client relationship, nurses may help instill hope into their clients or community to relieve psychological stress to assist in the healing process. The concept of healing when applied to nursing is a process of moving the client and community toward wholeness or a state of well-being. The term *heal* means to become whole or to make sound in restoring a person's health (American Heritage Dictionary, 1992). Wholeness implies a person is more than just a physical being or entity, but a multidimensional human. A person has a body–mind–spirit relationship interacting holistically with one's internal and external environment. Healing is a process of becoming restored or whole. Nurses facilitate healing through their interactions with clients or communities. For healing to occur, there must be a balance of unconditional acceptance between the nurse and the client as a whole person. The transformation of becoming whole is what Quinn (1997) identifies as the right-relationship among one or more levels of the human system. Right-relationship is defined "as any pattern of organization within the system that supports, encourages, allows, or generates actualization and self-transcendence—at any and all levels" (Quinn, 1997, pp 2–3). Nurses play a critical role in the process of assisting communities, families, and individuals in the process of becoming whole through facilitating right-relationships.

The development of the right-relationship is not an ethical or moral judgment, but a pattern of organization that generates self-transcendence or self-actualization (Quinn, 1997). In the postmodern world, physics has just begun to explore the new sciences of chaos theory, string theory, or dynamic systems theory. These new theories, for instance, may demonstrate how healing implies a balanced harmonic relationship between humans and their environment similar to the sounds of a symphony. The musical tones may resonate among the life forces in the human system in unpredictable patterns similar to those visualized through a kaleidoscope of colored glass as opposed to our modern theories of science, where everything is predictable, reducible, and reproduces clear pictures of reality with predetermined outcomes. Life forces are a part of the human whole with an essential but unknown connection between the body, mind, spirit, and environment. The art of nursing involves developing a sense of connectedness between clients, communities, and the nurse that resonates this harmonic relationship. For healing to occur, there needs to be a balance of unconditional acceptance of the client/community by the nurse.

The ability to heal may be expanded to communities as a whole. If you imagine communities made up of systems connected to form a natural healing web, nurses could create synergistic healing partnerships among individuals, families, and communities similar to energy flowing through electrical wires. The environment has a special place in the development of human relationships (Quinn, 1992). The energies within the environment according to Rogers (Falco & Lobo, 1995) are "pandimensional." Environmental energy fields are integral parts of human life patterns. In a healing web, nurses could integrate different worldviews to create a holistic perspective, one that values diversity of culture and humanness in forming partnerships with multiple community systems. A nurse working in a healing environment would want to look at what is creating disharmony within a community and pattern the environment to promote health and community well-being. Through communication and formulating partnerships among community systems, nurses may pattern the environment to develop healing partnerships or right-relationships. Relationships created within a natural healing web would allow for the development of extraordinary states of consciousness for true community healing to take place.

People are living systems, a part of a universal system, who maintain organizational systems in order to balance their lives. A person or community is more than just a system created from subsystems, but a complex whole whose energies are in constant interaction with the universe. The energy to heal is within each person and community and is part of the universal energy that surrounds a person. Nurses are fundamentally responsible for facilitating relationships that promote a sense of connectedness for healing to occur.

A harmonic balance created through healing relationships has not been the dominant paradigm of our health care system. The concept of healing differs philosophically from the medical paradigm of curing. A focus on the integration of wholeness in the healing process could transform health care from a curing model to a healing model, or to a system that is truly humanistic. The integration of healing in health care might transform our system into one where communities, families, or individuals are treated as a whole rather than a subsystem of parts where only one piece of the puzzle is "fixed" at a time.

In curing, a disease may be eliminated, but the body–mind–spirit imbalance may remain unchanged. We can be cured yet still perceive we are sick and thus remain in an unhealed state. The healing process occurs on a multidimensional level affecting all aspects of the body or community regardless of whether it has been "cured." The process of healing affects all levels of the human system from emotions to the body–mind–spirit relationship. The potential for healing is inherent in every community and every human being, and is always possible through the development of a connected relationship. A change in one part of our human systems leads to changes in other systems, the direction of which may be unknown in a healing model.

Community nurses have the potential to transform community systems into healing-caring environments. Figure 5–2 displays a model of the concepts of healing and the interactions between the nurse and community. Communities are composed of many core groups and subsystems in the community-as-partner model. Community nurses assist community members in the healing process by transforming relationships. If relationships are limited or confined to the elements of the biomedical model of health care based on curative measures, communities will not maximize their human potentials to become proactive for healing processes and outcomes. Although the biomedical model strives for predictable outcomes in curing disease, people may not be healed in the process. If nurses do not develop right-relationships with communities, community members may not be able to maximize their potential to become empowered. Community nurses who practice in a healing framework strive to develop a sense of connectedness or right-relationships with community members. Nurses who practice in a healing environment embrace multiple theories of knowing or understanding. Relationships built on the healing model embrace diversity where outcomes may be creative or unpredictable but are right for the community as a whole.

There is growing sentiment in this country for health care that would treat Americans like whole individuals rather than as fragmented parts. In a national health care study by Astin (1998) examining why Americans are looking for alternative health care choices, the reason most frequently cited includes a search for health care that is more congruent with their own values, beliefs, and philosophies related to life and health. With growing sentiment toward a more holistic approach to health care, a revolutionary crisis, or what Kuhn (1996) terms *a paradigm shift*, may be occurring. Nursing is in a prime position to articulate a model to the world that could transform health care in the next millennium to a healing paradigm; one that advocates safeguarding clients against abuses and violations of their rights.

In the traditional biomedical approach to health care, community health care workers have viewed community members as sources for data gathering or recipients of care. The conventional approach to health care has been paternalistic, resulting in fragmented or unwanted programs with community mem-

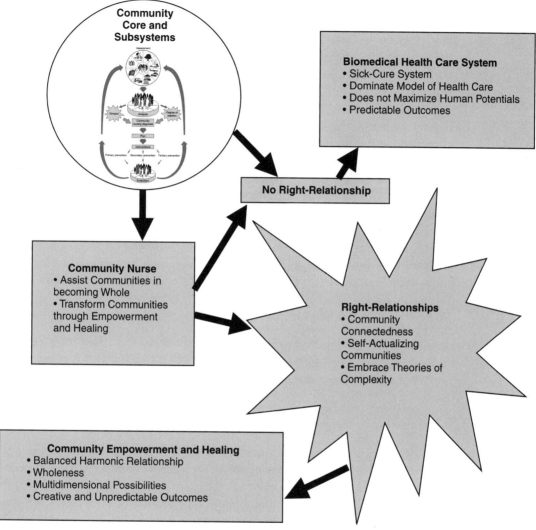

Figure 5–2. Model for community empowerment and healing.

bers as passive participants. Community health partnerships emphasize active participation by community members and health care workers not only from a variety of disciplines but from every relevant segment of society. The goal for community health care workers, then, should be to empower community members to visualize their needs and actively participate in planning and implementing needed change.

Transforming Communities Through Empowerment

How can nurses transform communities to expand their healing resources? Empowerment enhances the possibilities for people to create change through the healing process. Empowerment is an avenue for communities to gain control of resources and transform inequities of power through social change. Education is a process for social action to transpire by organizing people to gain control over their lives and community resources. Nurses work to empower communities not for domination or control of people, but rather to promote the development of others to promote change.

Dialogue is a critical element for community transformations to occur. All voices in a community are important. Paulo Freire (1997), a Brazilian educator, contributed philosophic and theoretical writings on empowering people through education to reverse the dehumanization and objectification of oppressed people. His concerns deal primarily with class oppression, but his philosophies have been applied to empowerment of professions such as nurses, feminist theory, and vulnerable populations among communities at risk for poor health. Exemplars of community empowerment identified by Wallerstein (1992, p 198) include:

> . . . achieving equity of resources; having both equity and the capacity to solve problems; identifying their own problems and solutions; increasing participation in community activities leading to improved neighborhoods, a stronger sense of community, and personal and political efficacy; and developing a participatory social action model to increase the effectiveness of natural helping systems and support proactive behaviors for social change.

Community partnerships develop through a process of empowerment. Partnerships are flexible systems of power structures established through negotiated efforts to distribute power among participants whose purpose is to improve the overall health or well-being of a community. Four characteristics of an empowered community (conceptualized from Paulo Freire's [1997] *Pedagogy of the Oppressed*) follow:

- Faith in people
- Trust established through dialogue
- Hope in positive transformations benefiting the community as a whole
- Discussions grounded in critical thinking without fear of repercussions by those who are in power

Freire hypothesizes that dialogue or communication between people is the key to empowerment. Each of the empowerment characteristics is discussed below.

Faith in people implies that all people have the *potential* to provide a voice in community affairs. Without faith, Freire (1997) proposes, there can be no dialogue, and dialogue cannot exist without love for the world and for people. Love is a fundamental priority for the foundation of dialogue and cannot exist in a world of domination where people are oppressed. Faith in humanity encourages a commitment between community members to create and transform the bonds of human communities and interconnect those who live on the fringes or are the most vulnerable to the whole of society. Vulnerability implies individuals or communities who are camouflaged in our society, such as the homeless, chronically disabled, immigrants, or low-income single parents. Vulnerable populations are at great risk in society for harm to occur and are often those with the least social capital. The risk encountered by the vulnerable is generally not voluntary or under their control. The more risk encountered, the more vulnerable the person or population becomes. Vulnerability leads to symptoms of victimization, alienation, helplessness, or powerlessness, all opposite approaches to empowerment.

Freire (1997) believes that faith in people through dialogue is a primary component in transforming those who are most vulnerable to the empowered, but we cannot have dialogue without *trust*. Trust in people is founded on the principles of truth and integrity in our words. False or feeble faith in one's intentions or actions does not create trust. Many well-intentioned community projects have failed through false leadership of people saying one thing or designing projects for their own personal reality, ignoring those the project is intended to serve, or performing actions not congruent with their behaviors.

Hope through dialogue is another vital component of empowerment (Freire, 1997). Hope engenders a sense of inner strength in people that propels them to act, mobilize forces, and envision a better tomorrow. Hope empowers a person to move beyond present difficulties and see a future with possibilities. Hope is all encompassing in providing people protection against despair and gives them strength, as well as determination to live, when misfortunes in life occur. Empowerment through hope inspires an ability to imagine another perspective. Without hope, dehumanization or hopelessness may result, causing silence or denial of the truth, leading to impoverishment or injustice of being denied the fruits of society. Empowerment through hope is not an entity of imagination acquired while sitting still, but rather a transformational process fought for with conviction. As long as you remain hopeful, you may endure failures and proceed with hope of eventual success. Empowerment is not an instant transformation, but a slow process of weaving thin threads of society together through dialogue like a spider weaves a web.

We have examined the significance of trust, faith, and hope, all "soft" concepts that relate closely to the components of developing healing relationships.

There is one essential component to empowerment that we have not discussed and that is critical thinking. It is through the process of critical thinking and evaluation that people are empowered. For empowerment and communication to be successful, people must engage in critical thinking, continually evaluating and reevaluating the premises behind their thoughts (Freire, 1997). Reality is a dynamic process of change as new technologies and discoveries transform the human environment. People need to be free to exchange ideas, weighing the positive and negative impacts of change on society or communities. As new realities emerge, people must critically evaluate their world and not remain blind or naive to those who are most vulnerable in our communities. Naive thinking justifies maintaining the "status quo" or the continual oppression of those who are at the greatest risk for harm to occur. For social inequalities to change, we must develop new abilities through education to influence others and transform our communities.

The doors of communication between people must always remain open for critical thought. Empowerment is gained through critical dialogue and reflection of critical thought, not necessarily from what is known. It is a process of going from the known to the unknown and reflecting on the possible, with hope for a better tomorrow. Without critical dialogue, true learning ceases to exist and only knowledge is passed between the empowered and the oppressed, not wisdom. Critical thinking encourages the transformation of knowledge into wisdom for those who are most vulnerable. The wisdom gained through critical thought, faith, trust, and hope in humanity may transform social structures from ones of oppression to powerful communities with a voice (Figure 5–3).

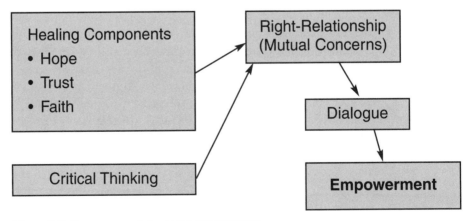

Figure 5–3. Key components for social transformation.

Empowering Communities Through Healing

Empowerment and healing are both synergistic processes and outcomes. Community nurses are responsible for caring for and supporting communities, families, and individuals as they respond to health, violence, or dissonance within society. Nurses are skilled in compassionate caring and the application of scientific knowledge and technology. We are also skillful at humanistic universal–psychosocial–spiritual interactions that support our clients and empower them in the change process. The nurse's role as a healer does not directly create change in others but creates the processes or conditions for change to occur. For compassion and healing care to be sustained, the communities we work with must be willing to care for themselves and to be capable of the process. Communities must be willing to awaken their healing capacity from within. The capacity for healing a community that is faced with a horrific act of violence and senseless loss of life by extremists on the fringes of society, for instance, may stimulate but not necessarily *cause* healing. The psychological scars communities face as the result of sudden acts of violence may persist unless the causes of the social imbalances are resolved. Healing is an intrinsic capacity of the community, and, as health care professionals, nurses have the potential to facilitate the healing process to balance the inequities faced by those with the greatest risk for social harm to occur.

Nurses need to awaken the healing capacity within themselves to facilitate the process of healing others. "Awakening the healer within, however, requires us to face both the limitations and the miracles of our humanness and our work with balanced perspective" (Wells-Federman, 1996, pp 14-15). We need to care for ourselves as human beings, balancing our commitment to practice with the need to heal others. Effective healing can transpire only through our own self-awareness to take responsibility for making change in our lives that will contribute to the well-being of others. Nurses, as universal–psychosocial–spiritual beings, have the unique capacity to understand healing interventions as well as the ability to look beyond the symptomatic causes of disharmony in our communities, placing nursing in a unique position to empower communities to change through healing interactions.

A HEALING CONSCIOUSNESS

The emergence of a healing consciousness where communities envision a mind–body–spirit connection with humanity can only occur through dialogue. Dialogue provides the critical mass for community transformations to take place. The process of empowerment through dialogue enables communities to see their inequities and transform their environment through healing interventions. "The spirit of dialogue involves an openness to new ideas" (Koerner & Bunkers, 1994, p 51). The spirit of openness implies people are open to listen to others and negotiate with an understanding of opposing viewpoints. Empowerment is a process of hope, trust, faith, and critical thinking based on mutual concerns and love for other human beings. Empowerment is a dualistic interactive process involving investment in understanding yourself and others and a willingness to impact change for the betterment of humanity.

The process of promoting a healing consciousness in communities parallels Freire's (1997) process of human liberation of oppression through education. Education, according to Freire, should provide a human awakening of consciousness or what he calls *"conscientizacao."* The awakening of the spirit develops through processes of reflection and critical thinking between the teacher and the students (Figure 5–4). The open exchange of ideas through dialogue does more than just pass old knowledge in justifying the inequities in communities; it provides new insight to the understanding of political, social, and economic forces of oppression. In the modern Western paradigm of the world, "a person is merely in the world, not with the world or with others; the individual is spectator, not re-creator" (Freire, 1997, p 56).

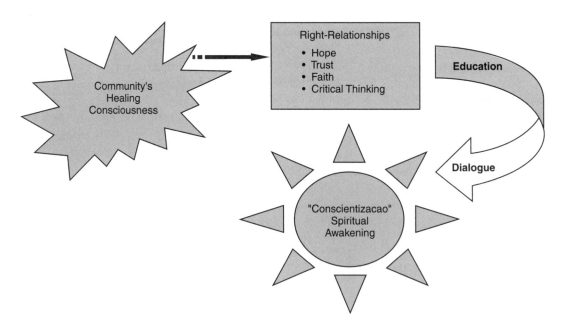

Figure 5–4. Promoting a healing consciousness in communities.

In the postmodern paradigm of a healing consciousness as a model for nursing, only our imaginations and our own fears limit reality. Empowerment and healing are touchstones essential to the nursing process. Nursing is a profession based on mutual understanding of clients, families, and communities. Healing provides the force of liberation to empower communities to reconcile forces of oppression and transform the human consciousness to awaken our capacities for humility, love, and reciprocal cooperation. For healing and empowerment to emerge as a new consciousness in the next millennium, community nurses must engage in active, critical dialogue that promotes understanding, mutual cooperation, and critical reflection of community aspirations. Nurses may institute global change through application of the concepts of healing and empowerment in our own communities to help them become whatever they dream or hope for.

TRANSFORMATION OF GLOBAL COMMUNITY

Empowerment and healing are essential elements to transform our global community. The transformation process of empowering a community through the integration of healing relationships by community nurses has the potential to change the global environment of health care and promote healthy environments for all. The community development approach to health care involves empowerment participation with the application of healing practices by all members of society regardless of culture, social status, gender, or ethnicity. As the world shrinks through global electronic communication, we are exposed daily, through the news media, to inequities in our global environment. We are able to witness first-hand the adversities of famine, drug abuse, unemployment, genocide, murder, and lack of health care worldwide. Community nurses must not remain blind to these inequities, but advocate transforming our societies into healing communities based on principles of trust, hope, love, and faith in humanity.

Our unique vantage point as nurses is our ability to communicate, dialogue, and form partnerships with large numbers of clients, families, and communities. Nurses are in a prime position to chart a new course for the delivery of health care and the resolution of social injustices for the world's disenfranchised based on principles of empowerment and healing. Nurses should assume the roles of "social activists" as conceptualized by Chopoorian (1990), a nurse environmental theorist. Social activism is a process of awakening the human consciousness to the political world around us.

It means being clear on what the dominant ideology is in our culture, how it operates, and whose interests it serves. It requires using our observations to make connections with larger societal issues. It means making the public aware of how problems in the clinical world are related to society. It requires that we form alliances
with co-workers, patients, neighbors, and consumer groups in order to bring issues
before community leaders, political figures, press, and government bodies. It means
that we bring our knowledge of people and their problems and concerns to the attention of others. It means that we are willing to take the risk to speak out against injustice of any kind. It means that we make connections between the suffering that we see
in our world with the suffering of people all over the world. (Chopoorian, 1990, p 35)

EMPOWERING A COMMUNITY THROUGH
PARTICIPATORY RESEARCH

Participatory research is a method community nurses may employ in empowering a community to focus on health problems. It is research done in collaboration with health professionals and community members. In instituting participatory research programs, nurses help communities identify, understand,
find solutions, and determine common goals in resolving community problems. Participatory research is a form of emancipatory inquiry that addresses
inequities and injustices in health and society (Drevdahl, 1995; Henderson,
1995; Lindsey & McGuinness, 1998). Participatory research is a consciousness-
raising action employing both critical and feminist theories. It incorporates conversations that produce both collaboration and self-awareness between nurses
and their community (Drevdahl, 1995).

The methodology of participatory research incorporates scientific research,
education, and political action developed primarily out of the works of Freire
(1997). Critical theory and feminist theory are important components underlying the emancipatory process. Critical theory emphasizes a critical analytic
approach to discussing social problems by active reflection and synthesis
through continuous dialogue. Behaviors may be changed through questioning
the learner and providing feedback. In understanding the social and political
patterns of oppression, community members may be able to emancipate themselves from oppressive power structures (Gortner, 1997). Feminist theory
shares many of the humanistic values of nursing based on concepts of caring,
intuitiveness, and valuing others' world views and experiences (Dunlap, 1994;
Meleis, 1997). A feminist perspective provides a powerful language to enhance
our understanding or to provide insights for social change.

Nurses are challenged to awaken the spirit of social change among those
who are most vulnerable in our communities. Emancipatory inquiry provides
a framework to expand the political consciousness of the disenfranchised in a

community. The problems examined through emancipatory inquiry are those that community members believe are important and not necessarily those identified by health professionals in the community. Participatory research is problem-focused or context-specific research centered on a particular problem involving all participants. Participatory research is similar to action research in which each person or group engaged in the process is committed to improvement through continuous interaction among dialogue, research, action, reflection, and evaluation (Hart, 1996). Individuals are active participants in change and are not passive objects. Through participatory research, community members can gain skills to critically think and analyze the health concerns of their community. "The goal of emancipatory inquiry is neither prediction nor understanding, but emancipation, both within the research process and within society" (Henderson, 1995, p 60).

Henderson (1995) identifies five ways participatory research differs from traditional research methodologies. One, the people engaged in the study are involved in all phases and processes of the research from the design to implementation and analysis. There is a reciprocal relationship between those being studied and those involved in the study. Two, participatory research places emphasis on different ways of knowing beyond scientific ways, such as through the use of intuition or generalized human experiences. Three, the research focuses on empowerment strategies and developing power relationships by focusing on the inequities between those who are being researched and the researchers. The opening of dialogue between the researcher and the researched is an empowerment process incorporated within the research process, but not necessarily the focus of the research as frequently described in nursing research. A conscious awakening occurs by acknowledging the inequities of power relationships between the parties involved and allows for investigation into the imbalances of power as part of the research process. Four, participatory research involves knowledge generation and sharing of ideas to raise awareness between the researcher and the researched creating both new data and theory. Five, the outcomes focus on social and political change in realigning power distributions within communities. The goal of participatory research is social change, not just the advancement of new scientific knowledge. Emancipatory inquiry is designed to have a direct effect on the lives of all participants in the research process not just the researcher. "In participatory nursing research, individuals become empowered to explore the links between the inequities in society and their own impaired health situations and to take action when these links are uncovered" (Henderson, 1995, p 64).

Lindsey & McGuinness (1998) identified several significant themes of participatory research in a qualitative study examining the community participation process. First, there must be planning for the participation. A considerable amount of time should be spent in advance planning and developing effective communication strategies involving key community stakeholders. Preparation is critical for success. Second, an infrastructure for community involvement must be established. The essential structural components include developing of steering committees, facilitating the meetings, involving community members, timing of activities, maintaining commitment, and finalizing the project. Steering committees are designed to maximize community input and are composed of those knowledgeable about the issues, committed to community participation, and able to articulate diverse points of view. The project's design should maximize the number of volunteers from the community, involving them directly in the data gathering, analysis, and dissemination of information. Participatory research is not a quick fix to problems. It involves considerable time and community commitment. Strategies should include ways to maintain enthusiasm and motivation toward the research project, such as dividing the project into small, achievable tasks with defined target dates for completion. Interest in the project may be maintained by giving continuous feedback on the progress of the research, acknowledging achievements, and ensuring the meetings are fun. When barriers are encountered, alternative strategies are proposed to provide community members with the motivation to keep going. In concluding the research project, the information is shared with the community in a forum where community groups and the major stakeholders committed to effecting future change meet to discuss and exchange their experiences. These are all helpful components community nurses may use in the development, implementation, and completion of participatory research projects.

Community nurses are the eyes, ears, and nose of what is going on in a community. We have considerable credibility in the community as health professionals. Our clinical and educational experiences guide us in assessing the pulse of our surroundings. We have numerous tools for implementing change in the community environment based on theory and experience. Nurses have strong interpersonal communication skills, understand the importance of client–nurse relationships, are willing to learn from others, and know how to maximize the health resources of a community. Through our professional encounters with clients, we learn to solve problems almost intuitively and attempt to fix them before harm occurs. Our solutions are not always the right answer if the end result is not congruent with the views or beliefs of those affected. A better solution is to empower the community to resolve its problems while at the same time expanding the community's healing resources. Participatory research is an excellent method for nurses to implement change, even on a small scale.

An example of participatory research by the community health nurse might be your recognition of the importance of informing clients of influenza vaccines for seniors during the flu season while working at a senior center checking blood pressures in a low-income, African-American neighborhood. In talking with clients, you may find that very few in this community have had flu shots, but many have friends who died last year or were seriously ill from influenza. The seniors seem very concerned in light of many news broadcasts predicting a major flu epidemic. You assess that this may be an important health issue to bring up at the monthly board of directors of the senior center meeting next week.

On the way back to the local public health department, you decide to stop by the epidemiology department to examine the community statistics related to influenza over the past few years. In analyzing the data, it is evident low-income seniors in the county had a death rate 50% higher than in other areas. The death rate for seniors living near the senior center where you were taking blood pressures was significantly higher than the rest of the city. The data also indicate that there is an overall higher death rate for senior African Americans within the county. You feel compelled to act because this is a significant health problem where nursing might make a difference.

Over the next week, you do a literature search and put together a proposal to present to the senior center's executive board members to develop a partici-patory research influenza immunization program with the support of the pub-lic health department. You reflect on how to make your proposal successful, knowing there are several barriers. A potential barrier identified is to make the program culturally sensitive to the African-American community. Many sen-iors around this senior center have limited access to health care, lack trans-portation, and have minimal understanding of the importance of influenza vac-cinations. Your literature search, as well as the experience of your practice, reveals some key issues related to the African-American communities. Religion is central in their lives; cultural beliefs and health practices are often underuti-lized, regardless of their impact on well-being; and family support networks and informal health care systems play important roles in maintaining health during periods of stress or crises (Russell & Jewell, 1992). The community health diagnosis for this proposal might be: decreased influenza immunization rate of senior African Americans living in this community related to (1) cultur-al barriers, (2) low socioeconomic status, (3) attitudes, and (4) lack of resources for health promotion and disease prevention, as manifested by statistical evi-dence of high mortality rates and low immunization rates.

Your proposal includes a conceptual framework for increasing the effec-tiveness of an immunization program for the senior center based on the com-ponents of the "community-as-partner model" (Anderson & McFarlane, 1996). The plan incorporates African-American cultural values relating to health and illness practices. The strategies include three main components. One involves increasing the active participation of community members from the senior center in the program design, implementation, and evaluation process. The second includes strategies to tap into the established formal and informal community networks, and the third is structuring the plan to be culturally sensitive with the assistance of the executive board of the senior center as well as religious leaders in the community.

A fundamental component to your proposal is how to empower senior African Americans to receive their flu immunizations through health promotion. Health promotion entails motivating the community, families, and individuals toward obtaining their optimum state of well-being, health, or happiness. The strategies should encourage the best quality of life with goals toward continuous improvement in the overall health of the community. The health status of a community is directly related to the individual health-related behaviors and environmental conditions and is indirectly affected by environmental factors, which influence health behaviors (Brown, 1991). Communities can directly influence their health status by targeting individual health-related behaviors and can change health-damaging environments to health-promoting environments. Brown states, "The ultimate objective of community action for health promotion must empower people to improve their individual and collective health" (p 455).

Three essential elements of health promotion identified by Brown (1991) involve (1) encouraging individuals to change and sustain personal behaviors that prevent disease and promote healthy lifestyles, (2) encouraging health-promoting behaviors that discourage health-damaging behaviors of individuals, and (3) creating an environment that promotes health by eliminating health hazards from the physical environment. According to Brown, most health promotion programs focus on encouraging individuals to change their health behaviors, but seldom look at empowering people to change the lifestyle or environment that shapes their behavior and influences their lifestyle. The goal is to increase the number of seniors immunized against the flu, and the objectives are to assist seniors to overcome their fears of immunizations, increase seniors' knowledge about the flu, increase their political power, and improve their physical health. The community-as-partner model, the concepts outlined for developing a participatory action research plan, and Brown's theory of health promotion are several tools community nurses can use to promote change.

With the approval of the executive board of the senior center, the nursing interventions to meet the objectives of the immunization project are focused on participatory research emphasizing education and focus group community interaction. The strategies addressed in the focus groups to make the program successful highlight clarification of information on flu immunizations, stressing healthy outcomes, keeping the message culturally sensitive, and decreasing fears of the vaccine.

The missing component in our discussion on developing a participatory research program for our immunization project is the ethic of connectedness or developing the right-relationship with the senior African-American community members. We have mentioned the critical component of cultural sensitivity, but we need to focus our energies on building healing relationships in the process of participatory research. The relationships nurses develop in the processes of human interactions are critical to the success of all community programs. We cannot ignore the political, social, environmental, cultural, and economic relationships among all community members. How we interact with communities on all social levels has an impact on our ability to provide voice to those who are most vulnerable in our society. Community nurses are morally responsible to provide a voice that maintains a dialogue of healing or caring and builds a dynamic of empowered connectedness within the community-as-partner model.

CONCLUSION

Community nurses are ideal change agents for emancipating health care in the next millennium. We are the critical conscience of health in the community. Nurses make up the greatest numbers among health professions, but for the last century our powers have not been realized. It is time for us to chart a new course committed to emancipatory goals of feminist and critical theories that engage in consciousness raising to address power imbalances. Empowerment is a process, not an object that can be purchased or consumed. It is a process that grows like a tree from its roots upward. Empowerment is not just a program nurses create, but a process enabled by community health nurses to transform thinking through dialogue in reconstructing a healing environment for all. Only through continued activism can nurses expose the social injustices that continue to contribute to powerless communities. Through community empowerment and healing, nurses can provide a moral voice to inspire change to regain our historical roots as vanguards of the community.

REFERENCES

American Heritage Dictionary of the English Language. (1992). (3rd ed.). New York: Houghton Mifflin.

Anderson, E.T. (1991). A call for transformation. *Public Health Nursing, 8*(1), 1-2.

Anderson, E.T. & McFarlane, J. (1996). *Community as partner: Theory and practice in nursing* (2nd ed.). Philadelphia: Lippincott-Raven.

Astin, J.A. (1998). Why patients use alternative medicine results of a national study. *JAMA, 279*(19), 1548-1553.

Behringer, B. & Richards, R.W. (1996). The nature of communities. In R.W. Richards (Ed.), *Building partnerships educating health professionals for the communities they serve* (pp. 91-120). San Francisco: Jossey-Bass.

Brown, E.R. (1991). Community action for health promotion: A strategy to empower individuals and communities. *International Journal of Health Services, 21*(3), 441-456.

Chopoorian, T.J. (1990). The two worlds of nursing: The one we teach about, the one that is. *NLN Publications, 15*(2351), 21-36.

DeJong G. (1979). Independent living: From social movement to analytic-paradigm. *Archives of Physical Medicine and Rehabilitation, 60*, 435-446.

Drevdahl, D. (1995). Coming to voice: The power of emancipatory community interventions. *Advances in Nursing Science, 18*(2), 13-24.

Dunlap, M. (1994). Is a science of caring possible. In P. Benner (Ed.), *Interpretive Phenomenology Embodiment, Caring, and Ethics in Health and Illness* (pp. 27-41). Thousand Oaks, CA: Sage.

Falco, S.M. & Lobo, M.L. (1995). Martha Rogers. In J.B. George (Ed.), *Nursing theories: The base for professional nursing practice* (pp. 229-248). Norwalk, CT: Appleton & Lange.

Freire, P. (1997). *Pedagogy of the oppressed.* (New Revised 20th-Anniversary Edition ed.). New York: Continuum.

Gortner, S.R. (1997). Nursing's syntax revisited: A critique of philosophies said to influence nursing theories. In L.H. Nicoll (Ed.), *Perspectives on Nursing Theory* (3rd ed., pp. 357-371). Philadelphia: Lippincott-Raven.

Hart, E. (1996). Action research as a professionalizing strategy: Issues and dilemmas. *Journal of Advanced Nursing, 23*(3), 454-461.

Henderson, D.J. (1995). Consciousness raising in participatory research: Method and methodology of emancipatory nursing inquiry. *Advances in Nursing Science, 17*(3), 58-69.

Koerner, J.G. & Bunkers, S.S. (1994). The healing web: An expansion of consciousness. *Journal of Holistic Nursing, 12*(1), 51-63.

Kritek, P.B. (1995). Negotiating at an uneven table. In L. Marcus (Ed.), *Renegotiating Health Care Resolving Conflict to Build Collaboration* (pp. 207-236). San Francisco: Jossey-Bass.

Kuhn. T.S. (1996). *The structure of scientific revolutions* (3rd ed.). Chicago: The University of Chicago.

Lindsey, E. & McGuinness, L. (1998). Significant elements of community involvement in participatory action research: Evidence from a community project. *Journal of Advanced Nursing, 28*(5), 1106-1114.

Meleis, A.I. (1997). *Theoretical Nursing: Development & Progress* (3rd ed.). Philadelphia: Lippincott-Raven.

_____ (1992). Community participation and involvement, theoretical and empirical issues. *Health Services Management, 5*(1), 5-6.

Quinn, J.F. (1997). Healing: A model for an integrative health care system. *Advanced Practice Nursing Quarterly, 3*(1), 1-6.

_____ (1992). Holding sacred space: The nurse as healing environment. *Holistic Nursing Practice, 6*(4), 26-36.

Rifkin, S.B. (1986). Lessons from community participation programs. *Health Policy and Planning, 1*, 240-209.

Rifkin, S.B., Muller, F., & Bichmann, W. (1998). Primary health care: On measuring participation. *Social Science and Medicine, an International Journal, 26*(9), 931-940.

Roberts, S.J. (1998). Health promotion as empowerment: Suggestions for changing the balance of power. *Clinical Excellence for Nurse Practitioners, 2*(3), 183-187.

Russell, K.J. & Jewell, N. (1992). Cultural impact of health-care access: Changes for improving the health of African Americans. *Journal of Community Health Nursing, 9*(3), 161-169.

Spector, R.E. (1996). *Cultural diversity in health and illness* (4th ed.). Stamford, CT: Appleton & Lange.

Wald, L. (1915). *The house on Henry Street.* New York: Henry Holt.

Wallerstein, N. (1992). Powerlessness, empowerment, and health: Implications for health promotion programs. *American Journal of Health Promotion, 6*(3), 197-205.

Watson, J. (1995). Nursing's care-healing paradigm as exemplar for alternative medicine? *Alternative Therapies, 1*(3), 64-69.

Wells-Federman, C.L. (1996). Awakening the nurse healer within. *Holistic Nursing Practice, 10*(2), 13-29.

World Health Organization. (1978, September). *Report of the International Conference on Primary Health Care,* held in Alma Ata, USSR. Geneva, Switzerland: Author.

INTERNET RESOURCES

Critical Thinking
www.sonoma.edu/cthink

Cultural Information
www.healthlinks.washington.edu/clinical/ethnomed

Judith C. Drew

CHAPTER

CULTURAL COMPETENCE IN PARTNERSHIPS WITH COMMUNITIES

6

Being the other is feeling different; it is an awareness of being distinct; it is consciousness of being dissimilar. Otherness results in feeling excluded, closed out, precluded, even disdained and scorned. . . . On the one hand being the other frequently means being invisible . . . or inevitably seen stereotypically. For the majority, otherness is permanently sealed by physical appearance. For the rest, otherness is betrayed by ways of being, speaking, or of doing. (Madrid, 1988, pp 10–11, 16)

Arturo Madrid tells his story of being different, its significance, and its consequences. His poignant expressions of "otherness" are wakeup calls for us. Our sensitivities may be sharpened if we consider that, in any place, at any time, we might just be an "other."

OBJECTIVES

This chapter focuses on the concepts basic to cultural interpretations of differences among people, how those differences are revealed in client–provider interactions, and how awareness, understanding, and changes in our sensitivity and functioning can make us and our institutions more culturally competent.

After studying this chapter, you should be able to

- Discuss the concepts of diversity, ethnicity, culture, and cultural health care systems.
- Acknowledge the influence of culture and ethnicity on health beliefs, illness behaviors, and client–provider relationships.
- Rediscover your own cultural identity and its role in shaping who you are.
- Value the significance of culturally competent providers and institutions.

INTRODUCTION

Since 1965, changes in immigration patterns and birth rates have influenced US population demographics. Experts suggest that the population of diverse racial and ethnic groups will continue to grow at a rapid rate through the middle of the 21st century, when descendants of European whites will become a designated minority (Congress & Lyons, 1992). As a result of these trends, health care providers will interact more frequently with clients of diverse ethnic affiliations whose health beliefs, languages, and life experiences differ greatly from their own. Diversity is a fact of human existence and must be celebrated. Celebrating diversity comes from an awareness of one's own ethnic and cultural backgrounds, an understanding of how they influence everyday life, and an appreciation for the rich beauty that the tapestry of American peoples exhibits.

Beyond awareness and understanding, health care providers must develop skills to work with culturally diverse clients, their families, and communities. Many believe that these skills are learned rather than innate and that they require commitment and nurturing. Such an imperative also suggests that programs and services be designed so that they are available, acceptable, and appropriate to the cultures they seek to serve (Adams, 1990). This "cultural competence" demands that practitioners and delivery systems understand a client's, family's, and even a community's perception of their health needs (Campinha-Bacote, 1995; Cross, 1987), including their health status and acceptable sources of help during vulnerability and illness. This chapter presents concepts that will assist you in building cultural competence, beginning with an enlightened awareness of diversity, ethnicity, and culture, and illustrating their influence on individuals' and communities' health and illness beliefs and practices. Self-assessment and an analysis of client–provider interactions are presented as learning experiences with implications for practice. After all, successful health promotion intervention strategies and outcomes depend on our abilities to competently reach and work with the diverse communities we serve.

DIVERSITY, ETHNICITY, AND CULTURE

Derived from the Latin *divertere*, diversity implies the condition of being different or having differences. There is no attempt made here to imply a ranking, ordering, or prioritizing of differences; they simply exist. How we look at and deal with differences in human attributes can either build bridges or construct barriers with individuals in and across groups and communities. Rather than thinking of differences as sources of conflict, we should view them as part of a whole process of social and individual identity. A celebration of differences can become commonplace when we understand that the principal strengths on which our country is built suggest a tolerance for individual uniqueness and a collective creativity.

Recognizing that each of us differs in what we think is functional in our lives, we must understand that those who act differently from the mainstream are not deficit in something or "disadvantaged"; they are rich in a different culture and are "other-advantaged" (Dervin, 1989; Lyons, 1972).

In daily practice, nurses are providing care to patients and families who represent our global communities. Yet, we know little about the basic cultures, beliefs, and values that shape our clients' health and healing beliefs and behaviors. Asking clients to teach us about themselves will extend to others our sensitivities about being different and will empower others to share their own awareness. Taking the time to value both the differences and commonalities across ethnic and cultural groups will provide us with valuable insights into the human experience and enable us to build bridges between providers and the growing numbers of diverse clients.

Given current population reports, it is estimated that one out of every four persons in the United States is a member of an ethnic minority (May, 1992). In its purest form, the term *minority* implies a condition of difference based on enumerating an identifiable characteristic. Wirth (1945, p 347) has suggested that a minority is "a group of people who, because of their physical or cultural characteristics, are singled out from others in the society in which they live, for differential and unequal treatment, and who therefore regard themselves as objects of collective discrimination." Health care providers need to appreciate the special histories of ethnic minority groups, how their identities are preserved, their variant subcultures, and their unique coping structures—all of which have been challenged by change, exploitation, and prejudice (Moore, 1971). Despite consistent attempts to improve health care to ethnic minorities, statistics reveal that white European-Americans still have higher life expectancy rates at most ages (Devore & Schlesinger, 1991). We still have a long way to go to improve services to groups of Americans who are at great risk. To do this, we must understand that there may be differences in health and healing beliefs between care providers and care recipients. Those differences are rooted in heritage, ethnicity, and culture, but they represent potential barriers to healing relationships.

Whether ethnicity is associated with minority or majority populations, ethnic groups are composed of persons who share a unique cultural background and social heritage that is passed from one generation to another. Ethnicity should be understood as a social differentiation that engenders in us a sense of self-awareness and exclusivity, a sense of belonging. Our ethnicity gives us a membership in a distinct social group and differentiates us from those in other groups. Our distinction is often based on such cultural criteria as a common ancestry, shared history, a common place of origin, language, dress, food preferences, and participation in rituals, networks, clubs or activities (Holzberg, 1982). For example, when members of an Italian-American family gather at a wedding, the nature of the celebration expresses the ethnic culture in many ways. The ceremony and the formalities of receiving witnesses and guests are unique to each group and are representative of "the way things are done." At the celebration that follows the exchanging of vows, the guests may feast on antipasto, linguini, chicken marsala, and cappuccino. Soon after, the accordion player might strike up the tarantella, an Italian folk song. Young and old alike may grasp hands and promenade as they laugh and sing. Late in the evening, the elders may be heard sharing stories about "the old country" with excitement and pride. Although members of this group may have emigrated at different times and may have been born in America, they share common bonds based on native language, history, and values. The passing of these beliefs, values, knowledge, and practices takes place through the rituals of sharing and participating in cultural events and celebrations.

It may be helpful to think of your own ethnic culture. What group(s) do you identify with and why? What are your common bonds? What cultural rituals do you celebrate and with whom? What are the purposes and meanings of your gatherings and celebrations? What types of things are shared and learned when people get together? What types of foods are prepared for the event? Are there dances, special rites, or ceremonies? Each of us can probably identify several shared beliefs, values, and practices that make us members of unique collectives, and many of us strive to preserve our rich cultures and histories by passing them on to each successive generation. Foods, languages, and other bonds of common ancestry are the cultural aspects of ethnicity that serve to offer consistency and structure to life, and provide individuals with abilities to interpret life events as significant and meaningful (Royce, 1982).

In health and illness, an ethnic group's shared beliefs, symbols, and customs serve as common reference points that members use to judge the appropriateness of their decisions and actions (Kleinman, 1978). However, attention must be given to the variations within and between generations that are sometimes attributed to acculturation, socioeconomic status, and education (Congress & Lyons, 1992). Caution should be taken by all health care providers not to generalize beliefs and practices to every member of an ethnic group or culture (Campinha-Bacote, 1995). Although ethnicity captures the larger cultural component of human experiences, we must not permit our awareness of a culture to erode its members' individual identities and dignity.

CULTURE, HEALTH AND ILLNESS, AND NURSING

Ethnic culture is the medium through which an individual's beliefs, standards, and norms for health and illness behaviors are structured, learned, shared, practiced, and judged. Cultural beliefs give meaning to health and illness experiences by providing the individual with culturally acceptable causes for illness, rules for symptom expression, interactional norms, help-seeking strategies, and determining desired outcomes (Harwood, 1981; Kleinman, 1980). For example, when you awake before school with a dryness in your throat and cramps in your stomach, several beliefs about what could be wrong and how you should act in response to what is wrong are set into action. What is causing this to happen to me? What can I do about it? Should I stay home from school? Whom should I call to help me? What will people think if I stay home today? The answers to these questions and the actions you take are learned and are influenced by the experiences you have had with your family and the larger ethnic aggregate. In some cultures, a special home remedy tea can be taken for specific complaints of dry throat and cramps and going to work or school is an expectation. Other cultural groups may expect you to be visited by a healer, stay home from work or school, and tell no one else about your problem.

Noted psychiatrist and anthropologist, Arthur Kleinman, studied members of many diverse ethnic groups to gain an understanding of the links between cultural beliefs and health and illness behaviors and actions (Kleinman, 1980). The findings of his studies are especially helpful in guiding community practitioners who interact with clients in their homes and various types of community institutions. He found, like other researchers, that cultural beliefs based in shared meanings, values, and norms are the basic guidelines people use for recognizing that something is wrong, interpreting what it might be, and organizing a plan of appropriate actions (Kleinman, 1986). For example, before action is taken in response to a problem, individuals and family members must first agree that the symptoms represent a problem. Next, there is an examination of all possible and probable causes, which may range from behaviors and foods to violations of cultural norms. Once a cause is identified, a plan of action is made and appropriate treatment is determined. In addition, how we act when we are "ill" is determined by our ethnic culture. Some cultures have specific norms for sick role behavior, whereas other cultures suggest that you continue to carry out your everyday role to the best of your abilities. In this overall illness recognition and management process, cultural beliefs influence the reasons the client formulates to explain the illness, the language and terms used for communicating the health problem, the choice of whom one talks to about the problem, the range of acceptable healing alternatives, how choices are made, and expectations for treatment outcomes (Helman, 1984; Kleinman, 1980; Mechanic, 1986).

For those of us in the nursing profession, culturally sensitive health care continues to be a central focus of a holistic and humanistic philosophy that guides our practice (Aamodt, 1978; Leininger, 1978; Munet-Vilaro, 1988). Because nursing is defined as the diagnosis and treatment of human responses to actual or potential health problems (American Nurses Association, 1980), the role of cultural beliefs in guiding a client's health practices and responses to illness episodes is an important nursing concern (Whall, 1987).

The healing goals of culturally sensitive care can only be achieved through conscious efforts at gaining knowledge of different groups' ways of explaining, understanding, and treating health problems. Certainly gaining this knowledge and putting it to use will take some time, but it is important for practitioners to learn the strategies presented in this chapter for eliciting from clients their cultural models for health, illness, help seeking, and healing.

CULTURAL HEALTH CARE SYSTEMS

Basic to successful interactions between clients and providers is the understanding that we are all different from one another, with different ethnic and cultural backgrounds, and, therefore, different health and illness beliefs and practices. There's that word again: "different." But despite our differences, we come together at a mutually agreed on place to achieve a common goal: to maintain or regain health. The dilemma presented here is that health means different things to each of us; we recognize it and measure changes in it differently, act in diverse ways when faced with these changes, and seek different methods for achieving healing outcomes. The settings where we meet and interact with each other may take on different veneers and titles, but they are all what Kleinman calls "cultural health care systems" (Kleinman, 1980). The simple fact that culture influences health and illness beliefs and behaviors serves as a constant reminder to us that wherever clients and providers interact, there is a system, and it is influenced by the beliefs, values, norms, and standards that each of us brings to it. Cultural health care systems are made up of individuals experiencing and treating illness and the social institutions where interactions between clients and providers take place (Kleinman, 1980; Kleinman, 1986). Each cultural health care system can have several recognized sectors. The three sectors Kleinman's model addresses are referred to as popular, folk, and professional. Typically, the popular sector is composed of ordinary people, families, groups, social networks, and communities. The lay practitioners and healers comprise the folk sector, whereas the professional sector is composed of the licensed health professionals (Kleinman, 1980). Let us look at these sectors in some detail.

Popular

The popular sector of cultural health care systems is made up of informal healing relationships that occur within one's own social network. Although the family is at the nucleus of this sector, health care can take place between people linked by kinship, friendship, residence, occupation, or religion (Helman, 1984). In the United States, there are as many versions of the popular sector as there are ethnic cultures. In neighborhoods where many ethnic groups have settled, popular sectors of health care systems are found to have several different ways of managing health, illness, and healing.

In the popular sector, the process of defining oneself as ill begins with a self-diagnosis confirmed by significant others based on the implicit standards of what it means to be well (Angel & Thiots, 1987; Eisenberg, 1980; Helman, 1984). Consequently, a person is defined as ill when there is agreement between self-perceptions of impairment and the perceptions of those around him (Helman, 1984; Weiss, 1988). The social, ethnic, and cultural values on which the illness judgment is based focus on the experience of discomfort, failure to function as expected, and a change in physical appearance. Whether a symptom is recognized as significant or normal is also influenced by the occurrence, persistence, and prevalence of the symptoms among group members (Angel & Thiots, 1987; Helman, 1984).

Once a symptom is recognized as significant, decisions about appropriate healing actions must be made. These decisions are also usually based on beliefs, standards, and norms passed along from previous generations. For example, decisions about seeing a physician for a health problem, as opposed to taking care of the symptoms at home, are made by the affected individual in collaboration with family and the social network. If the symptom is commonly observed in other members of the family or community and home remedies have successfully treated the problem, then going to the physician is not a priority. Within this sector, both the care recipient and the network counselors share similar assumptions about the observed symptoms and recommended healing strategies. Therefore, misunderstandings are rare, and the healer's credentials are based on experience rather than professional education and licensure (Chrisman, 1977; Kleinman, 1980).

Folk

The folk sector of cultural health care systems includes the interaction between a client and sacred and secular healers. Most healers share the same basic cultural values and beliefs as their constituents. In many cases, family members and others in the social network work alongside the client and the healer to discover and treat the problem. Sources of holistic health problems are believed to include relationships the client has with other people, with the natural environment, and with supernatural forces (Helman, 1984).

Treatment rituals and strategies are prescribed to correct disequilibrium and to promote healing. Healers have little formal training, although some have served an apprenticeship with another, more accomplished healer. Most are believed to receive healing powers through family position, inheritance, signs, revelations, or gifts (Lewis, 1988).

Within the folk sector, illnesses are defined as syndromes from which members of a group suffer and for which their culture provides a cause, a diagnosis, preventive measures, and regimens of healing (Rubel, 1977). It is very important that beliefs about causes of illnesses be compatible with selected treatments. In some cases, family and folk healers may be the only persons who can effectively recommend or perform healing rituals. For example, some Hispanics believe that *susto* results from a traumatic experience or that sickness is a punishment from God. Susto or *fright* is an emotional response to a traumatic experience. It is recognized by some Latina peoples as an illness that includes the loss of one's spirit from the body. Symptoms include crying, loss of appetite, listlessness, insomnia, nightmares, and withdrawal. Susto requires treatment by a curandero whose healing rituals attempt to get the individual's spirit back into the body. Sometimes complementary and supportive treatment from a psychiatrist is sought (Rivera & Wanderer, 1986; Ruiz, 1985). Working with clients and families to learn acceptable forms of healing for these problems is imperative.

Professional

The professional sector of cultural health care systems is made up of organized health professionals who are formally educated and legally sanctioned (Kleinman, 1980). Unlike the popular and folk sectors, the clients and the providers in the professional sector typically differ in their social and cultural values, beliefs, and assumptions. Based on these differences, as well as the unfamiliar surroundings and rules of the institutions where care is given in the professional sector, the client–provider relationship may be one of mistrust, suspicion, and conflict.

Although many collaborative, complementary, and alternative models of healing are gaining popularity, practices in the professional sector remain dominated by a biomedical disease and treatment orientation. A biomedical orientation suggests that disease is a physiologic and psychological abnormality.

This view is exclusive of and counter to the popular, holistic view of illness as a meaningful experience perceived and constructed in sociocultural context (Allan & Hall, 1988; Angel & Thiots, 1987). Some of us have prepared a home remedy for a sore throat problem or have applied a poultice to relieve a headache or a persistent cough. These are examples of actions taken, in the popular sector, in response to symptoms that are interpreted as part of a meaningful illness experience. In the professional sector, these same symptoms may be viewed as significant threats to health.

DECISION MAKING

People who become ill make choices about whom to consult in the popular, professional, or folk sectors of the cultural health care system. There is overwhelming evidence to suggest that those choices are influenced by the individual's subjective definition of the illness, its meaning, and its expected course (Fabrega, 1974). Attitudes toward different types of providers and decisions about whom one should seek for help vary according to how the symptom is interpreted and what it means to that person as a significant life event.

Forming these decisions is also a function of shared, family, and culture-based learning (Mechanic, 1982). Remember back to your childhood and a significant episode of not feeling well.

- Who decided what was wrong with you?
- What were the interpretations of your symptoms?
- Who made the decision about what to do for you?
- With whom did this person consult?
- Did the meanings of your symptoms and who was consulted have anything to do with the selected treatments?
- What were the expected outcomes from your treatments?
- How were those outcomes evaluated?

Just as important as finding answers to your own health, illness, and healing beliefs and practices is investigating the significance of these factors and processes in your clients' illnesses.

In developing a help-seeking pattern, most people establish a therapeutic network, which may include informal relationships with people and providers from some or all of the three sectors of cultural health care systems. Different types of providers, including family members and folk healers, may be used concurrently or in sequence depending on the client's perception of the cause of the problem, course of the illness event, and desired healing outcomes (Angel & Thiots, 1987; Helman, 1984; Kleinman, 1980; Mechanic, 1982).

Typically, people make their help-seeking choices based on prior learning, symptom significance, compatibility between the philosophies of the sectors, and evaluation of the treatment outcome (Blumhagen, 1982; Chrisman, 1977; Kleinman, 1980; Young, 1982). It seems logical that clients, in the process of seeking help, may involve a network of potential consultants ranging from informal structures in the nuclear family to select laypeople and professionals (Friedson, 1961; Roberts, 1988).

CONFLICT AMONG SECTORS

Given our diverse cultural backgrounds, we should not be surprised to find that research across many health-related disciplines provides evidence that barriers, conflicts, and misunderstandings among the system's sectors are, in part, related to the differences in cultural beliefs about illness causation and management (Chavez, 1984; Roberson, 1987).

Although we may never have viewed conflicts through Kleinman's (1980) perspective before, we have all encountered conflicts between providers and clients. We may have even been the clients! Have you ever gone to the physician only to find that he or she recommended a treatment that was not what you expected? Have you ever found that a medication prescribed by the physician is something that you would rather not take? None of us is a stranger to these types of conflicts. Even after students in undergraduate and graduate nursing programs are offered a greater knowledge of ethnicity and culture, the conflicts in beliefs and practices between sectors and resultant barriers to effective health care remain unresolved. The lack of progress in reducing barriers can be linked to professional providers' relative inattention to the popular sector of cultural health care systems. Have you ever heard a professional provider say, "This client is difficult" or "This client is noncompliant with his medicines and he won't follow his diet"? Perhaps you have made such comments yourself without thinking that what has been prescribed or recommended may not be compatible with the client's beliefs about treatment and healing. The problem could be more basic than a mere treatment conflict; perhaps the client and provider have incongruent beliefs about what is wrong and what caused the symptom of illness. In the popular or folk sector, illness is sometimes thought to be a somatization of a client's uneasiness with either a stressful relationship, the natural environment, or supernatural forces. This is an example of how cultural beliefs about the cause and management of an illness provide the client with a foundation for interpreting the illness experience as meaningful.

Because belief systems in the popular and folk sectors have often been termed as "unorthodox," "lay," "subjective," or "nonscientific" (Roberson,

1987) and have been associated with non-Western societies, a client's preference for such healing practices has been dismissed by some professional health care givers. This is problematic because if recommended treatments do not fit the cause, then the client may not follow suggested protocols.

If these problems are to be resolved, we need to understand and accommodate the ideologies and practices of diverse individuals. Professional providers must consider the significance of the illness interpretations and meanings for the clients we treat, thus facilitating a more comfortable and secure client–provider relationship. We must focus on the popular sector if working relationships are expected to have successful outcomes. Conflicts, misunderstandings, and barriers to effective health care will be reduced only by commitment to gain knowledge about the popular sector, where health beliefs and health practices are activated (Kleinman, 1980) and where 70% to 90% of all illness episodes are recognized and treated (Zola, 1972). The nursing profession's commitment to health and holism and its capacity to understand complex sociocultural responses to real and potential health problems make it the most logical choice for a professional segment element to act as a client advocate in facilitating interactions between the sectors. Appropriate advocacy must be based on the ability to understand the popular sector's realities and to translate and negotiate between the system's sectors with the goal of reducing barriers to culturally sensitive care (Chrisman, 1977). In doing so, nursing will lead the charge for cultural competence among providers and will model the application of those attributes for health care institutions.

Without a doubt, differences are sources of conflict and misunderstanding in client–provider relationships (Angel & Thiots, 1987; Blumhagen, 1982). A detailed understanding of cultural health care systems will provide us with many reasons for the existence and resolution of real and potential barriers between providers and laypeople in the care-giving process. Beyond a basic understanding of the ingredients for conflict, this paradigm of differences should be used by providers, partners, and communities as a guide for becoming culturally competent.

THE CULTURALLY COMPETENT PROVIDER

Cultural competence implies an awareness of, sensitivity to, and knowledge of the meaning of culture and its role in shaping human behavior (McManus, 1988). If culture, broadly defined, is socially transmitted beliefs, values, ways of knowing, and patterns of behavior characteristic of a designated population group (Kleinman, 1980; Wood, 1989), then cultural competence is the ability to express an awareness of one's own culture, to recognize the differences between oneself and others, and to adapt behaviors to appreciate and accommodate those differences (Dillard, Andonian, Flores, Lai, MacRae & Shakir, 1992). Culture includes more than race and ethnicity and may include a person's gender, religion, socioeconomic status, sexual orientation, age, environment, family background, and life experiences.

Cultural competence depends on the development of an attitude among health care providers. It is a process that begins with one's willingness to learn about cultural issues, proceeds with the commitment to incorporate at all levels of care the importance of culture, and is operationalized by making adaptations in services to meet culturally unique needs. Although some practitioners may have specific knowledge of the languages, values, and customs of other cultures, the most challenging tasks are understanding the dynamics of difference in the helping process and adapting practice skills to fit the client's cultural context.

Developing an awareness and acceptance of cultural differences is required as a first step in the process of becoming a culturally competent individual (Cross, Bazron, Dennis & Issacs, 1989; McManus, 1988). Many ethnic minorities have beliefs and practices about health, illness, and treatment that differ significantly from the Western, scientific medical paradigm around which the US health care delivery system is structured (Devore & Schlesinger, 1991; Eisenberg, 1980). However, negatively labeling people because the provider believes them to differ from him/her and the mainstream is unacceptable. Differences must be explored and understood so barriers to seeking health care can be reduced. Understanding differences begins with an awareness that they exist and continues with a willingness to accept them. In the sections that follow, there are suggestions for exercises to enhance your awareness of your own culture.

CULTURAL AWARENESS EXERCISES

A major component of cultural competence is an acknowledgment and awareness of one's own culture and a willingness to explore one's own feelings and biases. Each person is responsible for building an awareness of how culture influences his or her own ways of thinking and making decisions. Included in this awareness must be an acknowledgment of how day-to-day behaviors reflect cultural norms and values perpetuated by our families and larger social networks. To develop this awareness, Hutchinson (1989) suggests that we ask ourselves several questions that will direct our exploration of our cultural heritage and how our daily interactions are influenced by that culture. Sample questions include the following:

- What ethnic group, socioeconomic class, religion, age group, and community do I belong to?
- What about my ethnic group, socioeconomic class, religion, age, or community do I wish I could change and why?
- What experiences have I had with people different from me? What were those experiences like and how did I feel about them?
- What is there about me that may cause me to be rejected by members of other cultures or ethnic groups?
- What qualities do I have that will help me establish positive interpersonal interactions with persons from other cultural groups?

One strategy used in teaching diversity awareness to health professions students is a cultural assessment project that serves as a purposeful self-examination and an exercise in appreciating differences. The project asks you to begin by identifying your own cultural beliefs and values about health and illness, education and vocation, foods, religion, and role expectations. (You can do this now as you read this section.) Once identified, think through your responses and make notations about how you remember being taught about some of those values, practices, expectations, habits, and traditions.

- Where and how was knowledge about your heritage passed on to you?
- Who are the persons in your network responsible for influencing and shaping the lives of the young people?

Proceed with this project by seeking out someone known to you but who has a background, heritage, or ethnicity different from your own.

- Ask that person's permission for an interview and ask them the same things you asked yourself in establishing your basic cultural richness.
- When you have the data you set out to compare with your own, sit down and analyze what sociocultural similarities and differences the two of you have.

This exercise is particularly beneficial to the beginner who has not ventured into self-awareness projects from a cultural beliefs and values perspective. Having analyzed similarities and differences, proceed with your analysis and focus on predicting potential areas of conflict between the two views as well as the positive, congruent strengths. These may be as simple as food preferences and celebrated holidays or as complex as preferred vocations, generational hierarchies, and healing rituals. You may complete the practice assignment by asking the following question:

- What potential strengths in similarities between us should I build on to begin interactions with this client?

As the cultural project points out, all interacting parties bring with them unique histories, communication styles, and learned expectations. Together, these contribute to potential misunderstandings and misinterpretations that manifest the dynamics of difference. Therefore, strategies of relating with clients must include eliciting information about their health and illness practices, as well as basic ethnic and cultural norms. Specific knowledge about the culture is necessary for the relationship to be structured within the helping framework. Bringing down barriers and facilitating the negotiation of individualized plans of care will support positive health outcomes for all clients. The ultimate goal in planning collaborative approaches to illness treatment and healing is to preserve the dignity of the client and to foster health promotion and healing programs that are likely to meet with adherence because they support rather than offend the clients. Additional information about eliciting the client's cultural health and illness beliefs follows later.

ELICITING HEALTH AND ILLNESS BELIEFS

We have explored the idea that cultural health beliefs are the major determinants of a person's recognition and management of an illness experience. Although these beliefs exist independently of and prior to a given episode of illness (Kleinman, 1980), they are activated when one has to cope with and explain a particular experience or situation (Blumhagen, 1982; Gillick, 1985). Therefore, as practitioners, we should expect that it is appropriate to elicit cultural health beliefs when (and not before) an illness experience becomes a reality. According to several researchers, time and experience with an illness are necessary for the client to work the set of beliefs into a functioning set of reasons for the illness, directions for sick role behavior, and options for achieving healing (Blumhagen, 1982; Chrisman, 1977; Good & Good, 1981). Understanding ethnic interpretations of health and illness enables the practitioner to further clarify the sources of beliefs from which clients formulate their illness realities (Roberson, 1987).

This process begins with eliciting the client's subjective explanations for the cause, duration, and characteristics of symptoms. Further discussion with the client should include exploring the client's expectations for acceptable treatments, outcomes of the treatment, and the substance of the client–provider interaction (Berlin & Fowkes, 1983). Kleinman's (1980) original set of questions are adapted by Randall-David (1989) to ask clients their perspectives about health and illness experiences. Attention to the answers to these questions further increases the cultural competence of the provider:

- What do you think caused your problem?
- Why do you think it started when it did?
- How long do you think it will last?
- What have you done about your problem?
- With whom did you discuss your problem?
- What kind of help and from whom would you like to receive help for your problem?
- How will you know when your problem is getting better?

Additional questions formulated by this author for purposes of conducting explanatory model research include:

- What do you call your problem?
- What worries you most about having this problem?
- How did you come to know that you were having a problem?

Answers to these questions may take time and will take a conscious effort to collect and use. However, the process is well worth the time and commitment as we gain a greater understanding and respect for all clients' health beliefs and practices. This understanding can lead to both improved client–provider relationships and treatment outcomes. An analysis of the answers to these questions and much introspection will enable health care providers to understand the complexities of cross-cultural interactions.

ADAPTING SKILLS

Providers must develop critical skills so that cultural assessments can be elicited and appropriate sociocultural care can be delivered in conjunction with prescribed treatment interventions. This implies a contextual understanding that treating the illness and understanding what it means to the individual are as important as working to resolve the disease process (Kleinman, 1988). Although nurses study communication strategies as part of their educational preparation, the cognitive skills necessary to understand another's cultural beliefs and backgrounds need cultivation, refinement, and practice.

Sound physical and psychosocial assessment skills, sensitive interviewing skills, active listening, neutral body language, and self-awareness are the basic attributes required of culturally competent providers. Several of these attributes can be built using the contents of this chapter, but it is expected that the practitioner will seek out continuing education that will expand the skills necessary for thorough data collection. For example, physical assessment of people of color may be a learning need for some, whereas spending more time in a cultural self-assessment and an analysis of potential conflicts between the providers and their clients may be a priority for others.

Active listening, which is a learned skill that requires a lot of practice and critique, is a necessary component of sensitive interviewing. It is helpful if you can audiotape a "client" interview that employs role playing so you and a colleague can critique your style. Use the following questions to evaluate your progress toward becoming a skilled interviewer:

- Am I using slang or jargon that is only understood by other professionals?
- Are the questions I ask presented so rapidly in sequence that the client has no time to think and organize a response?
- Do I paraphrase a question so many times that it has lost its original intent?
- Are the questions I ask so long that the focus is diluted beyond recognition?

Sometimes the reasons our questions seem to go unanswered are related to our interviewing skills, styles, and competencies. For example, are you comfortable with pauses or do you have the need to always hear a speaking voice, even if it is your own? Are you asking appropriate follow-up questions that will probe a client's response to an earlier question? It is important for you to value what the client is saying. Active listening and planning appropriate responses are a sure way of accomplishing the task.

You must also learn how to present yourself with neutral body language during interactions with clients. Not everyone likes being touched or having someone else in their space. Although we may think touch is important in healing, remember it may not be culturally appropriate to the clients we serve.

In addition to physical assessment data, eliciting patient and family explanations of health status and illness realities helps providers take the patient's perspective seriously in organizing clinical care strategies. In turn, the provider's effective communication style assists patients and families in making more useful judgments of when to enter into treatment, with which practitioners, for what treatments, and at what ratio of cost and benefit (Kleinman, 1988). It is imperative to approach health teaching and self-care training with the attitude that providers and patients are collaborators and are working toward the same goals of positive outcomes for the patient and the family. Negotiation among patients and providers over conflicts in explanations, interpretations, and understandings can reduce barriers to effective care and instill in the patient the provider's respect for alternative viewpoints and preferences. These strategies work together to close the gap between the patient and the provider (Kleinman, 1988) and are necessary to increase access to care and improve health for our entire nation.

THE AGENCY

Cultural awareness, sensitivity, and competence are necessary accomplishments for all health care providers as well as the delivery systems of which they are a part. It makes no sense to have culturally competent practitioners in settings that are culturally ignorant. In services to individuals, families, and communities, culturally competent systems of care must acknowledge and incorporate the importance of culture, appreciate the dynamics of difference, and make a commitment to adapt services to meet unique needs (Issacs & Benjamin, 1991; Roberts, 1990). Culturally competent programs and services will respect their clients' cultural beliefs as well as the staff members' beliefs and include in their mission statements goals to maintain and improve the self-esteem and the cultural identity of employees and clients.

Several types of movements toward agency-level cultural competence have been reported in the literature. When success is measured by community acceptance and use, some agencies are recognized as more successful than others. McManus (1988) reports that a simple outreach model may be rejected by ethnic minority groups because service agencies frequently deliver to diverse communities the same services offered to mainstream groups. This approach is perceived by many to be a form of color-blindness that maintains barriers rather than removes them. A more meaningful and successful approach to agency cultural competence is mainstream support of local programs and services that employ and use staff who have similar cultural backgrounds to those for whom the services are intended (Barrera, 1978; Gallegos, 1982). This means that multilingual and multicultural services should be offered in some neighborhoods and communities. A needs assessment must be employed to identify the types of services and the systems of service delivery that are most acceptable and efficient (Angrosino, 1978).

For many existing agencies and delivery systems, structures, services, and competencies must be modified or created to be consistent and compatible with the cultures they encounter in their client populations. Culturally competent services, systems, agencies, and practitioners possess the capacity to respond to the unique needs of populations whose cultures differ from dominant or mainstream America.

An awareness that racial, ethnic, and minority groups have different needs, have been underserved, or have underutilized available services has created an interest in agency cultural competence. Assessing the types of services identified as wanted and needed by target populations is crucial to the reception and use of services by people with culturally diverse backgrounds. Agencies striving for cultural competence must be able to accept the values of the community's ethnic cultures, and develop and refine services and skills for working with the local population (McManus, 1988).

SUMMARY

Educators and providers must remember that ethnicity provides a sense of belonging to people in a pluralistic society; a celebration of differences in identity, strength, and survival. An understanding of ethnic culture is functional for coping with and appreciating differences. Research supports the roles of heritage and identity in influencing people's behaviors and attitudes and the perpetuation of ethnicity throughout generations. Cooperation with and respect for others with different heritages rather than eradication of differences, stimulation of conflict, and goals for sameness must be the focus of future practice and research. Cultural competence is an imperative for health promotion, healing, and successful outcomes for illness experiences. Many of the skills needed by providers are in place and available for enrichment through awareness, specialty and continuing education, and careful listening to what our clients teach us.

REFERENCES

Aamodt, A. (1978). The care component in a health and healing system. In E. Bauwens (Ed.), *The anthropology of health*. St. Louis, MO: C.V. Mosby.

Adams, E.V. (1990). *Policy planning for culturally comprehensive special health services*. Rockville, MD: United States Department of Health and Human Services, Maternal and Child Health Bureau.

Allan, J.D. & Hall, B.A. (1988). Challenging the focus on technology: A critique of the medical model in a changing health care system. *Advances in Nursing Science, 10*(3), 22–34.

American Nurses Association. (1980). *Nursing: A social policy statement*. Kansas City, MO: Author.

Angel, R. & Thiots, P. (1987). The impact of culture on the cognitive structure of illness. *Culture, Medicine, and Psychiatry, 2*, 465–494.

Angrosino, M.V. (1978). Applied anthropology and the concept of the underdog: Implications for community mental health planning and evaluation. *Community Mental Health Journal, 1-4*(4), 291–299.

Barrera, M. (1978). Mexican-American mental health service utilization: A critical examination of some proposed variables. *Community Mental Health Journal, 14*(l), 35–45.

Berlin, E.A. & Fowkes, W.C. (1983). A teaching framework for cross-cultural health care: Application in family practice. *Western Journal of Medicine, 139*(6), 934–938.

Blumhagen, D. (1982). The meaning of hypertension. In N.J. Chrisman & T.W. Maretzki (Eds.), *Clinical applied anthropology: Anthropologists in health science settings*. Boston, MA: Reidel.

Campinha-Bacote, J. (1995). The quest for cultural competence in nursing care. *Nursing Forum, 30*(4), 19–25.

Chavez, L.R. (1984). Doctors, curanderos, and brujas: Health care delivery and Mexican immigrants in San Diego. *Medical Anthropology Quarterly, 15*(2), 31–37.

Chrisman, N. (1977). The health seeking process: An approach to the natural history of illness. *Culture, Medicine, & Psychiatry, 1,* 351–377.

Congress, E.P. & Lyons, B.P. (1992). Cultural differences in health beliefs: Implications for social work practice in health care settings. *Social Work in Health Care, 17*(3), 81–96.

Cross, R.L. (1987). Cultural competence continuum. *Focal Point: The Bulletin of the Research and Training Center to Improve Services for Seriously Emotionally Handicapped Children and Their Families, 3*(1), 5.

Cross, T., Bazron, B., Dennis, K., & Issacs, M. (1989). *Towards a culturally competent system of care, Volume I.* Washington, DC: Georgetown University Child Development Center, CASSP Technical Assistance Center.

Dervin, B. (1989). Audience as listener and learner, teacher, and confidante: The sense-making approach. In R.E. Rice & C.K. Atkin (Eds.), *Public communication campaigns.* Newbury Park, CA: Sage.

Devore, W. & Schlesinger, E. (1991). *Ethnic-sensitive social work practice.* New York, NY: Macmillan Publishing.

Dillard, M., Andonian, L., Flores, O., Lai, L., MacRae, A., & Shakir, M. (1992). Culturally competent occupational therapy in a diversely populated mental health setting. *The American Journal of Occupational Therapy, 46*(8), 721–726.

Eisenberg, L. (1980). What makes persons patients and patients well? *American Journal of Medicine, 69*(2), 277–286.

Fabrega, H. (1974). *Disease and social behavior: An interdisciplinary perspective.* Cambridge, MA: The MIT Press.

Friedson, E. (1961). *Patient's view of medical practice.* New York, NY: Russell Sage.

Gallegos, J.S. (1982). Planning and administering services for minority groups. In M. Austin & W. Hersey (Eds.), *Handbook of mental health administration: The middle manager's perspective* (pp 87–105). San Francisco, CA: Jossey-Bass.

Gillick, M.R. (1985). Commonsense models of health and disease. *New England Journal of Medicine, 313*(11), 700–703.

Good, B. & Good, M.J. (1981). The meaning of symptoms: A cultural hermeneutic model for cultural practice. In L. Eisenberg & A. Kleinman (Eds.), *The relevance of social science for medicine.* Boston, MA: Reidel.

Harwood, A. (1981). *Ethnicity and medical care.* Cambridge, MA: Harvard University Press.

Helman, C. (1984). *Culture, health, and illness: An introduction for health professionals.* Boston, MA: Wright.

Holzberg, C.S. (1982). Ethnicity and aging: Anthropological perspectives on more than just the minority elderly. *The Gerontologist, 22*(3), 249–257.

Hutchinson, I. (1989). *Strategies for working with culturally diverse communities and clients.* Bethesda, MD: The Association for the Care of Children's Health, Maternal and Child Health Bureau.

Issacs, M. & Benjamin, M. (1991). *Towards a culturally competent system of care, Volume II: Programs which utilize culturally competent principles.* Washington, DC: Georgetown University Child Development Center, CASSP Technical Assistance Center.

Kleinman, A. (1988). *The illness narratives: Suffering, healing, and the human condition.* New York, NY: Basic Books.

_____. (1986). Concepts and a model for the comparison of medical systems as cultural systems. In C. Currer & M. Stacy (Eds.), *Concepts of health, illness, & disease: A comparative perspective.* New York, NY: Berg.

_____. (1980). *Patients and healers in the context of culture.* Berkeley, CA: University of California Press.

_____. (1978). Clinical relevance of anthropological and cross-cultural research: Concepts and strategies. *American Journal of Psychiatry, 135*(4), 427–431.

Leininger, M. (1978). *Transcultural nursing: Concepts, theories, and practices.* New York, NY: Wiley.

Lewis, M.C. (1988). Attribution and illness. *Journal of Psychosocial Nursing, 26*(4), 14–21.

Lyons, J. (1972). Methods of successful communication with the disadvantaged. In *Communication for change with the rural disadvantaged.* Washington, DC: National Academy of Sciences.

Madrid, A. (1988). Diversity and its discontents. *Black Issues in Higher Education, 5*(4), 10–18.

May, J. (1992). Working with diverse families: Building culturally competent systems of health care delivery. *The Journal of Rheumatology, 19*(33), 46–48.

McManus, M. (1988). Services to minority populations: What does it mean to be a culturally competent professional? *Focal Point: The Bulletin of the Research and Training Center to Improve Services for Seriously Emotionally Handicapped Children and Their Families, 2*(4), 1–17.

Mechanic, D. (1986). The concept of illness behavior: Culture, situation, and personal predisposition. *Psychological Medicine, 16*(l), 1–7.

Mechanic, D. (Ed.). (1982). *Symptoms, illness behavior, and help seeking.* New York, NY: Prodist.

Moore, J. (1971). Situational factors affecting minority aging. *The Gerontologist, 11,* 88–93.

Munet-Vilaro, F. (1988). The challenge of cross-cultural nursing research. *Western Journal of Nursing Research, 10*(1), 112–115.

Randall-David, E. (1989). *Strategies for working with culturally diverse communities and clients.* Bethesda, MD: The Association for the Care of Children's Health.

Rivera, G. & Wanderer, J. (1986). Curanderismo and childhood illnesses. *The Social Science Journal, 23*(3), 361–372.

Roberson, M. (1987). Folk health beliefs of health professionals. *Western Journal of Nursing Research, 9*(2), 257–263.

Roberts, R. (1990). *Developing culturally competent programs for families of children with special needs.* Washington, DC: Georgetown University Child Development Center, Maternal and Child Health Bureau.

Roberts, S.J. (1988). Social support and help seeking: Review of the literature. *Advances in Nursing Science, 10*(2), 1–11.

Royce, A.P. (1982). *Ethnic identity: Strategies of diversity.* Bloomington, IN: Indiana University.

Rubel, A.J. (1977). The epidemiology of a folk illness: Susto in Hispanic America. In D. Landy (Ed.), *Culture, disease, and healing: Studies in medical anthropology* (pp 119–128). New York, NY: Macmillan.

Ruiz, P. (1985). Cultural barriers to effective medical care among Hispanic-American patients. *Annual Review of Medicine, 36,* 63–71.

Weiss, M.G. (1988). Cultural models of diarrheal illness: Conceptual framework and review. *Social Science & Medicine, 27*(1), 5–16.

Whall, A. (1987). Commentary. *Western Journal of Nursing Research, 9*(2), 237–239.

Wirth, L. (1945). The problem of minority groups. In R. Linton (Ed.), *The science of man in the world crisis.* New York, NY: Columbia University Press.

Wood, J.B. (1989). Communicating with older adults in health care settings: Cultural and ethnic considerations. *Educational Gerontology, 15,* 351–362.

Young, A. (1982). The anthropology of illness and sickness. *Annual Review of Anthropology, 11,* 257–285.

Zola, I.K. (1972). Culture and symptoms: An analysis of patients' presenting complaints. *American Sociological Review, 5,* 141–155.

INTERNET RESOURCES

Here are a few of the many websites that provide information about cultural issues and cultural competence.

www.omhrc.gov
This is the home page for the Office of Minority Health Resource Center, U.S. Department of Health and Human Services. It offers access to news, databases, publications, funding resources, employment opportunities, events and conferences, a resource persons network, Federal Register notices, and press releases.

www.air.org/cecp/cultural
This is a specific page dedicated to cultural competence and sponsored by the Center for Effective Collaboration and Practice. It offers links to sources that provide definitions of cultural competence, why it is important, how it benefits children, and where you can find more information.

www.diversityRx.org
Diversity Rx is sponsored by the National Conference of State Legislatures (NCSL), Resources for Cross Cultural Health Care (RCCHC), and the Henry J. Kaiser Family Foundation of Menlo Park, CA. Its goals include promoting language and cultural competence to improve the quality of health care for minority, immigrant, and ethnically diverse communities.

Beverly C. Flynn   CHAPTER

HEALTH POLICY FOR HEALTHY CITIES AND COMMUNITIES

7

OBJECTIVES

This chapter focuses on the importance of healthy public policies for healthy communities, while building on the concepts of primary health care.

After studying this chapter, you should be able to

- Understand the basic elements of healthy public policy.
- Describe the process of policy development.
- Appreciate the importance of the community health nurse's role in the promotion of healthy public policy.

INTRODUCTION

The concept of health policy that is presented in this chapter has been called healthy public policy in the literature (Evers, Farrant & Trojan, 1990; Hancock, 1985; Milio, 1990; Pederson, Edwards, Kelner, Marshall & Allison, 1988) and is particularly focused on promoting health in communities. Healthy public policy was cited in the *Ottawa Charter for Health Promotion* (WHO, 1986b) as the most important action to promote health. The characteristics of healthy public policy and healthy cities and communities are consistent with primary health care as presented in Chapter 1. This chapter explores the conceptual foundations of health promotion and healthy public policy with application to the healthy cities and communities movement. Opportunities for nursing in relation to the future development of healthy public policy and healthy cities and communities are suggested.

WORLD CONFERENCES ON HEALTH PROMOTION AND HEALTHY PUBLIC POLICY

Four world conferences provided supporting documents for health promotion and healthy public policy. The 1978 Declaration of Alma Ata adopted the goal of health for all by the year 2000 through the primary health care approach (WHO, 1978). Implicit in the health for all strategy was a new concept of health promotion that combined lifestyle change with policy and environmental improvement. Since the middle 1980s, there has been increasing attention to the concept of health promotion.

The second world conference was held in Ottawa, Ontario, Canada, and produced the *Ottawa Charter for Health Promotion* (WHO, 1986b). Conference participants agreed that health promotion exceeds the activities of the health sector. Nine prerequisites for health were cited as peace, shelter, education, food, income, a stable ecosystem, sustainable resources, social justice, and equity. Five interdependent action areas for effective health promotion, in order of priority, were identified as the following:

- Building healthy public policy in all sectors and at all levels
- Creating supportive environments so it is easier to be healthy
- Strengthening community action with self-help and social support
- Developing personal skills as people take responsibility for their own health
- Reorienting health services toward promoting health and preventing disease

The third world conference was held in Adelaide, Australia, on the theme of healthy public policy. Conference participants accepted the position that health was a fundamental right and a social investment. The conference proceedings recommended that governments promote health by linking economic, social, and health policies. The need for equity in health and the development of new partnerships with business, trade unions, nongovernmental organizations, and community groups were also suggested (WHO, 1988).

The fourth international conference on health promotion was held in Jakarta, Indonesia, in 1997, the first held in a developing country. The five priorities for health promotion in the 21st century that were cited in the *Jakarta Declaration* (WHO, 1997) are:

- Promote social responsibility for health
- Increase investments for health development
- Consolidate and expand partnerships for health

- Increase community capacity and empower the individual
- Secure an infrastructure for health promotion

These world conferences have led to new thinking about how health promotion can lead to healthier people. Each conference provided substantial material for discussion and debate as to how the basic principles of primary health care, health promotion, and healthy public policy can be harnessed for the future.

HEALTH PROMOTION

Historically, the concept of health promotion has focused on the concept of helping people promote health through personal lifestyle change (Minkler, 1989). The emphasis was on the role individuals can play in modifying their behaviors to improve their health status. Consistent with this approach is the fact that much of the research on health promotion also focused on individual behavioral change with a similar impact on public policy development (Milio, 1981). Hancock (1986) noted that the focus on individual responsibility for health contributes to victim blaming.

The newer concept of health promotion was clarified in the *Ottawa Charter for Health Promotion* (WHO, 1986b, p 1):

> Health promotion is the process of enabling people to increase control over, and to improve, their health. To reach a state of complete physical, mental and social well-being, an individual or group must be able to identify and realize aspirations, to satisfy needs, and to change or cope with the environment. Health is, therefore, seen as a resource for everyday life, not the objective of living. Health is a positive concept emphasizing social and personal resources, as well as physical capacities. Therefore, health promotion is not just the responsibility of the health sector, but goes beyond healthy life-styles to well-being.

This definition of health promotion recognized the social, economic, and political determinants of health. Robertson & Minkler (1994) summarized the characteristics of this definition to include the following:

- A broad definition of health and its determinants
- The incorporation of social and political approaches
- Individual and collective empowerment
- Community participation in identifying problems and solutions

In their examination of health promotion, Robertson & Minkler (1994) noted that these characteristics often have multiple meanings. They suggested that these meanings need careful scrutiny for the science of health promotion to develop.

HEALTHY PUBLIC POLICY

The concept of healthy public policy is based on the principles of primary health care in reaching the goal of health for all and health promotion policy (WHO, 1978; WHO, 1986a). Principles of health promotion policy include being multisectoral in scope, ecologic, responsible for increasing health-promoting options, multifaceted, complementary to health services, and participatory. In 1985, the *Canadian Journal of Public Health* reported the proceedings of a conference on healthy public policy (Canadian Journal of Public Health, 1985). Hancock (1985) noted that healthy public policy is based on a multisectoral approach, community involvement, and appropriate technology, three of the components of the WHO primary health care approach. He clarified that healthy public policy is concerned with creating a healthy society, following an appropriate technology approach to health, being holistic and future oriented, and questioning the givens about how society could be structured to promote health. As noted earlier, the *Ottawa Charter for Health Promotion* (WHO, 1986b) identified healthy public policy as one of the five action strategies for health promotion. Through healthy public policy, health can be placed on the agenda of policy makers so they can recognize and be held accountable for the health consequences, not just the economic considerations, of their policy decisions. Furthermore, healthy public policy can foster greater equity by ensuring safer and healthier products, services, and environments.

In 1988, the Adelaide conference on healthy public policy generated recommendations by emphasizing community involvement and cooperation among sectors based on the concept of primary health care (WHO, 1988). The main goal of healthy public policy is to create supportive environments for people to lead healthy lives, making the healthy choices the easier choices for citizens.

Pederson et al. (1988) concurred with these definitions but also noted that healthy public policy included a focus on issues of equity in health. Key elements of healthy public policy are focusing on the determinants of health, where health is created; discovering which investment produces the largest health gains; determining which strategies will promote equity and narrow the gap in health status; and allocating public resources on the basis of these elements (WHO, 1993). Pederson et al. (1988) refer to healthy public policy as public policy for health, considering health in the broad ecologic sense. Kickbusch (1992) noted that healthy public policy is built on a proactive concept of health that shifts "policy priorities to get action on health where it really matters."

In a discussion document, WHO (1992) suggested three categories of healthy public policy. These were policies concerned with health promotion, disease prevention, and provision of health care services; social, educational, and cultural concerns; and economic and environmental concerns that include industrial development, transportation, and housing. Examples of healthy public policies are farm and food policies to develop improved health promotion options for consumers and producers; smoking control policies such as banning advertisements, limiting smoking in public places, and restricting sales; and income maintenance such as family and housing allowances, unemployment insurance, and maternity benefits (Milio, 1985).

For healthy public policy to become a reality, additional knowledge is needed. Kickbusch (1992) suggested that knowledge of the positive and negative health impacts of policy, knowledge of the policy process, and knowledge of health measurement are needed to guide the development of healthy public policy.

Healthy public policy is upstream thinking that is concerned with primary prevention. The challenge for change lies with communities at the local level. There is strong support for moving public health into the policy arena (Institute of Medicine, 1988; Stoto, Abel & Dievler, 1996). Public health professionals are expected to work with elected officials within the political arena of public health. The healthy cities and communities movement advocates for a new type of health policy that focuses on health promotion consistent with these expectations for public health.

Healthy Cities and Communities

The concepts presented under health promotion and healthy public policy have guided the development of the healthy cities and communities movement. Duhl (1986) was the first to cite the requirements for a healthy city. He noted that the city must respond to its developmental needs, cope with system and member breakdowns, have the ability to modify itself and meet its changing needs, be competent so that local residents use it, and educate its residents. Citizens can take actions to create a more healthy city through responding to symptoms, dealing with underlying issues, and taking specific actions such as creating consensus through community-wide responses.

Milio (1990) viewed the emerging healthy cities movement as the new public health, by clarifying that "there can be no health without community." She recognized that the principles of the *Ottawa Charter for Health Promotion* (WHO, 1986b) guide the new public health by making the health-promoting choices easier than the health-damaging choices. Furthermore, Milio visualized healthy cities as creating a political reservoir on which to advance the new public health.

The healthy cities and communities movement exemplifies these concepts in practice. Prominent features of this movement include recognizing the multiple determinants of health, involving multiple sectors and broad citizen participation, developing community partnerships, focusing on local assets and needs, and developing systems change to reduce the inequalities in health.

The healthy cities and communities movement started to gain strength with the WHO Healthy Cities Project in Europe, beginning in 1986. Currently, healthy cities and communities may be found in every region of the world. The literature indicates that healthy cities and communities aim to provide a clean and safe physical environment that is ecologically stable and that offers community residents access to prerequisites to health and a diverse, vital, and innovative economy (Hancock & Duhl, 1988). Healthy cities and communities are both political and process oriented. Healthy cities and communities advocate for change at the local level through public–private partnerships. They aim to promote equity, sustainable and supportive environments, community participation, and improved health and quality of life at the local level (Tsouros, 1990).

The healthy cities process involves many stages in mobilizing the community in reaching its goals (Flynn & Ivanov, 2000). These necessary stages include:

- Orienting the community to health promotion and the healthy cities and communities process
- Building local partnerships and establishing community commitment
- Developing the community structure for health promotion, including the healthy city and coordinating council to steer the process and subcommittees to work on specific action priorities
- Leadership development in relation to health promotion, healthy public policy, and healthy cities and communities
- Community assessment of local assets and needs
- Community-wide planning for health, including priority setting and strategic planning for local health action
- Community action for health in terms of program and policy development
- Providing data-based information to policy makers to facilitate the development of, and advocate for, healthy public policy
- Monitoring and evaluating the impact of programs and policies in terms of the community's health

WHO (1992) suggested that healthy cities and communities need to keep three considerations in mind in promoting the development of healthy public policies: (1) defining health gains of policies that respond to the local political culture; (2) participating in policy discussions across community sectors; and (3) developing clear policy priorities that have potential broad economic and social impact as well as opportunities for support and change.

Local policies are concerned with three phases: policy formulation or development, policy adoption, and policy implementation. It has been suggested that the ten-step policy cycle provides a model for healthy cities and communities to identify potential opportunities to influence policy development at the local level (WHO, 1992). This cycle is depicted in Table 7–1.

TABLE 7–1 ■ Model Ten-Step Policy Cycle for Healthy Cities and Communities

Step	Description
Agenda setting	Involves identifying community health problems and assets that suggest opportunities for action. Within healthy cities and communities, there is concern about equity and access to prerequisites for health, healthy lifestyles and environment, and health care.
Issue filtration	Involves selecting health issues for more extensive analysis in order to define the significance and characteristics of the problem. Healthy cities and communities coordinating councils and committees, because of their broad look at community assets and problems, are in key positions to select these issues and to inform community policy makers, such as city council, of the selections made.
Issue definition	Involves defining health problems in more precise terms as well as the economic and social factors involved. Healthy cities and communities can use their contacts with expertise in the community, such as universities and colleges, the local health department and community groups, to employ specialized knowledge and skills. It is important to quantify and describe the significance of problems and their contributing factors.
Problem forecasting	Involves projecting the development of the problem in terms of future scenarios. Healthy cities and communities need knowledge of the policy intentions of local administrators in order to develop problem forecasting.
Setting objective and priorities	Involves the development of expected results and outcome indicators for priorities selected by the healthy cities and communities and local policy makers.
Options analysis	Involves an exploration of strategies to achieve the objectives. The multisectoral approach of healthy cities and communities provides opportunities for different organizations to contribute to the development of options. Different sectors can address a single policy issue in different ways. Also, examples of strategies used by other healthy cities and communities can be models to generate local options.

Continued

TABLE 7–1 ■ Model Ten-Step Policy Cycle for Healthy Cities and Communities (Continued)

Step	Description
Policy adoption	Involves discussion and decision making by policy makers, such as the city council. Healthy cities and communities coordinating councils or committees may make formal presentations to policy makers who also will need to consider the allocation of resources for their policy decisions.
Policy implementation, monitoring, and control	Involves putting the policy into practice. After policy maker approval, implementation actions will be designed by local departments and other organizations, and responsibility and resources will be assigned. A system to monitor implementation progress also needs to be established along with the decision-making process to assess whether the performance is meeting expectations. The healthy cities and communities coordinating council or committee can provide or help identify technical support in establishing a system for monitoring implementation.
Evaluation and review	Involves assessing whether the policy has been successful in achieving its objectives and at an acceptable cost. Healthy cities and communities can identify expertise to assist in the following ways: helping raise awareness of the health effects of current policy; providing examples of innovative practices in other communities; and providing advice on health impact assessments.
Policy maintenance and termination	Involves the decision-making process of whether the policy is continued, terminated, or replaced, depending on its impact on health. Healthy cities and communities can advocate for support of policy decisions or for a reexamination of policies.

The ten-step policy cycle provides healthy cities and communities many options to consider in their work in healthy public policy development. In addition, there are also actions the coordinating council can take that may facilitate the various steps of the policy process. The following actions provide the tools for advocacy for healthy public policy (WHO, 1992):

- Using political links to build awareness of current and emerging policy issues
- Using data to provide continuous environmental scanning useful in addressing unresolved policy questions
- Building capacity in strategic planning and policy analysis
- Developing comprehensive local health plans
- Developing methodologies for locally relevant health impact assessments
- Issuing periodic health status reports for policy makers, the media, and the public
- Promoting well-documented innovative approaches to address health issues

HEALTH POLICY ACTIONS OF HEALTHY CITIES AND COMMUNITIES

The literature clearly suggests that the principles related to health promotion and healthy public policy are being implemented by healthy cities and communities. But, how are healthy cities and communities implementing these principles? What health policy actions have they instituted? What is the impact of these policy actions on the community's health?

Flynn & Ray (1999) used a self-administered questionnaire to survey healthy cities coordinators in 1995–1996, and the results included 183 healthy cities in different regions of the world. The displayed material summarizes the health policy actions of these healthy cities. It is interesting to note that these policy actions focused on the environment and population groups at risk to health problems. The data also confirmed the use of a broad definition of health.

In a review of the first 5 years of the Healthy Cities Project in Europe, it was found that cities used the following common approaches to policy change (Draper, Curtice, Hooper, & Goumans, 1993):

- Adopting position statements and advocating resolutions on health issues
- Facilitating the adoption of policies
- Facilitating the formulation and adoption of city health plans
- Advocating assessments of the impact of city policies on health

This report further highlighted a number of case examples of health policy actions of healthy cities. In this early stage of reporting of European healthy

---

Health Policy Issues Identified by 183 Healthy Cities

Drugs and alcohol
Environment
Maternal and child health
Nutrition
Tobacco
Traffic
Women's health
Youth

cities, a number of cities developed city health plans, including Eindhoven, The Netherlands; Pecs, Hungary; Rennes, France; Seville, Spain; and Vienna, Austria. Goumans & Springett (1997) examined the evidence from ten healthy cities in the Netherlands and the United Kingdom and concluded that substantive policy change had not taken place. They suggested that, in most cases, healthy cities initiatives were still projects and not policies.

However, specific case examples found in the literature suggest health policy changes have occurred. For example, in Gothenburg, Sweden, a comprehensive policy on the care for elderly has been reported that includes enabling people to remain in their own homes, developing group housing with access to 24-hour medical care for those who cannot remain at home, providing readily available home help, refining clinical care at geriatric and psychogeriatric clinics, and encouraging skilled primary care (Draper et al., 1993).

Healthy City Toronto (Canada) has indicated a network of policy initiatives that aim to make the city healthy. These policy initiatives include safety and justice, equality and access, and long-term environmental planning (Toronto Healthy City Initiatives, 1997). For example, the city council endorsed a community safety strategy for the city in 1995, bringing together various city sectors to coordinate staff and resources and reduce duplication of services. Another example was the Toronto Mayor's Committee on Community and Race Relations. This broad-based committee worked to combat racism and hate-motivated crime; addressed the needs of lesbian and gay populations and promoted tolerance and acceptance of these groups; improved police–minority relations, employment equity, and access to services for diverse populations; and advocated for youth employment. Efforts were also reported to improve the environment through city recycling policies.

In the United States, New Castle Healthy City in Indiana advocated for policy change at two levels. One was to advocate for a no-smoking ordinance that was passed by the city council. Another was to present health risk data to the county commissioners and advocate in support of a new health educator position in the local health department. Both of these policies were passed by policy makers.

Networks across healthy cities are being formed to address broader policy issues. For example, in Europe Multi-City Action Plans (MCAP) have developed that link healthy cities concerned with common health problems. Examples include tobacco, acquired immunodeficiency syndrome (AIDS), and women's health. MCAP cities agree to share technical knowledge and experiences and work together to promote healthy public policy. In the United States, the Coalition for Healthier Cities and Communities has gained momentum with an emphasis on promoting community dialogues, statewide networks, and information exchange. In Latin America, healthy cities are called healthy municipalities. Healthy municipalities networks are forming within and across the healthy communities in the province of Quebec, Canada, and Brazil, and healthy cities and communities in Indiana, United States, and Costa Rica and Honduras.

From these examples, there is evidence that healthy cities and communities have facilitated and advocated for healthy public policy as proposed by WHO (1992). These examples suggest that healthy cities and communities have adopted position statements and resolutions on health issues, facilitated the adoption of policies, facilitated the formulation and adoption of city health plans, used political links to build awareness of current and emerging policy issues, used data in addressing unresolved policy questions, and developed comprehensive local health plans. However, there is no scientific evidence on the health impact assessments of these health policy actions and limited evidence documenting the effectiveness of healthy cities and communities models and networks being developed.

OPPORTUNITIES FOR NURSING

There are numerous opportunities for nursing in relation to future development of healthy public policy and healthy cities and communities. Nurses need to understand the evolving concepts of health promotion and healthy public policy. We can read the research and related literature on these concepts and we can attend health promotion, healthy public policy, and healthy cities workshops and conferences. There is considerable information available on the Internet, and nurses can become skilled "surfers" and read conference documents found there.

Nurses can also become involved in healthy cities and communities locally or initiate the process where it has not be implemented. We have many skills that are useful in program planning and policy development. We can help adapt or develop healthy cities and communities initiatives that are appropriate locally. We can advocate for healthy public policy through our unique knowledge of communities and the health of people by participating in the ten-step policy cycle presented earlier.

Nurses can work with other disciplines in research development that can facilitate the healthy cities and communities process. Nurses can promote involvement of the community in action research. Action research can involve community leaders in identifying information that can help them in their decision making for policy change (Flynn, Ray & Rider, 1994; Rains & Ray, 1995). There is little research that focuses on the practical issues that healthy cities and communities encounter in implementing the health promotion and healthy public policy principles. Knowledge needs to be developed on the theory underlying healthy cities and communities and healthy public policy. Nurses can help develop research methodologies that measure the health effects of healthy public policies and to document the effectiveness of healthy cities models and networks being developed. There is a need to develop indicators of successful healthy public policy and healthy cities and communities. Little is known about the effects of the community context on the implementation of healthy cities and communities and healthy public policy. Information is needed about the complexities of local health decision making in healthy cities and communities. More needs to be known about the processes through which decisions are made and influenced.

These are just some examples of the opportunities nurses have to facilitate the development of healthy public policy and healthy cities and communities. These examples are consistent with the ten-step policy cycle and the stages of the healthy cities and communities process described in this chapter.

SUMMARY

The concepts of health promotion and healthy public policy have been presented with application to healthy cities and communities in different regions of the world. Nurses, particularly community health nurses, have the knowledge and skills necessary to work with the community as a partner in facilitating community health promotion, healthy public policy, and healthy cities and communities in the next millenium.

REFERENCES

Canadian Journal of Public Health. (1985, May/June). *76*(Supplement 1), entire issue.

Draper, R., Curtice, L., Hooper, J., & Goumans, M. (1993). *WHO healthy cities project: Review of the first five years (1987–1992).* Copenhagen, Denmark: WHO Regional Office for Europe.

Duhl, L.J. (1986). The healthy city: Its function and its future. *Health Promotion, 1*(1), 73–76.

Evers, A., Farrant, W., & Trojan, A. (Eds.). (1990). *Healthy public policy at the local level.* Boulder, CO: Westview Press.

Flynn, B.C. & Ivanov, L. (2000). Health promotion through healthy cities. In M. Stanhope & J. Lancaster (Eds.), *Community health nursing* (5th ed.). (pp 349–359). St. Louis, MO: Mosby.

Flynn, B.C. & Ray, D.W. (1999). *Predictors of healthy cities programs and policies.* Unpublished manuscript, Institute of Action Research for Community Health, Indiana University School of Nursing. Indianapolis, IN.

Flynn, B.C., Ray, D.W., & Rider, M.S. (1994). Empowering communities: Action research through healthy cities. *Health Education Quarterly, 21*(3), 395–405.

Goumans, M. & Springett, J. (1997). From projects to policy: Healthy cities as a mechanism for policy change for health? *Health Promotion International, 12*(4), 311–322.

Hancock, T. (1986). Lalonde and beyond: Looking back at a new perspective on the health of Canadians. *Health Promotion, 1,* 93–100.

_____. (1985). Beyond health care: From public health policy to healthy public policy. *Canadian Journal of Public Health,* 76(Suppl 1), 9–11.

Hancock T. & Duhl, L. (1988). *Promoting health in the urban context.* Copenhagen: Denmark: FADL Publishers.

Institute of Medicine. (1988). *The future of public health.* Washington, DC: National Academy Press.

Kickbusch, I. (1992, June 10). *Healthy public policy.* Plenary presentation, Copenhagen Healthy Cities Conference 9–12 June 1992, WHO Regional Office for Europe, Copenhagen, Denmark.

Milio, N. (1990). Healthy cities: The new public health and supportive research. *Health Promotion International,* 5(4), 291–297.

_____. (1985). Healthy nations: Creating a new ecology of public policy for health. *Canadian Journal of Public Health,* 76(Suppl 1), 79–87.

_____. (1981). *Promoting health through public policy.* Philadelphia, PA: Davis Company.

Minkler, M. (1989). Health education, health promotion and the open society: An historical perspective. *Health Education Quarterly,* 16(1), 17–30.

Pederson, A.P., Edwards, R.K., Kelner, M., Marshall, V.W., & Allison, K.R. (1988). *Coordinating healthy public policy: An analytic literature review and bibliography.* Ottawa, Canada: Minister of National Health and Welfare.

Rains, J.W. & Ray, D.W. (1995). Participatory action research for community health promotion. *Public Health Nursing,* 21(4), 256–261.

Robertson, A. & Minkler, M. (1994). New health promotion movement: A critical examination. *Health Education Quarterly,* 21(3), 295–312.

Stoto, M.A., Abel, C., & Dievler, A. (Eds.). (1996). *Healthy communities: New partnerships for the future of public health.* Washington, DC: National Academy Press.

Toronto Healthy City Initiatives. (1997, Autumn). *Newsletter of the healthy city office.* Toronto, Ontario, Canada.

Tsouros, A. (Ed.). (1990). *World Health Organization healthy cities project: A project becomes a movement.* Copenhagen, Denmark: FADL Publishers.

World Health Organization. (1997). *The Jakarta declaration on leading health promotion in the 21st century.* WHO Geneva and Ministry of Health, Republic of Indonesia. Geneva, Switzerland: Author.

_____. (1993). *City action for health.* WHO Regional Office for Europe. Copenhagen, Denmark: Author.

_____. (1992, June 4). *Making health public policy in cities, discussion document.* WHO Regional Office for Europe. Copenhagen, Denmark: Author.

_____. (1988). *Report on the Adelaide conference, healthy public policy.* WHO European Office for Europe and Department of Community and Health Services, Australian Commonwealth, Copenhagen and Adelaide: Author.

_____. (1986a). *Health promotion.* Copenhagen, Denmark: Author.

_____. (1986b). *Ottawa charter for health promotion.* WHO Regional Office for Europe. Copenhagen, Denmark: Author.

_____. (1978, September). *Report of the International Conference on Primary Health Care,* held in Alma Ata, USSR. Geneva, Switzerland: Author.

INTERNET RESOURCES

www.ahcpr.gov/
Agency for Health Care Policy and Research

THE PROCESS OF COMMUNITY AS PARTNER

Elizabeth T. Anderson

CHAPTER

A MODEL TO
GUIDE PRACTICE

8

OBJECTIVES

Models that serve as guides for nursing practice, education, and research have become important tools for community health nurses. This chapter, in which we begin our examination of the nursing process as applied to the community as partner, focuses on the use of one nursing model to guide practice.

After studying this chapter, you should be able to

- Define *model* and *nursing model*.
- Describe the purposes of a nursing model.
- Begin to use a nursing model in practice.

INTRODUCTION

Although nursing models have been in existence since the beginnings of the profession, it was not until the 1960s that they were systematically identified, studied, and explicitly applied to practice. Boundaries are needed to define areas of concern for nursing, and a conceptual "map" of the nursing process is a necessary guide for action. This is particularly true when the nursing practice focuses on the entire community. The community-as-partner model provides us with both the map and the boundaries and will be used throughout this chapter.

MODELS

A conceptual model is the synthesis of a set of concepts and the statements that integrate those concepts into a whole. A nursing model can be defined as a frame of reference, a way of looking at nursing, or an image of what nursing encompasses. A nursing model is a representation of nursing, not a reality. Other types of models that are used to represent realities are model airplanes, blueprints, chemical equations, and anatomic models.

A model with which nurses identified for many years was the medical model; that is, a disease-oriented, illness- and organ-focused approach to patients, with an emphasis on pathology. However, reliance on the medical model excludes health promotion and the holistic focus that is central to nursing. Additionally, important aspects of care, such as psychological, sociocultural, and spiritual areas, are not included in the medical model. Thus, a nursing model should encompass all aspects of health care needs and incorporate long-range goals and planning.

As a representation of reality, a model can take numerous forms. Because they describe nursing, all nursing models are narrative; that is, words are the symbols that are used by nurses to define how they view their practice. And although all nursing models are described in words, many are clarified further through the use of diagrams or illustrations. The use of such images allows the model builder to show relationships and linkages among the concepts in the model. Diagrams are an efficient and effective way of depicting nursing models. The diagram is often thought of as the model itself, with accompanying text then seen as the elaboration or explanation of the model.

The method chosen to depict a nursing model reflects the model builder's own philosophy and preference; no one method is accepted as the best. There are, however, certain components that must be included in any model of nursing. Table 8–1 presents these essential elements.

There is general agreement that four concepts are central to the discipline of nursing: *person, environment, health,* and *nursing. (Concepts* are defined as general notions or ideas and are considered to be the building blocks of models.) How each of the four concepts is defined will both dictate the organization of the model and be illustrated in that model. For example, health may be defined on a continuum with wellness at one end and death at the other, as a dichotomy wherein one is seen as well or ill, as the outcome of numerous biopsychosocial and spiritual forces, or as the interaction of these same forces. In the medical model, *health* has been defined traditionally as the absence of disease. Figure 8–1 depicts four ways to view health and illustrates these definitions.

TABLE 8–1 ■ Essential Units of a Nursing Model	
Essential Unit	**Description of Unit**
A goal of action	The mission or ideal goal of the profession expressed as the end product desired (a state, condition, or situation)
A descriptive term for the patient population	That concept that best isolates who or what is acted on to achieve a goal; that is, those aspects of the person (as patient) or the organization or those aspects of their functioning toward which attention is to be directed; the target of action
The actor's role	A descriptive label that indicates the nature of the nurse's (the actor's) actions on patients
Source of difficulty	The origin of deviations from the desired state or condition
Intervention focus	The kind of problems found when deviations from the desired state occur; the kinds of disturbances in patients that are to be prevented or treated. Mode is the major means of preventing or treating such problems (the kinds of levers that can be used to change the course of events toward the desired end).
Consequences intended	Outcomes of action that are desired, stated in more abstract or broader terms than the mission, or including significant corollaries of the intended outcomes. Unintended outcomes may follow and may or may not be desirable.

(Data from Riehl, J.P. & Roy, C. [1980]. *Conceptual models for nursing practice* [2nd ed.], p. 2. New York: Appleton-Century-Crofts; from unpublished lecture notes of D. Johnson, UCLA, Fall 1975.)

Notice that the diagrams vary widely, reflecting the fundamental differences among these views of health.

What, then, are the uses of a model of nursing? Think for a moment of what a nursing model is to you and how a model might be useful in your practice. Although you may not have formulated your own model of nursing, you have been influenced greatly in your education by the model or models on which your nursing curriculum is based. Does your faculty subscribe to one particular nursing model? Just as the choice of a model creates a basis for curriculum planning and decisions, a model can also provide a basis for practice.

What is nursing to you? If you can express an answer to that question, you have begun to describe your model of nursing. A nursing model serves the following purposes:

- Provides a map for the nursing process
  - Gives direction for assessment (What do you assess?)
  - Guides analysis

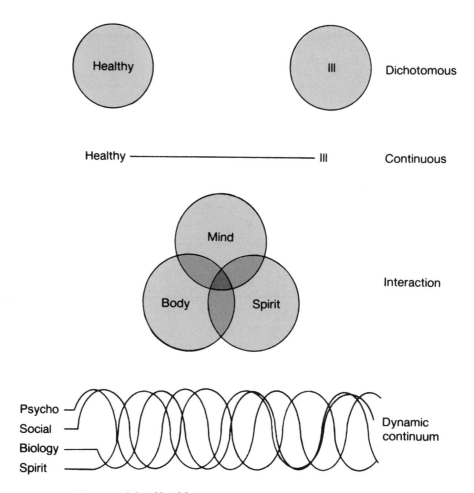

Figure 8–1. Four models of health.

- • Dictates nursing diagnoses
- • Assists in planning
- • Facilitates evaluation
- • Provides a curriculum outline for education
- • Represents a framework for research
- • Provides a basis for development of theory

A model is nothing more—or less—than an explication of nursing. A model not only describes what is but also provides a framework for making decisions about what *could be.*

COMMUNITY-AS-PARTNER MODEL

Based on Neuman's model of a total-person approach to viewing patient problems (1972), the *community-as-client model* was developed by the authors to illustrate the definition of public health nursing as the synthesis of public health and nursing. The model has been renamed the *community-as-partner model* to emphasize the underlying philosophy of primary health care.

Consider the community-as-partner model (Figure 8–2). There are two central factors in this model: a focus on the *community* as partner (represented by the community assessment wheel at the top, which incorporates the community's people as the core) and the use of the *nursing process*. The model is described in some detail to assist you in understanding its parts so you may use it as a guide to your practice in the community. Refer now to Figure 8–3 for the following discussion.

The *core* of the assessment wheel represents the *people* that make up the community. Included in the core are the *demographics* of the population as well as their *values, beliefs,* and *history*. As residents of the community, the people are affected by and, in turn, influence the eight subsystems of the community. These subsystems are physical environment, education, safety and transportation, politics and government, health and social services, communication, economics, and recreation.

The solid line surrounding the community represents its *normal line of defense*, or the *level of health* the community has reached over time. The normal line of defense may include characteristics such as a high rate of immunity, low infant mortality, or middle-class income level. The normal line of defense also includes usual patterns of coping, along with problem-solving capabilities; it represents the *health* of the community.

The *flexible line of defense*, depicted as a broken line around the community and its normal line of defense, is a "buffer zone" representing a dynamic level of health resulting from a temporary response to stressors. This temporary response may be neighborhood mobilization against an environmental stressor such as flooding or a social stressor such as an unwanted "adult" bookstore. The eight subsystems are divided by broken lines to remind us that they are not discrete and separate but influence (and are influenced by) one another. (Remember that one of the principles of ecology is that everything is connected to everything else. This also applies to the community as a whole.) The eight divisions both define the major subsystems of a community and provide the community health nurse with a framework for assessment.

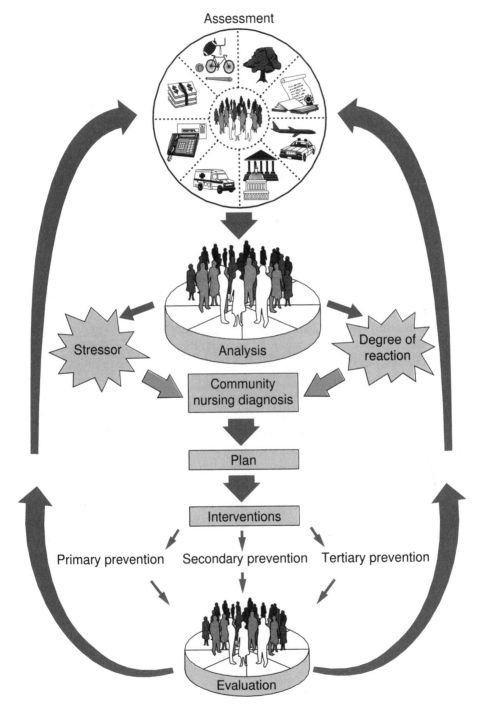

Figure 8–2. Community-as-partner model.

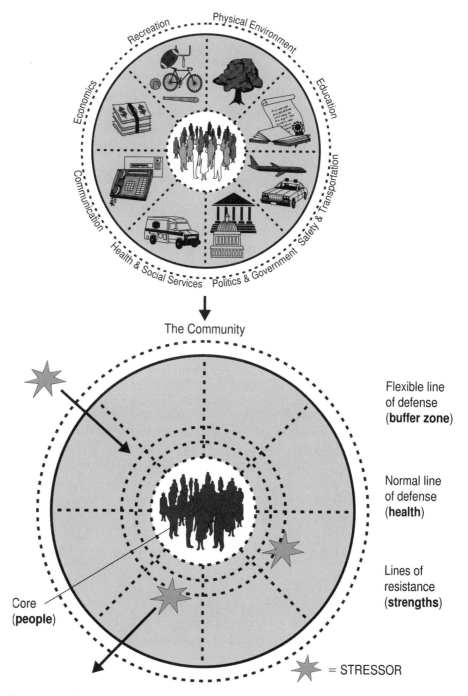

Figure 8–3. The community assessment wheel, featuring lines of resistance and defense within the community structure.

TAKE NOTE

Take a moment to examine the selection of subsystems that have been identified. Can you think of any that have been omitted? Think of the community where you live. What examples of each subsystem can you identify?

Within the community are *lines of resistance,* internal mechanisms that act to defend against stressors. An evening recreational program for young people implemented to decrease vandalism and a free-standing, no-fee health clinic to diagnose and treat sexually transmitted diseases are examples of lines of resistance. Lines of resistance exist throughout each of the subsystems and represent the community's *strengths.*

Stressors are tension-producing stimuli that have the *potential* of causing disequilibrium in the system. They may originate outside the community (eg, air pollution from a nearby industry) or inside the community (eg, the closing of a clinic). Stressors penetrate the flexible and normal lines of defense, resulting in disruption of the community. Inadequate, inaccessible, or unaffordable services are stressors on the health of the community.

The *degree of reaction* is the amount of disequilibrium or disruption that results from stressors impinging on the community's lines of defense. The degree of reaction may be reflected in mortality and morbidity rates, unemployment, or crime statistics, to name a few examples. Stressors and degree of reaction become part of the community nursing diagnosis. For example, a problem may be increased rate of respiratory illness (a degree of reaction) related to air pollution (a stressor).

TAKE NOTE

The outcome of a stressor impinging on a community is not always negative. Often it is positive. For example, in the face of a crisis, people may band together and develop a community group to deal with the crisis. This group may continue to function after the crisis is over—strengthening the community and continuing to contribute to its "health." (Advocacy for gun control laws after the shooting at Columbine High School in Colorado is an example of a positive outcome following a stressor.)

ASSESSMENT

The community's core and subsystems, its lines of defense and resistance, its stressors, and its degree of reaction comprise assessment parameters for the community worker who views the community as partner. Analyzing data on these parameters with the community leads to the *community nursing diagnosis.* Note the similarities and differences between a nursing diagnosis of an individual and a community nursing diagnosis depicted in Table 8–2.

Response	System/Function	Source of Situation	Manifestation of Problem
TABLE 8–2 ■ Nursing Diagnosis: Comparison of Individual and Community Focus			
Individual			
Patient behavior	Biopsychosocial-spiritual	Etiology	Symptoms from head-to-toe assessment
Example: Alteration in status	Oral integrity	Loose-fitting dentures	Oral pain; redness in mucosa; 10-cm open sore, and so on
Community			
Degree of reaction	Community subsystem	Stressor	Systems assessment (eg, rates)
Example: Increased	Respiratory disease	Air pollution	Increased hospital admissions for respiratory problems; higher rate of chronic obstructive pulmonary disease readmissions

TAKE NOTE

The term *community health diagnosis* is preferred over community nursing diagnosis for three reasons: It is holistic and does not imply that only a nurse can address the identified problem; it underscores that work in the community is by nature inter- and intradisciplinary (not even confined to health professions but incorporating many others); and it places the emphasis once again on the community, which is the focus of our practice. For the purposes of planning nursing interventions, however, do use community nursing diagnosis.

DIAGNOSIS AND PLANNING

The community health diagnosis gives *direction* to both nursing's goals and its interventions. The goal is derived from the stressors and may include the elimination or alleviation of the stressor or strengthening of the community's resistance through strengthening the lines of defense. By stating the degree of reaction, the nurse can plan interventions to strengthen the lines of resistance through one of the prevention modes.

INTERVENTION

In this model, *all* nursing interventions are considered to be preventive in nature. *Primary prevention* is the nursing intervention that aims at strengthening the lines of defense so stressors cannot penetrate to cause a reaction or at interfering with a stressor by taking action against it. An example of primary prevention is the immunization of preschoolers to increase the percentage of immunized children in the community. *Secondary prevention* is applied after a stressor has penetrated the community. Interventions support the lines of defense and resistance to minimize the degree of reaction to the stressor. Conducting a breast cancer screening (breast self-exam and mammography) and referral program is an example of secondary prevention. Such a program is aimed at early case finding to reduce the degree of reaction (such as the severity of the cancer when found). *Tertiary prevention* is applied after the stressor penetrates and a degree of reaction has taken place. There has been system disequilibrium, and tertiary prevention is aimed at preventing additional disequilibrium and promoting equilibrium. For example, a school fire has occurred and a large number of children are suffering from shock (physical and emotional). Teams of specialists (including community health nurses) are brought in to provide appropriate therapies and long-term follow-up as needed to reestablish equilibrium in the community and prevent additional problems in the children.

TAKE NOTE

In the school fire example, both tertiary and primary prevention are illustrated— tertiary, by providing appropriate therapy to prevent further trauma to the children due to this fire, and primary, by strengthening the children's coping mechanisms should another traumatic event occur in the future.

EVALUATION

Feedback from the community provides the basis for evaluation of the community health nurse's interventions just as involvement of community persons in all steps of the nursing process ensures relevance to the community. Often, the parameters that were used for assessment are also used for evaluation. For example, after the immunization program, did the percentage of immunized preschoolers increase? How many persons with breast lumps were identified and referred for medical care? What was the long-term effect of the school fire? Were the children reassimilated into their classes? Were fire codes investigated? Were additional precautions (eg, increased fire drills, replacement of flammable materials) instituted in the schools? Such is the process of working with the community as partner. Interconnections, overlap, and interdisciplinary considerations are the rule rather than the exception.

SUMMARY

Consider the community-as-partner model (see Figure 8–2) once more. The goal represented by the model is system equilibrium, a healthy community, and includes the preservation and promotion of community health.

TAKE NOTE

Health may not be a primary goal of the community (although it may be that of the community health nurse). It is, however, an important resource for the community to meet its goals. Realizing that we do not always share the same goals is important for anyone working in the community and must at least be considered (if not reconciled) as we plan, implement, and evaluate programs aimed at improving health.

The model's target (the patient, in an individual-focused practice) is the total community, the aggregate, and, as such, includes individuals and families. The nurse's *role* is to assist the community to attain, regain, maintain, and promote health—that is, to act as a facilitator, catalyst, and advocate for health—so the community is empowered to regulate and control its responses to stressors that are the source of difficulty. The *intervention focus* is the actual or potential disequilibrium or an inability of the community to function. The *intervention mode* is comprised of the three levels of prevention: primary, secondary, and tertiary. The consequences intended in this model include a strengthened normal line of defense, increased resistance to stressors, and a diminished degree of reaction to stressors by the community. Congruent with the principles of primary health care, it is the community's competence to deal with its own problems, strengthen its own lines of defense, and resist stressors that dictates the interventions. Let us now begin the process.

REFERENCES

Neuman, B.N. (1972). A model for teaching total person approach to patient problems. *Nursing Research, 21*(3), 264–269.

SUGGESTED READINGS—MODEL EXAMPLES

Buckner, W.P., Miner, K.R., Kreuter, M.W., & Wilson, M.G. (Eds.). (1992). PATCH: Community health promotion: The agenda for the '90s. [Special Edition]. *Journal of Health Education, 23*(3).

Green, L.W. & Kreuter, M.W. (1991). *Health promotion planning: An educational and environmental approach.* Mountain View, CA: Mayfield Publishing Co.

Kretzmann, J.P. & McKnight, J.L. (1993). *Building communities from the inside out: A path toward finding and mobilizing a community's assets.* Evanston, IL: Center for Urban Affairs and Policy Research, Northwestern University.

Lowry, L. (1998). *The Neuman systems model and nursing education: Teaching strategies and outcomes.* Indianapolis, IN: Sigma Theta Tau International, Center Nursing Press.

Minkler, M. & Wallerstein, N. (1997). Improving health through community organization and community building: A health education perspective. In Minkler, M. (Ed.), *Community organizing and community building for health* (pp. 30–52). New Brunswick, NJ: Rutgers University Press.

Pender, N.J. (1996). *Health promotion in nursing practice* (3rd ed.). Stamford, CT: Appleton & Lange.

Elizabeth T. Anderson **and** Judith McFarlane

COMMUNITY ASSESSMENT

9

OBJECTIVES

Preceding chapters have focused on the foundational concepts of primary health care, epidemiology, ecology, culture, ethics, empowerment, and policy. Community-focused models were introduced in Chapter 8 to guide you in the process of working with the community. This chapter and the four that follow focus on the *application* of the nursing process to the community. Consequently, the objectives will be practice oriented.

After studying this chapter, you should be able to complete a community health assessment using one selected model.

INTRODUCTION

Community assessment is a process; it is the act of becoming acquainted with a community. The people in the community are partners and contribute throughout the process. Our nursing purpose in assessing a community is to identify factors (both positive and negative) that impinge on the health of the people in order to develop strategies for health promotion. As Hancock and Minkler (1997, p 140) point out, "For health professionals concerned with . . . community building for health, there are two reasons for [conducting] community health assessments: information is needed for change, and it is needed for empowerment." We will use the community assessment wheel (Figure 9–1) as a framework for the assessment. (For a specific assessment guide for industry, see Appendix A. Appendix B includes the completed assessment of one industry.)

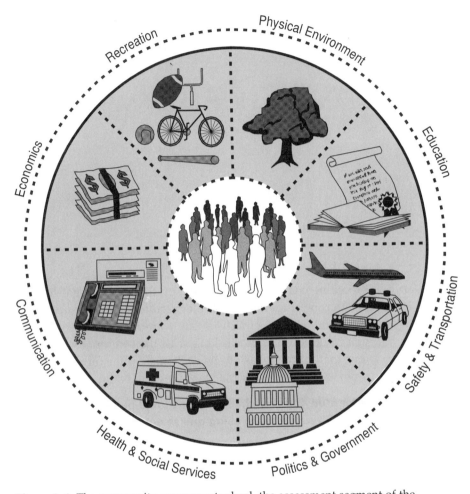

Figure 9–1. The community assessment wheel, the assessment segment of the community-as-partner model.

TAKE NOTE

Community assessments are not done in a vacuum. You are probably already familiar with some aspects of the community by virtue of your involvement in caring for people who reside there, perhaps in a clinic or a nearby hospital. In addition, this is not a solo job; many people will contribute to the assessment, so try not to get discouraged by the seeming enormity of the task. Tackle it in increments.

(*To the reader:* Regarding information contained in tables, our intention is to provide you with numbers, percentages, rates, and so forth, along with their source. These figures, however, are for illustration only and do not reflect current data related to the areas where they are found. For your assessment, be sure to use the latest figures and include the date within the citation.)

COMMUNITY ASSESSMENT

Begin by identifying your community. Recall that a system is a whole that functions because of the interdependence of its parts. A community, too, is a whole entity that functions because of the interdependence of its parts, or subsystems. The community assessment wheel (see Figure 9–1) will be your overall framework while the assessment is facilitated by using the model in survey form. The survey, "Learning About the Community on Foot" (Table 9–1), was adapted from an earlier version of the "windshield survey" that has been expanded to include each component of the community assessment wheel. Note that the guide has three parts: (1) the community core, (2) the community subsystems, and (3) perceptions. In addition, there are columns for the listing of observations and data.

The community of Rosemont, comprised of Census Tracks (CT) 402 and 403, will be used to illustrate the use of the model in conducting a community assessment (as well as subsequent analysis, diagnosis, planning, intervention, and evaluation). Although we have chosen an urban community defined by census tracts, the guide can be used to assess any community regardless of size, location, resources, or population characteristics. It can also be used to assess a "community within a community," such as a school, an industry, or a business. Examples of these communities are included in Part III of this book. In addition, this guide can be used if you are assessing an aggregate; that is, a defined group within the community (for example, teenagers, battered women, the elderly, or children under age 5) by providing the *context* in which this group is found. The *process* of assessment, regardless of where it is applied, always remains the same.

TAKE NOTE

It may be that in your community health nursing course time limitations will not permit each student to complete an entire community assessment. In fact, it is a rare instance when an individual completes a community assessment alone. Community assessment requires teamwork. Therefore, teams of students may be assigned to assess one or two community subsystems. At the end of the course, each team will present its assessment, and the total community assessment may be completed. A similar situation may arise in agencies when health care providers who are from a variety of disciplines are assigned one aspect (one subsystem) of a community to assess.

I. Community Core	Observations	Data
1. History—What can you glean by looking (eg, old, established neighborhoods; new subdivision)? Ask people willing to talk: How long have you lived here? Has the area changed? As you talk, ask if there is an "old-timer" who knows the history of the area.		
2. Demographics—What sorts of people do you see? Young? Old? Homeless? Alone? Families? What races do you see? Is the population homogeneous?		
3. Ethnicity—Do you note indicators of different ethnic groups (eg, restaurants, festivals)? What signs do you see of different cultural groups?		
4. Values and Beliefs—Are there churches, mosques, temples? Does it appear homogeneous? Are the lawns cared for? With flowers? Gardens? Signs of art? Culture? Heritage? Historical markers?		
II. Subsystems		
1. Physical environment—How does the community look? What do you note about air quality, flora, housing, zoning, space, green areas, animals, people, human-made structures, natural beauty, water, climate? Can you find or develop a map of the area? What is the size (eg, square miles, blocks)?		
2. Health & Social Services—Evidence of acute or chronic conditions? Shelters? "Traditional" healers (eg, curanderos, herbalists)? Are there clinics, hospitals, practitioners' offices, public health services, home health agencies, emergency centers, nursing homes, social service facilities, mental health services? Are there resources outside the community but accessible to them?		

	Observations	Data
3. Economy—Is it a "thriving" community or does it feel "seedy?" Are there industries, stores, places for employment? Where do people shop? Are there signs that food stamps are used/accepted? What is the unemployment rate?		
4. Transportation and Safety—How do people get around? What type of private and public transportation is available? Do you see buses, bicycles, taxis? Are there sidewalks, bike trails? Is getting around in the community possible for persons with disabilities? What types of protective services are there (eg, fire, police, sanitation)? Is air quality monitored? What are the types of crimes committed? Do people feel safe?		
5. Politics and Government— Are there signs of political activity (eg, posters, meetings)? What party affiliation predominates? What is the governmental jurisdiction of the community (eg, elected mayor, city council with single member districts)? Are people involved in decision making in their local governmental unit?		
6. Communication—Are there "common areas" where people gather? What newspapers do you see in the stands? Do people have TVs and radios? What do they watch/listen to? What are the formal and informal means of communication?		
7. Education—Are there schools in the area? How do they look? Are there libraries? Is there a local board of education? How does it function? What is the reputation of the school(s)? What are major educational issues? What are the dropout rates? Are there extracurricular activities available? Are they used? Is there a school health service? A school nurse?		

Continued

	Observations	Data
TABLE 9–1 ■ Learning about the Community on Foot* (Apriendiendo acerca de la communidad a pie) (*Continued*)		
8. Recreation—Where do children play? What are the major forms of recreation? Who participates? What facilities for recreation do you see?		
III. Perceptions		
1. The residents—How do people feel about the community? What do they identify as its strengths? Problems? Ask several people from different groups (eg, old, young, field worker, factory worker, professional, minister, housewife) and keep track of who gives what answer.		
2. Your perceptions—General statements about the "health" of this community. What are its strengths? What problems or potential problems can you identify?		

Note: Supplement your impressions with information from the census, police records, school statistics, chamber of commerce data, health department reports, etc., to confirm or refute your conclusions. Tables, graphs, and maps are helpful and will aid in your analysis.
*Revised "Windshield Survey." Anderson, E.T. & McFarlane, J.M. (1988). *Community as client: Application of the nursing process.* Philadelphia, PA: J.B. Lippincott, pp 178-179, which also incorporates all aspects of the assessment wheel from Anderson, E.T. & McFarlane, J.M. (1995). *Community as partner: Theory and practice in nursing.* (2nd ed.) Philadelphia: J.B. Lippincott, p 178.

Assessment is a skill that is refined through practice. Everyone feels awkward and unsure as he or she begins (remember the first time you took a blood pressure?); this is normal. The first step is always the most difficult. It is time to take the first step.

COMMUNITY CORE

The definition of *core* is "that which is essential, basic, and enduring." The core of a community is its people—their history, characteristics, values, and beliefs. The first stage of assessing a community, then, is to learn about its people. In fact, partnering with people in the community is an integral part of working in the community. Table 9–2 lists the major components of the community core

TABLE 9–2 ■ Community Core Data	
Components	**Sources of Information**
History	Library, historic society
	Interview "old-timers," town leaders
Demographics	Census of population and housing
Age and sex characteristics	Planning board (local, city, county, state)
Racial distribution	Chamber of commerce
Ethnic distribution	City hall, city secretary, archives
	Observation
Household types by	Census
Family	
Nonfamily	
Group	
Marital status by	Census
Single	
Separated	
Widowed	
Divorced	
Vital statistics	State department of health (distributed through
Births	city and county health departments)
Deaths by	
Age	
Leading causes	
Values and beliefs	Personal contact
	Observation ("Learning about the Community
	on Foot")
	(To protect against stereotyping, avoid the library
	for this portion of the assessment.)
Religion	Observation
	Telephone book

along with suggested locations and sources of information about each component. Because every community is different, information sources available to one community may not be available to another.

The History of Rosemont

The Rosemont property was originally deeded to a Miss Ima Smith, who received a land grant of 3370 acres in 1827. For almost 100 years, the area remained as prairie, dotted with cattle ranches and small farms. In 1920, John Walker and William Bell formed a land corporation and began developing the Smith property. The first area that was improved and deed restricted was named Rosemont after a legendary town in Scotland. After development, Rosemont prospered and attracted newcomers to the area. Numerous prominent families made their homes in Rosemont, including a state governor, a Nobel laureate, and a president of the United States. However, during the economic depression of the 1930s and the years before and during World War II, a drastic decrease in building activities occurred. Many stately homes deteriorated and either became multifamily dwellings or were left to decay. Eventually, economic forces succeeded in breaking deed restrictions, and residential areas were forced to accept the introduction of industry and small businesses. As a result, property values plummeted, leaving quaint boutiques and antique shops to exist alongside an increasing number of nightclubs and nude modeling studios.

From 1950 to 1970, Rosemont witnessed the influx of a large population of young adults, commonly referred to as "hippies," who used the large, spacious homes for group living. This practice of congregate housing was also taken up by drug addicts and runaways. Rosemont gradually assumed the reputation of tolerating "nontraditional" lifestyles—a factor that precipitated an influx of a large population of gay men.

Because of lower property values and affordable rent during the mid to late 1970s, large groups of Vietnamese and Mexicans also settled in Rosemont. Simultaneously, established families and single professionals, weary of the lengthy commute from suburbia to the inner city, began returning to Rosemont—a trend that continues today. Today, older homes are being refurbished, businesses are being revitalized, and pride, once lost, is being reclaimed.

Demographics and Ethnicity

Tables 9–3 and 9–4 set forth age, sex, race, and ethnicity data for CT 402 and CT 403 as well as for the nearest city and county. Gathering data on city, county, state, and nation affords comparisons that may be important for the analysis. (The census lists only numbers of people; you must calculate percentages.) Tables 9–5 and 9–6 list data on family types and marital status.

TAKE NOTE

During the next step of the nursing process (in other words, analysis), you will need data about the other comparable entities, so collect all needed data now.

TABLE 9–3 ■ Population Age and Sex Characteristics for CT 402, CT 403, City of Hampton, and Jefferson County

Age (years)	CT 402 Males	CT 402 Females	CT 402 Total %	CT 403 Males	CT 403 Females	CT 403 Total %	Hampton Number	Hampton Total %	Jefferson County Number	Jefferson County Total %
Under 5 yr	370	362	10.6	29	11	0.6	123,150	7.8	189,246	8.4
5–19	1200	991	31.9	241	195	6.5	377,345	23.9	569,991	25.3
30–34	395	437	12.2	1965	911	42.6	514,705	32.6	716,431	31.8
35–54	837	970	26.2	1758	721	36.7	339,453	21.5	484,380	21.5
55–64	222	370	8.6	221	181	5.9	116,835	7.4	157,705	7
65 and over	270	450	10.5	175	349	7.7	107,361	6.8	135,176	6
Total	3294	3580	100	4389	2368	100	1,578,849	100	2,252,929	100

(Data from Census of Population and Housing, Selected Characteristics.)

	CT 402 Number	CT 402 Total %	CT 403 Number	CT 403 Total %	Hampton Number	Hampton Total %	Jefferson County Number	Jefferson County Total %
White	852	12.4	5,871	88.5	970,489	61.5	1,562,091	69.4
Black	3732	54.3	305	4.6	434,014	27.5	467,177	20.7
Asian/ Pacific Islander	1312	19.1	54	0.7	32,335	2.1	45,432	2
Hispanic	625	9.1	321	4.7	131,763	8.3	163,774	7.3
American Indian	242	3.5	38	0.6	3,203	0.2	4,923	0.2
Other	111	1.6	58	0.9	7,045	0.4	9,532	0.4
Total	6874	100	6,757	100	1,578,849	100	2,252,929	100

(Data from Census of Population and Housing, Selected Characteristics.)

TABLE 9–5 ■ Population by Family Types for CT 402 and CT 403

	CT 402 Number	CT 402 Total %	CT 403 Number	CT 403 Total %
Family	5706	83	2443	36.2
Nonfamily	1168	17	4103	60.7
Female-headed household	721		994	
Male-headed household	447		2189	
Group quarters			211	3.1
Total	6874	100	6757	100

(Data from Census of Population and Housing, Selected Characteristics.)

TABLE 9–6 ■ Persons Age 15 and Over by Sex and Marital Status for CT 402 and CT 403

Marital Status	CT 402			CT 403		
	Male	Female	Total %	Male	Female	Total %
Single	348	408	15.2	2418	1016	53.5
Married	1510	1498	60.1	796	768	24.4
Separated	120	245	7.2	113	72	2.8
Widowed	52	119	3.4	68	198	4.3
Divorced	294	407	14.1	572	397	15
Total	2324	2677	100	3967	2451	100

(Data from Census of Population and Housing, Selected Characteristics.)

Vital Statistics

Table 9–7 lists birth and death vital statistics for CT 402 and CT 403 as well as for the city and county. Using a similar format, Table 9–8 lists the leading causes of death. *Please note:* It is always preferable to report rates because you can then make comparisons. However, if you do not know the population at risk (the denominator), it isn't possible to calculate rates. These morbidity data do not allow the calculation of rates for that reason.

Values, Beliefs, and Religion

Part of the community core are the values, beliefs, and religious practices of the people. All ethnic and racial groups have values and beliefs that interact with each community system to influence the people's health. Review the chapter on cultural competence for methods to help you understand these cultural elements of the community. Notice that Table 9–2 cautions against the exclusive

TABLE 9–7 ■ Selected Birth and Death Vital Statistics for CT 402, CT 403, City of Hampton, and Jefferson County

	CT 402	CT 403	Hampton	Jefferson County
Births	210	117	30,726	56,865
*Deaths (rates)**				
Infant	7 (33)	2 (17)	372 (12)	698 (12.3)
Neonatal	5 (23)	2 (17)	245 (7.9)	471 (8.3)

*Rates are per 1000.
(Data from State Vital Statistics, Department of Health.)

TABLE 9–8 ■ Deaths by Selected Causes for CT 402, CT 403, City of Hampton, and Jefferson County*

Cause of Death	CT 402		CT 403		Hampton		Jefferson County	
	Number	Total %	Number	Total %	Number	Total %	Number	Total %
Heart disease	16	22.2	10	23.8	3,186	33.4	5,932	36
Malignant neoplasms	17	23.6	11	26.1	2,078	21.8	3,972	24.2
Cerebrovascular	6	8.3	2	4.7	690	7.3	1,213	7.4
Accidents	4	5.6	4	9.5	585	6.2	932	5.7
Emphysema, asthma, bronchitis	0	0	0	0	79	0.8	115	0.7
Diseases of early infancy	7	9.7	1	2.4	248	2.6	501	3
Homicides	6	8.3	1	2.4	592	6.2	831	5.1
Cirrhosis of liver	0	0	1	2.4	163	1.7	253	1.5
Pneumonia	2	2.8	1	2.4	210	2.2	365	2.2
Suicides	3	4.2	1	2.4	195	2	234	1.4
Diabetes mellitus	0	0	2	4.8	139	1.4	305	1.8
Congenital anomalies	0	0	2	4.8	99	1	245	1.5
Nephritis and nephrosis	0	0	0	0	13	0.1	26	0.2
Tuberculosis	1	1.4	0	0	17	0.2	28	0.2
All other causes	10	13.9	6	14.3	1,239	13	1,488	9.1
Total deaths, all causes	72	100	42	100	9,533	100	16,440	100

*Note: It is always preferable to report *rates* because you can then make comparisons. However, if you do not know the population at risk (the denominator), it isn't possible to calculate rates. These morbidity data do not allow the calculation of rates.
(Data from Hampton Vital Statistics, City of Hampton Health Department.)

use of the library for information about values, beliefs, and religious practices—the reason being that books and articles frequently offer broad generalizations to describe the practices of ethnic and racial groups (for example, the lifestyles of urban blacks) or discuss one practice of one ethnic group (such as breast-feeding practices of Mexican-born Hispanics). Each community is unique, with values, beliefs, and religious practices that are rooted in tradition and continue to evolve and exist because they meet the community's needs.

To validate the published, secondary demographic data, use your survey to establish the presence and geographic location of different racial and ethnic groups. It is during this phase—assessment of the physical system—that we

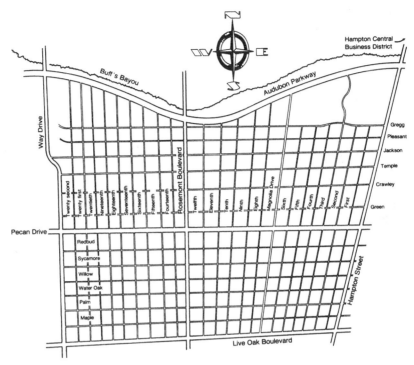

Figure 9–2. Rosemont Community streets and boundaries.

step into the community to learn and experience the values, beliefs, and religious practices of the community.

Our partner, the Rosemont community, is located within the City of Hampton and is in Hampton's central business district. It is bounded by Way Drive on the west, Buff's Bayou on the north, Live Oak Boulevard on the south, and Hampton Street on the east. Figure 9–2 is a map of the Rosemont community. Using the "Learning About the Community on Foot" survey (see Table 9–1) as a guide, we step into the community.

PHYSICAL ENVIRONMENT

Just as the physical examination is a critical component of assessing an individual patient, so it is in the assessment of a community. And just as the five senses of the clinician are called into play in the physical examination of a patient, so, too, are they needed at the community level. Table 9–9 provides the components of the physical examination, both of an individual and a community, and compares tools and sources of data for each.

TABLE 9–9 ■ Physical Examination Components and Sources of Data

Components	Sources of Data	
	Individual	**Community**
Inspection	All senses	All senses
	Otoscope	Windshield survey
	Ophthalmoscope	Walk through community
Auscultation	Stethoscope	Listen to community sounds/residents
Vital signs	Thermometer	Observe climate, terrain, natural boundaries, and resources
	Sphygmomanometer	"Life" signs such as notices of community meetings; density
Systems review	Head-to-toe	Observe social systems, including housing, businesses, churches, and hangouts
Laboratory studies	Blood tests	Almanac; census data
	X-rays	Chamber of commerce planning studies and surveys
	Scans, other tests	

Inspection

Rosemont Boulevard bisects the community and serves as a major north–south thoroughfare for residents traveling to or through the community. It is tree-lined and divided by a grassy median in sections. Many businesses, especially restaurants, are located along Rosemont Boulevard. Many of the restaurants are of the "specialty" type that serve quiche, sprout sandwiches, and herbal teas. Other businesses situated along the boulevard are gas stations, office buildings, art-supply stores, a veterinarian, small art galleries, a nursery, one Mexican *barbacoa* stand in a grocery store, florists, a bank, a pharmacy, and various shops specializing in leather goods, books, and handcrafted items. (See the Economics section of this chapter for a summary of business units.)

The major east–west thoroughfare through Rosemont, Pecan Drive, is also lined with businesses and, with fewer trees, presents a more urban face. At the east end can be seen nude modeling studios, small restaurants specializing in various ethnic foods (Greek, Pakistani, Mexican, Vietnamese, and Indian, to name a few), and numerous small art shops. The Rosemont Health Center, which is discussed later in this chapter, is located in this area. Further west on this street is a large theater that attracts many first-run productions. There are a couple of "adult" movie houses and the ubiquitous specialty restaurants (in this area, they are of the type that caters to the business or professional crowds—quiet tea rooms that play classical music). Along this street, too, are many large old houses, many of which have been converted into antique shops, flower shops, and other small stores. There is no large industry in Rosemont. Behind the two business-filled thoroughfares that divide the community, Rosemont can give one the feeling of having entered a different world. The streets are narrower, and some are cobbled; old oaks and pecan trees are abundant, and, in many areas, the branches of the trees meet over the streets to form protective canopies of green.

The streets (except the thoroughfares) are narrow, and most of them have sidewalks, as is typical of older neighborhoods in Hampton. In general, the streets and sidewalks are in good repair and free from debris; however, because there is little off-street parking, many residents park on the streets, so there is traffic congestion at the times when most residents are home (primarily nights and weekends).

Vital Signs

The climate of Rosemont (and the Hampton Standard Metropolitan Statistical Area [SMSA]) is mild and moderated by sea winds. Summers are hot (the temperature is 90°F or higher approximately 87 days a year) and humid (averaging 62%), but evenings are cool, and there is rarely a hard freeze in the winter. Flora, both temperate and tropical, abounds—live oaks, hibiscus, and pines may grow in one block, for example.

The terrain is generally flat, with little variation in grade. It is 20 feet above sea level. The only naturally occurring water in the area is Buff's Bayou, a concrete-lined "river" that serves to carry off excess rain and drainage to reduce chances of flooding in Hampton. The bayou ends in the Hampton Ship Channel, which leads to the sea.

Rosemont is the third most densely populated area in Hampton, with 14.4 people per acre. An area in CT 402 that contains the subsidized housing complex is the most densely populated in all of Hampton, with 221 people per acre (Census).

The variety of local stores reflects the diversity of interests in Rosemont. Posters advertising a meeting of the Gay Political Caucus share bulletin-board space with senior citizens' meetings, church announcements, educational programs at the community college's "Sundry School," Vietnamese relocation services, the community's STD (sexually transmitted diseases) Clinic, and a musical show by "El Barrio" from the Mexican-American area. Rosemont is a community of rich diversity, a microcosm of Hampton.

The churches of Rosemont also reflect its diversity—virtually all denominations are represented. From the large Methodist and Presbyterian churches on its borders to the small storefront churches for refugees, Rosemont contains resources for all major religious groups.

Systems

Most of Rosemont is developed; there is little space not in use. Four small neighborhood parks, a narrow strip along the bayou, and the land around the Community College are the "greens" available to the community (Figure 9–3), although most houses have well-kept lawns with trees and shrubs. Table 9–10 presents land use data for Rosemont.

The majority of houses in Rosemont are old, reflecting the early development of the area. Within certain sections, the houses resemble each other (for example, all one-story, wood frame houses with porches); however, there may also be great heterogeneity from one block to the next. In the northeast quadrant is a large subsidized housing area comprised of run-down apartments with broken windows and poorly kept streets, whereas in the southwest quadrant are houses that have been well maintained and remodeled. Also in the

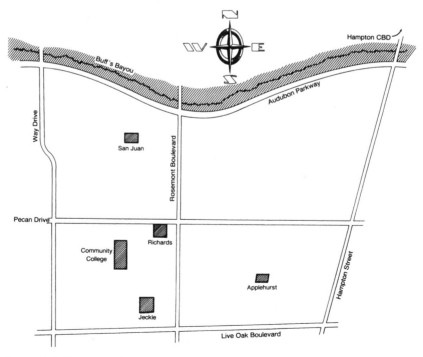

Figure 9–3. Rosement Community greens and parks.

TABLE 9–10 ■ Rosemont Land Use

Land Use	CT 402		CT 403	
	Number of Acres	Total %	Number of Acres	Total %
Single-family dwellings	161.2	28.03	95.4	31.78
Multifamily dwellings	46.4	8.06	46.5	15.49
Commercial	210.2	36.55	61.2	20.39
Industrial	44.9	7.8	0.2	0.06
Public	6.8	1.18	11.1	3.69
Open	52.9	9.2	53.2	17.72
Water	6.3	1.09	4.7	1.56
Undeveloped	46.3	8.05	14.6	4.86
Right-of-way	0	0	13.2	4.39
Total acres	575	100	300.1	100

(Data Book, Rosemont Community Development, City of Hampton, Planning Department.)

northeast is an area covering several blocks of what are called "shotgun hous-es" (the story is told that one can shoot a shotgun from the front door, and the shot will go out the back door); placed side by side, they are tiny and poorly maintained. See Table 9–11 for housing information.

During the day, most of the people seen on the streets move quickly and purposefully as though on business or an errand. Those who could be described as "strolling" are elderly people or young men, usually alone. Few children are seen during the day except in the schoolyards, which are not on the main thoroughfares. Dogs are heard to bark as one walks through the neigh-borhoods, and cats sun themselves in windows; however, few pets run loose in the area.

At night, Rosemont assumes a different flavor along Pecan Drive: All of the restaurants are open, and many have outdoor patios for serving. Smells of faji-tas, curry, exotic spices, and charbroiling fill the air. "The Strip," as Pecan Drive

TABLE 9–11 ■ Average Value of Housing and Rent for Years 1980 and 1990

	CT 403		CT 402		Hampton	
	1980	1990	1980	1990	1980	1990
Average value of housing	$58,432	$62,400	$25,777	$43,300	$49,630	$61,900
Average rent	$259/mo	$346/mo	$243/mo	$284/mo	$244/mo	$337/mo

(Data from Census of Population and Housing, Bureau of Census.)

is called, comes alive with sounds of rap, disco, country, and rock-and-roll, along with the stroking of a sitar or quiet strumming of a guitar.

Most of the clients in these restaurants and nude modeling "studios," according to residents, come from outside of Rosemont. Many are attracted by the food and some by the free-wheeling sex that is reputed to be available in the area.

Many of the residents express disdain for the Strip, calling it a "tourist attraction," and they believe it is contributing to the deterioration of Rosemont. They state that "outsiders" and "cowboys" exploit and prey on unsuspecting tourists and that the unsavory reputation of the area is not the fault of the people who live there. An absence of zoning laws has facilitated the establishment of some of the less-than-desirable businesses in the area.

The physical examination of Rosemont reveals it to be a community of contrasts: churches and nude modeling studios, subsidized city housing units and restored homes from a more affluent time, old people and young, white and black (and all shades between), quiet tree-lined streets and busy thoroughfares, sedate tea rooms and garish adult movie theaters, families and singles, and the rich and poor.

HEALTH AND SOCIAL SERVICES

One method of classifying health and social services is to differentiate between facilities located outside the community (*extracommunity*) versus those within the community (*intracommunity*). Once the health and social service facilities are identified, group them into categories, perhaps by type of service offered (for example, hospitals, clinics, extended care), by size, or by public versus private usage. Table 9–12 suggests a classification system as well as possible major components of each facility requiring assessment.

Extracommunity Health Facilities

Hospitals

Jefferson County has 50 hospitals with a total of 12,321 beds, of which 4,321 are in the Hampton Medical Center—a complex that includes all medical subspecialties as well as sophisticated diagnostic and treatment services. The Medical Center is located 7 miles from Rosemont. All patients admitted to the Medical Center must be referred by a physician; self-referral is not permitted. (Self-referral allows the individual independently to choose and acquire medical

TABLE 9–12 ■ Health and Social Services

Component	Sources of Information
Health Services	
Extracommunity or intracommunity facilities. Once identified, group into categories (eg, hospitals and clinics, home health care, extended care facilities, public health services, emergency care).	Chamber of commerce Planning board (county, city) Phone directory Talk to residents Interview administrator or someone on the staff Facility annual report
For each facility, collect data on 1. Services (fees, hours, and new services planned and those discontinued) 2. Resources (personnel, space, budget, and record system) 3. Characteristics of users (geographic distribution, demographic profile, and transportation source) 4. Statistics (number of persons served daily, weekly, and monthly) 5. Adequacy, accessibility, and acceptability of facility according to users and providers	
Social Services	
Extracommunity or intracommunity facilities. Once identified, group into categories (eg, counseling and support, clothing, food, shelter, and special needs).	Chamber of commerce United Way directory Phone directory
For each facility, collect data on areas 1–5 listed above.	

care.) Although existence of the Medical Center is common knowledge among Rosemont residents, few people know anyone who has sought or received care there. Numerous private hospitals are located in Jefferson County, most being in Hampton. All private hospitals require third-party reimbursement for services rendered. (Third-party reimbursement means payment for services by an entity other than the patient. For example, Medicare, Medicaid, insurance, and Workmen's Compensation are third-party reimbursers.) In addition to private hospitals, most communities use tax revenues to support at least one hospital for the general public. In Jefferson County, the public hospital is Jefferson Memorial.

Jefferson Memorial is a full-service facility located 5 miles south of Rosemont. Care units and clinics at Memorial include medical, surgical, pediatrics, maternity, gynecology, trauma and burns, psychiatry, and emergency rooms. People can self-refer to Jefferson Memorial. According to the director of the emergency room (ER), 290 people are seen daily in the ER (approximately 100,000 people annually). Of these, some 40% are admitted. Follow-up care is provided by Memorial's outpatient clinics. Memorial is supported by city and county taxes as well as by fees collected for services. The base charge for an ER visit classified as minor is $85.20; a visit deemed major costs $274.40. Health care provider fees, as well as treatments and diagnostic services are in addition to the base fee. All fees are on a sliding scale according to income and family size. Rosemont residents use Memorial but complain of lengthy waits of up to 8 hours and of having to undergo repeated assessments as they are moved from one health care provider to another. Hospital personnel recognize the lengthy waiting period and fragmentation of care, but they cite budget constraints and high staff turnover as major obstacles to improving care. No services have been discontinued at Memorial, and no new services or staff positions are budgeted for the next 2 years.

Private Care Providers, Group Practices, and Specialty Clinics

A full selection of general medical and specialty care is available in Jefferson County through private practitioners, group practices, and specialty clinics. Payment is usually third-party reimbursement. Two health maintenance organizations (HMOs) are located in Jefferson County. Rosemont residents with adequate finances use a variety of private practitioners and specialty clinics. The residents usually self-refer after a favorable recommendation from a neighbor, friend, or work colleague.

Public Health Services: The Health Department

To monitor, maintain, and promote the public's health, each state has a state health department and accompanying regional, county, and sometimes city health departments. National, state, and local tax revenues are used to support public health services. There exists a Hampton Health Department as well as a Jefferson County Health Department. Because Rosemont is within the city limits of Hampton, the services of the Hampton Health Department are assessed.

The Hampton Health Department offers all medical outpatient services through its seven satellite clinics. The Sunvalley Clinic, located 6 miles from Rosemont and closest to the area, provides the following services:

* Immunizations
* Well and ill infant, child, adolescent, and adult care
* Antepartum/postpartum care
* Family planning
* Nutrition counseling

- Screening and testing for genetic and acquired conditions such as sickle-cell anemia, diabetes, and phenylketonuria (PKU)
- Dental assessment, cleaning, and restoration
- Mental health counseling and referral
- Health education
- Maternal and infant home visitation after early hospital discharge (defined as earlier than 48 hours after delivery)
- Child abuse, battered spouse, and abandoned person counseling and referral
- STD screening and follow-up (including HIV testing)

Additional services include a pharmacy, laboratory, and radiation department. Payment for most services is on a sliding scale; remaining services are free to all city residents. Free services include immunizations as well as screening and treatment for STDs. The majority of Rosemont residents who use the health department attend antepartum or postpartum clinics. The staff nurse in the maternity clinic estimates that of the 75 women seen in the prenatal clinic each week, 20 to 25 are Rosemont residents.

The major service-delivery problem cited by nurses in the maternity clinics is the long waiting period (frequently 8 to 10 weeks) between a woman's initial request for an appointment and the scheduled appointment date. Because many women wait until they are 6 or 7 months pregnant to request antepartum care, the first available appointment time may be after the woman's expected delivery date. Consequently, a large number of women from Rosemont deliver at Jefferson Memorial having received no antepartum care. The administrator of the Sunvalley Clinic felt a top service priority to be additional education, support, and monitoring services for pregnant women and new mothers.

No services have been discontinued in the recent past. With regard to the question of services that are needed, the elderly were identified as a target group. Plans were under way to establish a nursing clinic for the elderly as well as a wellness program to be offered at day care for the elderly and at senior centers. There are presently more than 10 such facilities for seniors within the city of Hampton.

Numerous Rosemont residents use the health department services, especially the Sunvalley Clinic. Problems cited include lack of a direct bus connection to the clinic (three bus transfers are required) and "impersonal" service. Because patients are not assigned to a primary care provider, it is customary for them to see a different health care provider at each visit. Maternity patients have an additional concern. Each woman must make her own delivery arrangements, and frequently women who qualify for antepartum care at Sunvalley Clinic do not meet eligibility requirements for delivery at Jefferson Memorial.

Consequently, women must search for a facility that will admit them for labor and delivery. All too often, they are forced to deliver at home, a situation documented by Sunvalley nurses and confirmed by several Rosemont residents.

Home Health Agencies

The Visiting Nurses Association (VNA) of Hampton is the largest home health agency in Jefferson County. Services of the VNA include home health care by registered nurses, physical and occupational therapists, speech therapists, social workers, and home health aides. The VNA accepts paying clients and third-party reimbursements. Paying clients are charged on a sliding scale according to income and family size. Patients who are unable to pay a fee can request financial assistance from several community social service agencies such as the United Way.

Numerous other home health agencies are located in Hampton and Jefferson County. Although more limited in scope of service, all offer home health services and require fees or third-party reimbursement for payment.

Long-Term, Extended-Care, and Continuing-Care Facilities

There are two long-term facilities within 8 miles of Rosemont: the Pinewoods Rest Center and the Windsail Nursing Home. Each facility is classified as an intermediate-care facility and is licensed by the state health department. A profile of the services, resources, and characteristics of the residents for each facility is presented in Table 9–13. In addition, several hospitals offer extended-care services.

Emergency Services

The Poison Control Center provides information to individuals and health care providers on harmful substances and methods of assessment and treatment. The center provides educational materials and programs for schools and interested groups. Their easy-to-remember number is 1-POISON.

Medical Emergency Ambulance Service (MEAS) is financed by Hampton city taxes, public donations, Jefferson County contributions, and organized fund-raisers. The MEAS first-aid services are free and available 24 hours a day to all residents of Rosemont. (The MEAS operates in conjunction with the local fire stations. See the Safety and Transportation section of this chapter for a description of fire protection services.)

TABLE 9–13 ■ Services, Resources, and Resident Characteristics at Pinewoods Rest Center and Windsail Nursing Home During the Preceding Year		
	Pinewoods Rest Center	**Windsail Nursing Home**
Services	Convalescent nursing care; physical, occupational, and speech therapy	Convalescent nursing care
Full-time personnel	Six RNs, four licensed visiting nurses (LVNs), three nurse aides, one administrator	Three RNs, two LVNs, one nurse aide, one administrator
Licensed bed capacity	96	38
Patient days	33,524	12,965
Occupancy rate	0.96	0.93
Certified bed capacity*	96	38
Median age of residents	79	76
Average duration of stay	Four years	Six years

*Recommended occupancy rate for nursing home beds is 90%.
(Data from Jefferson County Planning Council, Pinewoods Rest Center, and Windsail Nursing record books.)

The MEAS closest to Rosemont has two ambulances; one is used daily, and the other serves as a backup. The MEAS averages 90 to 110 calls a month, with a response time of less than 8 minutes. (Table 9–14 presents specific reasons for ambulance service to people in Rosemont during the last 3-month period.) Calls are received through the central fire department and dispatched by radio to the nearest MEAS team. Each MEAS team consists of 26 people: 3 paramedics having completed 100 hours of classwork and 200 hours of hospital

TABLE 9–14 ■ Reasons for Medical Emergency Ambulance Service to Persons in Rosemont During the Preceding 3-Month Period	
Reason	**Total %**
Cardiac-related problems and cerebrovascular accidents	25
Falls and household accidents	19
Respiratory problems	12
Dizziness and weakness	12
Lacerations	11
Fractures and dislocations	9
Abdominal pain	7
Mental–psychiatric disorders	5

(Data from MEAS paramedics records.)

experience and 22 emergency medical technicians (EMTs) with basic paramedic training and additional experience in intravenous therapy and intubation. Both paramedics and EMTs are certified. In addition to emergency service, the MEAS team offers CPR and first-aid classes to community groups.

Special Services

Frequently, special facilities exist to serve specific groups such as the handicapped or retarded. After surveying the immediate extracommunity area, no such facilities were located within a 10-mile radius of Rosemont.

Intracommunity Health Facilities

According to the Health Systems Agency (HSA) of Jefferson County, CT 402 is a medically underserved area; CT 403 is not.

The type and number of practitioners offering health services in Rosemont are listed in Table 9–15. A need for gynecologic and obstetric services was frequently expressed by female residents. Numerous people cited the need for family practitioners as well as bilingual health care providers. (One of the nurse practitioners speaks Spanish, but none speaks Vietnamese.) Rosemont residents with financial resources tend to select from extracommunity medical services, whereas indigent residents rely on medical services within the community. All private practitioners require payment when services are rendered or third-party reimbursement; the nurse practitioners use a sliding scale to calculate fees. In addition to private practitioners, two clinics—the Third Street Clinic and the Rosemont Health Center—are located in Rosemont.

TABLE 9–15 ■ Practitioners in Rosemont

Type	Number
Dentist	6
General medical	1
Optometrist	2
Orthodontist	1
Osteopath	2
Podiatrist	1
Chiropractor	3
Nurse Practitioner	2

(Data from Windshield survey, chamber of commerce, and phone directory.)

Third Street Clinic

The Third Street Clinic was founded in 1968 by concerned citizens and church leaders in Rosemont. The clinic, located in the center of CT 402, was initially financed by public donations and church-sponsored fund-raisers. All professional time and supplies were donated. Today, the Third Street Clinic serves 30% to 40% of Rosemont residents and has an annual operating budget of $750,000, a reduction of $220,000 from 2 years ago. The majority of funds are from federal and state grants as well as from client fees and Medicare and Medicaid reimbursements. Although patients are charged according to a sliding scale, no one is denied care. Services provided at Third Street Clinic are summarized in Table 9–16. The clinic provides no acute or trauma care services. One part-time physician, two part-time nurses, one social worker, one administrator, and a clerk form the clinic's staff. Both nurses speak Spanish, but none of the staff speaks Vietnamese. Optometry students and supervising faculty provide services 1 day a week, and one nurse-midwife provides antepartum care two mornings a week. The clinic is open Monday through Friday, 8 AM to 5 PM. On average, 125 people are seen weekly. Medical professionals and citizens form the board of directors. According to the clinic's director, immediate medical needs for the residents of CT 402 include the following:

- Ill infant, child, adolescent, and adult assessment, treatment, and follow-up
- Dental assessment and restoration
- Counseling, referral, and, when possible, treatment for drug abuse and alcoholism
- Group health teaching, especially for pregnant women, parents of young children, and adolescents

TABLE 9–16 ■ Services and Number of People Served at Third Street Clinic

Service	Description	Patient Visits (Weekly Average)
Family planning	Physical exams, education, and prescriptions filled	24
Well-child examinations	Physical assessment, referral for illness, immunizations, and screening	19
Antepartum and postpartum	Physical assessment and monitoring	42
Optometry	Eye exams and prescriptions filled	9
Podiatry	Assessment and treatment	6
Chronic disease counseling and treatment	Treatment and care instructions for hypertension, diabetes, and cardiovascular conditions	31

- Wellness and self-care classes for all age groups
- Support groups for single parents and senior citizens

There are no consistent health education or counseling services. Transportation services from area neighborhoods to the clinic, as well as dental and home nursing care, were discontinued 2 years ago after grant reductions. The major problem confronting the clinic is the recruitment of health care providers, especially nurses and physicians. Clinic services cannot be expanded (or maintained at the present level) unless additional health care providers are recruited and retained.

Most Rosemont residents are aware of the Third Street Clinic, and many use the clinic's services routinely. The major impediment to clinic use is the 1- to 2-mile walk to the clinic for many residents (there is no direct bus connection for most people). Rosemont residents feel welcomed at the clinic, and low staff turnover has fostered positive relationships between the staff and the community. Residents did, however, express a need for additional services at the clinic.

Rosemont Health Center

The Rosemont Health Center, centrally located in CT 403, is a nonprofit clinic devoted to the diagnosis and treatment of STDs (including human immunodeficiency virus [HIV] infection). The clinic is open Monday to Saturday, 6 PM to 10 PM, and Sunday, 2 PM to 10 PM. The center reports 20% of the syphilis cases and 60% of the gonorrhea cases in Jefferson County. Approximately 600 patient visits occur monthly (200 new cases, 200 repeat cases, and 200 follow-ups). All 75 professional staff members are volunteers and donate 4 to 10 hours of service a month. The director of the clinic is employed part-time. The state donates penicillin, tetanus cultures, and Venereal Disease Research Laboratory (VDRL) tests. Initially, there were no fees for services. Now, a fee of $10 per visit is assessed to defray costs of equipment, rent, and utilities. (However, no person is denied care.) Ninety percent of the patients are gay men. Each patient is issued an identification number and card that is used with each visit. People in psychological crisis are referred to the city health department for counseling. Most patients drive or walk to the clinic.

The director of the health center discussed the immediate need for expanded counseling and support groups, especially for people who are HIV positive. A second need is for an orientation program and information update sessions for staff members, most of whom are former patients. The majority of patients are from the Rosemont area, although an increasing number of patients are commuting to the clinic from Hampton and surrounding Jefferson County. Patients surveyed in the waiting room rated the care as excellent; appointments are rarely canceled by patients.

Observations at the clinic revealed a warm, caring atmosphere where people were treated with respect and were provided privacy when needed. In addition, however, there were two open trash bags filled with syringes and attached needles and no visible emergency cart. There were no standard policy and procedure manuals and no posted protocol for an adverse treatment response (such as penicillin reaction) for the many volunteers who worked there.

Social Service Facilities

Because social service agencies are frequently located in office buildings, their location in the community may be difficult to determine during a windshield survey. It is preferable to use a directory such as the type compiled by the chamber of commerce or local planning board to begin identifying social service organizations relatively close to the community being assessed. If the community does not have a chamber of commerce, use the phone directory.

Extracommunity Social Service Facilities

Counseling and Support Services

The Hampton Comprehensive Counseling Center was founded in 1971 by concerned citizens of Hampton and Jefferson County for the purpose of providing counseling to adolescent drug users. Today, the center offers a comprehensive mental health program for all residents of Hampton. The center is located 2 miles south of Rosemont. Although people can self-refer to the center, most patients are referred from schools, clinics, and private practitioners. Fees are based on a sliding scale; third-party reimbursements are not accepted. Last year's operating budget was $800,000. The majority of revenues are from clients, although numerous churches and social service agencies sponsor individuals and families. The staff consists of six professionals and two clerks. Services are outlined in Table 9–17. An average of 300 patients are seen monthly. The director describes the patient population as white and middle to upper class, with more males than females. Most patients use private transportation to arrive at the clinic. No additional services are planned because the center staff believes they are adequately meeting the needs of the population. Rosemont residents queried were unaware of the existence of the counseling center, and no one knew of anyone having used the center, although all residents interviewed knew of several adolescent drug users.

The YMCA Youth Development Center borders Rosemont and offers a variety of educational and recreational programs. Adjacent to the "Y" is the

TABLE 9–17 ■ Services Offered at the Hampton Comprehensive Counseling Center

Service	Description
Diagnosis	Screening procedure for the mentally handicapped; recommends services required for clients' needs
Information and referral	Liaison teams coordinate services with state schools for the mentally retarded and state hospitals for the mentally ill
Counseling and therapy	Group and play therapy provided
Alcohol and drug abuse services	Counseling services
Psychiatric evaluation and medical services	Psychiatric department provides evaluations and medications for clients
Emergency service	Handles crisis calls 24 hours/day, 7 days/week
Education and consultation	Center staff works with other community groups, including schools, police, and social service agencies, to solve local problems

(Data from Hampton Comprehensive Counseling Center.)

YMCA Indo–Chinese Refugee Program, an agency that seeks to facilitate the resettlement of Asian immigrants. Major services include cultural orientation, job counseling and placement, and courses in English as a second language. The agency services have experienced a 200% increase in usage during the past 3 years. Presently, over 100 people use the facility daily. Although all four staff members are bilingual, this is too small a staff to meet the needs of the Vietnamese community—a large proportion of which lives in Rosemont. The staff believes the immediate need is for counseling and therapy programs for alcohol and drug abuse as well as teaching basic survival skills (for example, finding a job, housing, and medical care). The staff estimates that 40% to 50% of the Asians using their services are from Rosemont. Asian residents in Rosemont agree that the "Y" is responsive to their needs, but, when asked, they do acknowledge long waiting periods (sometimes weeks) for classes and counseling.

Clothing, Food, Shelter, and Basic Welfare Services

Most churches and synagogues in the area have a food pantry, and many can arrange emergency shelter and provide clothing and essential transportation services. People are usually helped on a walk-in basis, but sometimes the church is referred to a family or individual in need. In Hampton, a special organization, The Metropolitan Ministries, serves as an interfaith link between the religious communities of Hampton and community residents in need of social services. The Metropolitan Ministries acts to coordinate services, thereby avoiding duplication, and refers people to the program that can best meet their immediate needs.

TAKE NOTE

In most communities, churches must be contacted individually for a listing of services.

In addition to the churches and synagogues, numerous resale clothing shops are located in shopping areas close to Rosemont. Residents are very knowledgeable about available retail stores and actively promote preferred merchants.

The Jefferson County Welfare Department and the Hampton Welfare Department screen and process applicants for food stamps, housing subsidies, and financial aid checks. Each welfare department has a division of child protection that investigates reports of child abuse and neglect. The division provides casework services, foster home placement, and emergency shelter for women and children as well as parenting classes and child therapy groups. Welfare departments are financed by federal, state, and local tax revenues.

Special Services

The United Way lists 42 private and public-supported social service agencies located in Hampton or Jefferson County. The United Way directory includes identifying information for each agency, plus services and fees. Agencies on the roster include the Society to Prevent Blindness, American Lung Association, March of Dimes, Woman's Center, Paralyzed Veterans Association, and the International Rescue Committee.

TAKE NOTE

In your community assessment material, this would be an ideal location to append a list of social service agencies, along with identifying information (such as address, phone number, major services, and contact person). Brochures describing services, eligibility, and so on are useful to include as well.

Intracommunity Social Service Facilities

Two churches in Rosemont, South Main Methodist and Westpark Episcopal, have extensive social outreach programs, including preschool and day care services; benevolence funds for food, clothing, and shelter; and numerous support groups (for example, Parents Without Partners, Singles, and Solitaires). Westpark has a seniors' center open 8 AM to 6 PM daily. The seniors enjoy a variety of recreational and educational programs and a hot noon meal. In addition, volunteers are enlisted to assist with shopping and errands, minor home repairs, light housekeeping, and meals for fellow seniors who are permanently or temporarily incapacitated. Noticeably absent from Westpark were any support groups or programs directed at the large gay male population. When asked about this, staff members responded that "that problem does not exist in this community." South Main does offer a coffee klatch on Friday night and plans to offer additional services to the gay male population, although there is strong resistance from the older parishioners.

On the north side of CT 403 is Lambda Alcoholics Anonymous (AA), a program specifically for gay men and women, a group originally not allowed to join Alcoholic Anonymous. Lambda AA in CT 403 is an active group, with the present participation exceeding 200 people. All socioeconomic groups are represented in the meetings, and members take turns leading the support groups.

ECONOMICS

The economic subsystem includes the "wealth" of Rosemont—that is, the goods and services available to the community—as well as the costs and benefits of improving patterns of resource allocation. It should be evident that extra-community factors, such as the state of the US and world economies, affect in great measure the local economy. Nevertheless, intracommunity economic factors impinge on all other subsystems, so they must be included in the assessment. Table 9–18 lists the suggested areas for studying a community's economy, along with sources of the data. The census data can be used to summarize most of these economic indicators. Two key indicators of a community's economic "health" are the percentage of households below the poverty level and the unemployment rate.

Financial Characteristics of Households

The two census tracts that comprise the Rosemont community vary greatly in income characteristics. The census data show the median income for households in CT 402 to be $21,238, whereas in CT 403 it was $25,878. Table 9–19 lists the household income for the community and Hampton, comparing 1980 and 1990 figures.

Businesses

Several high-rise office buildings are located on the northern boundary of the area along the Audubon Parkway, including the National General Life Insurance complex of three towers, the new National Tower, the National

TABLE 9–18 ■ Economic Indicators and Sources of Information

Indicators	Source
Financial Characteristics	
Households	
Median household income	
% households below poverty level	
% households receiving public assistance	Census records
% households headed by females	
Monthly costs for owner-occupied households and renter-occupied households	
Individuals	
Per capital income	
% of persons who live in poverty	Census records
Labor Force Characteristics	
Employment Status	
General population (age 18+)	
% employed	
% unemployed	Chamber of commerce
% not participating in employment (retired)	Department of Labor
Special groups	Census records
% women working with children under age 6	
Occupational Categories and Number (%) of Persons Employed	
Managerial	
Technical	
Service	
Farming	Census records
Production	
Operator/laborer	
Union Activity and Membership	Local union(s) office

Service Corporation, and the Second Mortgage Corporation's building. Way-on-the-Bayou, a new office complex, is also being constructed at the corner of Way Drive and Buff's Bayou. These buildings all feature spacious landscaped grounds, modern architecture, and covered parking. Some of the residents of the area are employed in these offices; however, most employees, according to local residents, live outside of Rosemont.

The major area businesses include the Rose Milk Company factory at the northern edge of the area on Way Drive, the Sheet Metal Workers Union Local No. 54 at the corner of Way Drive and Jackson, and American Life Insurance Company on Green.

TABLE 9–19 ■ Income Indices for the Years 1980 and 1990 for CT 402, CT 403, and City of Hampton

Income Indices	CT 403		CT 402		Hampton	
	1980	1990	1980	1990	1980	1990
Median household income	$4,776	$21,238	$16,019	$25,878	$15,321	$29,378
% of all families with incomes below poverty level	53.7	18.3	5.4	13.3	7.1	14.2
% of female-headed households	49.2	NA	11.1	NA	15.4	12.7

NA = not available.
(Data from 1980 Census, Selected Characteristics; 1990 Census, Selected Characteristics.)

All of the main thoroughfares in the area are lined with locally owned businesses such as grocery stores, craft stores, antique shops, cleaners, and small restaurants (see the Physical Description section). In addition, these kinds of businesses are also dispersed throughout the area within the residential districts. The Hampton Lighting and Power Service Center is located near the northern edge of the area. Hampton's vehicle maintenance department and its street repair department are also located on West Pleasant in the northern part of the Rosemont area. There are also a considerable number of printing houses (probably the largest concentration in Hampton) on the northern edge of the area, as well as the broadcast studios of Channel 11 (KHAM-TV).

According to local residents, the economic impact of these businesses on the Rosemont area is minimal because most residents are employed outside of Rosemont, and, although they do patronize neighborhood convenience stores, they tend to shop for major purchases in other areas of the city. The residents also indicated that the vast majority of the businesses do not directly participate in the life of the community. Selected industries of the area are listed in Table 9–20.

TABLE 9–20 ■ Selected Industries in Rosemont

	CT 402		CT 403	
	Number	Total %	Number	Total %
Manufacturing	92	10	430	15
Wholesale and retail trade	450	48	1084	37
Professional and related services	387	42	1423	48
Total	929	100	2937	100

(Data from Census, Selected Characteristics.)

TABLE 9–21 ■ Rosemont Labor Force	CT 402	CT 403	Hampton
Persons 16 and over	4,580	6,470	1,189,136
Labor force	1,825	5,472	850,389
Percentage of persons 16 and over	39.8	85.4	71.5

(Data from Census of Population and Housing.)

When there are major businesses within a community that employ a substantial number of community residents, a thorough assessment is required. For an excellent guide to assess an occupational setting, see the Serafini (1976) article listed in the suggested readings at the end of this chapter.

Labor Force

Employment Status

As mentioned earlier, the unemployment rate is a key indicator of the economic "health" of the community. The labor force of a community is comprised of people 16 years of age and over. Table 9–21 summarizes key data relating to the workforce of the Rosemont community. The majority of workers are categorized under "private wage and salary," as shown in Table 9–22.

Occupation

General occupational categories are included in the census. Table 9–23 lists the occupations of the citizens of Rosemont.

TABLE 9–22 ■ Class of Workers, Rosemont	CT 402		CT 403	
	Number	Total %	Number	Total %
Private wage and salary	1219	67	4168	76
Government	326	18	664	12
Local government	238	13	307	6
Self-employed	42	2	333	6
Total	1825	100	5472	100

(Data from Census of Population and Housing.)

TABLE 9–23 ■ Occupations, Rosemont				
	CT 402		CT 403	
	Number	Total %	Number	Total %
Managerial and professional specialty	117	7.1	2238	42.1
Technical, sales, administrative support	198	12.1	1813	34.1
Service	724	44.2	560	10.5
Farming	28	1.7	11	0.2
Precision production	186	11.3	463	8.7
Operators, fabricators, laborers	387	23.6	230	4.3
Total	1640	100	5315	100

(Data from Census of Population and Housing.)

TAKE NOTE

Census occupational categories are quite general. To determine more precisely what sort of work is incorporated in a category, it is necessary to ask those who do the job or to look up the category in the Department of Labor publications.

Differences between the two census tracts that comprise Rosemont are clearly seen in the occupational makeup of the community. Whereas almost half of the workers in CT 402 are categorized under "service," a similar percentage of workers in CT 403 are classified under "managerial and professional specialty."

SAFETY AND TRANSPORTATION

Table 9–24 lists the major components of safety and transportation that affect the community.

Protection Services

Fire, police, and sanitation services are provided by the city of Hampton. Rosemont residents pay for these services through their city taxes. Therefore, these services are extracommunity, located outside the community of Rosemont.

TABLE 9-24 ■ Safety and Transportation

Indicators	Sources of Information
Safety	
Protection services	Planning office (city, county, and state)
Fire	Fire department (local)
Police	Police department (city and county)
Sanitation	
Waste sources and treatment	Waste and water treatment plants
Solid waste	
Air quality	Air control board (state, regional, and local offices)
Transportation	
Private	
Transportation sources	Census data: Population and housing characteristics
Number of persons with a transportation disability	
Public	
Bus service (routes, schedules, and fares)	Local and city transportation authorities
Roads (number and condition; primary, secondary and farm-to-market roads)	State highway department
Interstate highways	
Freeway system	
Air service (private and publicly owned)	Local airports (*Note:* Local airports are frequently owned and operated by city government.)
Rail service	In the United States, Amtrak is the primary source of intercity rail transportation

Fire Protection

The fire department and MEAS are combined in Hampton. (For a description of the MEAS, see the Health and Social Services section.) The fire station serving Rosemont maintains two fire trucks, one air boat (for evacuations during flooding), and 20 personnel. Firemen must complete 335 hours of basic certification courses. The fire captain reports a response time of less than 10 minutes. During the 90 days before the assessment, the station responded to 45 fires. This compares to 39 responses during the same period of the previous year. Forty responses were to homes—the major culprit being grease fires that started in the kitchen. Other leading causes of fires include lighted cigarettes and children playing with matches. In addition to responding to fires, personnel perform safety checks of homes; teach fire prevention classes to school and community groups; and distribute window stickers that specify the location of children, elderly citizens, and pets for emergency alert during a fire.

Police Protection

The police department serving Rosemont has a staff of 27 full-time employees, including 21 police officers and 6 civilians (4 dispatchers and 2 record clerks). Equipment includes five marked and four unmarked patrol cars, two motorcycles, and a complete computerized data storage and retrieval system. This station has one holding cell where people are detained until they can be transported to the Hampton Jail. According to the dispatcher, response time to Rosemont is 4 to 6 minutes. Crime statistics for CT 402 and CT 403 are presented in Table 9–25.

The most frequent crimes are burglaries and thefts, which the police captain believes are committed mainly by nonresidents of Rosemont. Speeding and driving while intoxicated (DWI) are also frequent crimes in Rosemont, although after the addition of two motorcycle police officers 2 years ago, the number of traffic accidents has decreased by 38%. The police department offers the following services to Rosemont residents:

- Housewatch—When residents are out of town, the police will check their house three times a day for up to 30 days.
- Identification—The police department loans an engraver to citizens who wish to engrave personal belongings. The department also provides household possessions registration and pamphlets on how to protect one's home from burglary.

TABLE 9–25 ■ Crime Statistics for CT 402 and CT 403

	1996		1997		1998		1999	
	CT 402	CT 403	CT 402	CT 403	CT 402	CT 403	CT 402	CT 403
Murder	5	3	7	7	8	6	10	3
Rape	24	19	22	18	27	11	34	17
Robbery	196	100	204	104	252	165	328	186
Aggravated assault	40	17	47	27	58	27	94	29
Burglary	263	288	274	279	295	321	345	339
Theft	403	462	423	371	397	384	384	363
Vehicle theft	103	144	113	214	112	232	109	327
Total	1034	1033	1090	1020	1149	1146	1304	1264

(Data from City of Hampton Police Department.)

- Fingerprinting—Fingerprinting is done and a record of the prints is provided to the person for personal identification as well as for immigration requirements. The police department is presently pursuing a special project, a citywide campaign to fingerprint all children and adolescents. A copy of the fingerprint record is given to parents, and the original remains with the police. After several weeks of radio and TV announcements, police personnel are now present at local shopping centers every weekend to explain and complete the fingerprinting process. This special project is in response to citizen concern and requests for police assistance in locating an increasing number of missing children.
- Animal Protection Officer—The City of Hampton has a leash and fence law for dogs. The animal protection officer picks up stray animals and detains them in the city kennel until the owner or an adopter can be found.
- Public Education—Crime prevention programs are offered to community and school groups.

Residents of Rosemont repeatedly voiced concern about their personal safety. Elderly citizens expressed fear of being mugged and related stories of friends who have been harassed and robbed during the day as they walked to and from local stores. (One grocery store owner reported that he has stopped cashing Social Security checks because so many patrons had been mugged after leaving his store.) The feeling of being a prisoner in one's own home was repeatedly expressed, as were questions regarding what people could do to protect themselves.

Gay men described experiences of perceived harassment by police as well as incidences of marked delay (up to 30 minutes) in police response time to requests for help. Residents reported that brawls, quarrels, and physical violence are becoming commonplace in Rosemont. The citizens are concerned for themselves and others; they want a safe place to live.

Sanitation

Water Sources and Treatment

The terrain of Rosemont is flat with minimal changes in elevation. Stagnant pools of water are common—a situation that promotes mosquito populations during the warm months. Drainage is toward the northeast and into Buff's Bayou, the only open stream in Rosemont. All storm water and sewage are gathered into Hampton's sewage system. There is no separate system for storm water disposal. As a result, raw sewage backs up during heavy rains, and residents complain of the smell and problems associated with toilets that cannot be flushed.

Sewage from Rosemont is treated at the 5th Street Plant. A sewage moratorium exists for Rosemont owing to overcapacity at the 5th Street Plant. Consequently, only single-family dwellings can be built on plotted lots. Builders requesting permits for multifamily dwellings are given the option of delaying building indefinitely or being assessed a fee based on projected occupancy of their building and the associated gallons of sewage that will be produced. The assessed fee is used to increase the capacity of the treatment plant. However, even if the assessed fee option is chosen, it may be 3 to 4 years before the permit is issued.

Potable (drinking) water for Rosemont comes from Lake Hampton, located 20 miles north of the city. Residents are concerned about possible contamination of the drinking water with lead and other heavy metals. There is no routine testing of the drinking water except to meet state health department requirements for chlorine content. Fluoride is not added to Rosemont's drinking water, and it is not present naturally.

Solid Waste

Garbage is collected twice weekly; residents state that the service and frequency are adequate. The major complaint is that illegal dumping of large items, such as refrigerators, stoves, and so forth, has increased, and, despite numerous calls to proper authorities, the trash is not cleaned up with any regularity. Parents are concerned that children attracted by abandoned machinery and appliances may be hurt as they explore. In addition, inoperable automobiles are abandoned in parking spaces on the streets, and months can pass before the cars are removed by the city.

Air Quality

The Federal Air Quality Act of 1967 provided for the establishment of air-quality control regions. Regional offices maintain an inventory of air-pollution sources and monitor air status. In similar fashion, individual states formed advisory boards that developed air-quality standards and long-range air-quality programs. Local air-monitoring stations sample and record information levels on such pollutants as ozone, carbon monoxide, sulfur dioxide, and nitrogen dioxide. In addition, some 30 to 40 suspended particles in the air (solids) are measured and recorded, as are certain gaseous substances (for example, ammonia).

To assess the air quality of Rosemont, the Air Control Board was contacted; its recent reports document a rise in air pollution, which is attributed to an increase in industrial growth and a high population density. Some 25 miles east of Rosemont is a large industrial complex, and, although the daily emissions from the industries are within acceptable limits, certain wind and temperature patterns act to compound emissions. This causes a visible yellow haze to form that shrouds Rosemont and surrounding communities many days of the year. Area residents complain of eye irritation and increased frequency of respiratory conditions. The chemical reactions that lead to the haze and the contribution of automotive and industrial emissions, as well as potential health effects associated with the haze, are unknowns presently being researched.

TAKE NOTE

Air pollution is a frequently used term; it means the presence of one or more contaminants in such concentration and of such duration that they may adversely affect human health, animal life, vegetation, or property.

Despite the pollution increase and industrial growth, there has been no significant increase in the amount of pollutants introduced into the atmosphere surrounding Rosemont. This is attributed to compliance of industries with the Air Control Board regulations and the permit system for new industries. Citizens can contest industry construction permits and through this process provide a forum for public opinion and objections that regulation boards take into consideration during the permit decision-making process. Citizens are also entitled to complain to the board regarding a specific industry's emissions; the board will then investigate and file a report.

During the past year, Rosemont has experienced three air stagnation advisories. Because the pollution concentration is greater than usual, people with respiratory conditions such as bronchitis and emphysema are advised to remain indoors and limit outside activities until the air stagnation clears.

TAKE NOTE

Air stagnation occurs when a layer of cool air is trapped by a layer of warmer air above it; the bottom air cannot rise and pollutants cannot be dispersed.

The board believes citizens are ill informed regarding the meaning of and the appropriate actions that should be taken during air stagnation advisories as well as each citizen's responsibility in minimizing pollution. For example, citizens seem unaware that transportation sources (such as automobiles and buses), not industry, are the major contributors of air pollution problems and that a citizen who burns leaves or trash is releasing tiny particles of matter into the air that can irritate the eyes, nose, and lungs. To promote public awareness and understanding, the local office makes presentations to organizations, schools, and citizen groups. Numerous public television and radio programs were planned for the year after the assessment.

Transportation

Private

The primary means of transportation in Rosemont include walking, bicycle riding, automobiles, Hampton city buses, Hampton city vans (special transportation for the elderly and handicapped), and school buses.

The major source of private transportation is the automobile. Table 9–26 presents the types of transportation used to commute to work, and Table 9–27 indicates the number of people 16 years of age or older who have a transportation disability. According to the census data, mean travel time to work for Rosemont residents is 17.7 minutes as compared to 26.6 minutes for Hampton residents.

Public

The major source of public transportation within Rosemont and surrounding communities is the Hampton bus system. The city provides east–west bus service at half-hour intervals during the day on Pecan Drive and Live Oak Boulevard. The same service is provided on north–south routes for Way Drive, Rosemont Boulevard, and Hampton Street. For people who qualify (such as the elderly and/or handicapped), the bus company provides door-to-door service from the person's home to essential services such as food shopping or medical care visits. The cost of this service varies from $0.50 to $1.00 per trip, according to geographic area. Although all users agree the service is reliable, it is only available Monday through Friday, 8:30 AM to 5:00 PM, and reservations are

TABLE 9–26 ■ Transportation Sources to Work That Are Used by Residents of CT 402 and CT 403

	CT 402		CT 403	
	Number	Total %	Number	Total %
Drive alone	1351	42.8	3279	63.8
Carpool	749	23.7	808	15.7
Public transportation	721	22.8	567	11
Walk	231	7.3	300	5.8
Other means	79	2.5	130	2.5
Work at home	27	0.9	58	1.2
Total	3158	100	5142	100

(Data from Census of Population and Housing.)

TABLE 9–27 ■ Noninstitutionalized Persons 16 Years of Age or Older by Transportation Disability Status for CT 402 and CT 403

	With Disability		Without Disability		Total	
	Number	Total %	Number	Total %	Number	Total %
Age 16–64						
CT 402	221	5.9	3495	94.1	3716	100
CT 403	15	0.3	5908	99.7	5923	100
Age 65 and Over						
CT 402	197	21.3	728	78.7	925	100
CT 403	55	10.5	469	89.5	524	100

(Data from Census of Population and Housing.)

required several days in advance—a requirement that is impossible to meet in situations such as during acute illnesses.

Roads

Jefferson County (of which Rosemont is a part) has adequate primary, secondary, and farm-to-market roads. In addition, several miles of a freeway system circle Hampton. Two major interstate highways transect Hampton, and the state highway department has budgeted $2 billion for highway construction and maintenance for Jefferson County over the next 20 years. Recently, the residents of Jefferson County voted for an additional tax devoted entirely to improving intracounty transportation. Rosemont residents complain of congested freeways and damaged roads that go without repair for months. The need was expressed for a road system that efficiently handles local traffic.

Air Service

Jefferson County has four small, privately owned airports. The City of Hampton owns and operates two airports; both provide national and international service.

Rail Service

Amtrak connects Hampton to other major cities in the state as well as to other states. There are no private or public commuter rail services within Jefferson County or Hampton.

POLITICS AND GOVERNMENT

Rosemont falls within the city limits of Hampton, which has a mayor-council form of government. There are 14 council members (5 at-large), one of whom represents Rosemont and nearby communities. Each serves a 2-year term. The city council meets at City Hall on the first Tuesday of each month. The meetings are open to the public, and Rosemont residents often attend.

The city council and mayor comprise the policy-making body as well as the administrative head of Hampton. Their duties include the following: maintaining competent staff to operate all city services (the health department and police, for instance), passing ordinances, and appropriating funds to carry out policies.

The councilman for District Three, which includes Rosemont, is James Browning. Councilman Browning was elected by a wide margin of votes and has been popular with the Rosemont community because he has spearheaded the fight against sexually oriented businesses (the "SOB Fight," as it is popularly called). This issue has not been settled, and the citizens are supporting Councilman Browning's reelection so he may continue the fight.

The active participation in the Hampton council of Councilman Browning is only one indicator of Rosemont's politics. There are several politically oriented organizations and civic clubs in the area, all of which seek to improve the quality of life in Rosemont and help to support intercommunity activities.

A brief synopsis of several organizations that are politically active in Rosemont is presented in Table 9–28. (Contact person, address, and phone number should be included in such lists but have been omitted from this description.)

Several other groups in the community are less visible and active unless an issue of particular interest becomes "hot." For instance, many voluntary agencies, such as the American Lung Association—Hampton Chapter, are located in the community and can be called on to assist specific campaigns (for example, smoking-prevention programs in the schools or antipollution campaigns aimed toward extracommunity sources). The Community Services Directory lists all such organizations both by interest (heart, lung, crime, and so on) and general area (Rosemont groups can usually be found under "Southwest, near downtown").

Political activism is evident throughout Rosemont: During election years, there are campaign posters everywhere; talk at gathering places (barbershops, grocery stores, bars) inevitably turns to politics; and numerous rallies are held in support of candidates or issues. In Rosemont, there appear to be two major political factions. Voting records show CT 403 residents to be more liberal than

TABLE 9–28 ■ Organizations Politically Active in Rosemont	
Organization	**Description**
Neartown Business Alliance (Founded 1949)	Owners of businesses in the area meet monthly and work to promote the area and its businesses. The alliance contributes to campaigns of supporters of Rosemont.
Gay Political Caucus (Founded 1964)	This is a very active and visible group. It works to influence elections through voter registration, campaign work, and education. It has been credited with the election or defeat of certain candidates. Membership is open to all interested in community improvement. It meets on third Tuesday, 7:00 PM.
Rosemont Firehouse (Founded 1973)	This is a coordination and referral group; it operates a 24-hour crisis hotline. It is sponsored by donations from most of the area's churches as well as the civic groups, and most of the workers are community volunteers.
Rosemont Watch (Founded 1978)	The Watch works to prevent crime in the area through education and visible activities such as "Block Awareness Week." It coordinates activities with the Hampton City Police. All citizens are encouraged to become involved. It meets monthly.
Seniors for a Safe Community (Founded 1980)	Comprised primarily of retired people (but open to all interested residents), this group was formed to address the problem of the mugging or robbing of senior citizens, especially on the days when Social Security checks arrived. The original small group has expanded, as have their goals, so that now they are actively involved in promoting a better quality of life for all in the community (with a special emphasis on the elderly). This group is active in the "SOB Fight" and also works closely with Rosemont Watch.

residents in CT 402. This may reflect the fact that CT 403 is comprised of more affluent, younger, and professional residents than is CT 402.

COMMUNICATION

Communication may be formal or informal. Formal communication usually originates outside the community (extracommunity) as opposed to informal communication, which almost always originates and is disseminated within the community. Salient components of formal and informal communication, as well as sources of data, are presented in Table 9–29.

Formal Communication

Hampton has one major newspaper, *The Hampton Herald*. Additional daily newspapers include a business journal, *Current Issues*; a black-oriented

TABLE 9–29 ■ Communications	
Components	**Sources of Information**
Formal	
Newspaper (number, circulation, frequency, and scope of news)	Chamber of commerce
	Newspaper office
Radio and television (number of stations, commercial versus educational, and audience)	Telephone company
	Yellow Pages
Postal service	Telephone book
Telephone status (number of residents with service)	Census data on phone use
Informal	
Sources: bulletin boards; posters; hand-delivered flyers; and church, civic, and school newsletters	Learning about the community on foot
	Talking to residents
Dissemination (How do people receive information?)	Survey
Word of mouth	
Mail	
Radio, television	

paper, *Progress*; one Spanish-language paper, *La Prensa*; and a Vietnamese tabloid. Hampton has 12 AM radio stations and 10 FM stations, 6 commercial TV stations, and 1 educational network. Cable television is available to Rosemont residents on a monthly subscription basis. Residents receive home mail delivery.

Informal Communication

Bulletin boards and posters dot community and municipal buildings in Rosemont. Posters are placed on trees and tacked to buildings throughout the community, and a rainbow of flyers can be seen tucked into fence and door crevices. Radio and television announcements herald forthcoming events and offer open forums on community issues. The Rosemont Civic Association publishes a bimonthly four-page newsletter to notify residents of upcoming meetings and social activities. Polls and surveys are a regular feature of the newsletter, which is distributed free to all residents.

Key informants within Rosemont include the Civic Association secretary, local ministers, and fire and police personnel as well as community civic board members. People can be seen "chatting" throughout Rosemont, and, when asked how information is received, they mention all of the above formal and informal sources.

EDUCATION

The general educational status of a community can be summarized using census data. Census information lists the number of residents attending schools, years of schooling completed, and percentage of residents who speak English. To supplement this broad assessment, information is needed about major educational sources (for example, schools, colleges, and libraries) located inside the community. Table 9–30 is a suggested guide for assessing a community's educational sources.

· · · · · · · · ·
TAKE NOTE

· · · · · · · · · · · ·

It is sometimes difficult to decide which educational sources to include in the assessment. Community usage is probably the single most important indicator. Primary and secondary schools attended by the majority of youngsters in a community, regardless of intra- or extracommunity location, are major educational sources and require a thorough assessment, whereas schools composed primarily of students from outside the community do not require such an extensive appraisal.

TABLE 9–30 ■ Education	
Components	**Sources of Information**
Educational Status	
Years of school completed	Census data—Social characteristics section
School enrollment by type of school	Census data—Social characteristics section
Language spoken	Census data—Social characteristics section
Educational Sources	
Intracommunity or extracommunity (collect data for each facility)	Local board of education
Services (educational, recreational, communication, and health)	School administrator (such as the principal or director) and school nurse
Resources (personnel, space, budget, and record system)	School administrator
Characteristics of users (geographic distribution and demographic profile)	Teachers and staff
Adequacy, accessibility, and acceptability of education to students and staff	Students and staff

Educational Status

Table 9–31 presents the years of schooling completed by adults in CT 402 and CT 403. In a similar format, Table 9–32 lists school enrollment by type of school, and Table 9–33 presents the number and percentage of community residents who speak English.

Educational Sources

Intracommunity—Temple Elementary School

Temple Elementary School is located on the corner of Pecan Drive and Magnolia Drive, close to the center of CT 402. Asphalt lots bound three sides of Temple; two are used for vehicle parking, and one is for play. A small patch of grass persists on the remaining side, a fenced-in area that contains several large trees, a swing set, and three teeter-totters. Several broken windows were seen, and no graffiti was noted. Temple is in its 64th year of continuous operation teaching grades kindergarten to eighth. Present enrollment is 924; 42% of the students are black, 33% are Asian, 18% are Hispanic, and 5% are white. Most of the children live in Rosemont and either walk to school or ride the school bus (provided for children living further than 2 miles from Temple).

TABLE 9–31 ■ Years of School Completed for CT 402, CT 403, and City of Hampton

	CT 402	CT 403	Hampton
Persons 25 years and over	3,459	4,948	888,269
Elementary			
0 to 4 years	611	26	41,695
5 to 7 years	665	164	66,775
8 years	409	101	37,373
High school			
1 to 3 years	800	278	136,179
4 years	661	914	240,320
College			
1 to 3 years	181	1,173	160,999
4 or more years	132	2,292	204,928
% high school graduates	28.2	88.5	68.3

TABLE 9–32 ■ School Enrollment and Type of School for CT 402, CT 403, and City of Hampton

	CT 402	CT 403	Hampton
Type of school			
Public nursery school	94	44	20,735
Private nursery school	77	44	15,427
Public kindergarten	194	14	21,863
Private kindergarten	25	14	4,833
Public elementary (1 to 8 yr)	1,258	186	198,367
Private elementary (1 to 8 yr)	10	136	18,440
Public high school (1 to 4 yr)	482	92	94,099
Private high school (1 to 4 yr)	12	25	7,154
College	92	922	78,472
Total enrolled in schools (age 3 years and over)	2,120	1,258	413,536

(Data from Census of Population and Housing.)

As part of the Hampton School District (HSD), Temple receives funding from the district revenues obtained from local property taxes, state coffers, and the federal budget. State monies to HSD are based on average daily attendance of students at each school. Most policies affecting Temple are formed and enforced by the HSD Board. The board is composed of eight nonsalaried people, each elected from one of eight regions in the school district. Each term of office is 4 years. Board member Jane Roberts represents Rosemont; at the time of assessment, she was in the second year of her 4-year term. Responsibilities of the HSD board include prescribing qualifications of employees, establishing salary schedules, setting goals and objectives for the district, establishing the policies to implement the goals and objectives, and evaluating the performance

TABLE 9–33 ■ Ability to Speak English for CT 402, CT 403, and City of Hampton

	Percentage Who Speak English Poorly or Not at All	
	Age 5–17	Age 18 Years and Over
CT 402	75.9	73.8
CT 403	11	19.3
Hampton	21.4	26.2

(Data from Census of Population and Housing.)

of the district in relationship to adopted goals and objectives. The General Superintendent is the administrative head of the board and is salaried and recruited by the Board.

PRINCIPAL

Temple's principal cited truancy and the related problem of academic failure as the school's major problems. According to office records, some 6% to 8% of the student body is absent each day, and most of those absent are not ill. Compounding the problem is the fact that many parents do not have telephones. As a result, it is not uncommon for a youngster to be absent for 2 or 3 days before parental contact is made. (In most cases, it is found that the parent assumed the child was in school.) The principal believed that truancy is most common among seventh and eighth graders, especially among Hispanic boys.

Regarding bilingual education for non–English-speaking students, the principal believes that all classes should be in English and that the presence of bilingual education at Temple only slows the progress of the children who are learning English. There are two bilingual teachers at Temple; they reported that they have a list of over 100 youngsters who have requested and have been assessed as needing the bilingual program.

TEACHERS

Teachers repeatedly stated the need for improved communication with parents. They believe that parents need to have current information about their child's learning needs and school performance as well as a knowledge of specific techniques for fostering academic achievement. (School policy allows for two 20-minute parent–teacher conferences yearly—a time allotment that was rated as extremely inadequate by the teachers.) The teachers reported that 22% of the student body at Temple failed last year. Major impediments to learning were listed as poor English-speaking skills and understanding of English, stressful home environments, and inadequate adult supervision at home. Teachers felt overwhelmed and frustrated; the average employment stay at Temple is 2 years.

SCHOOL NURSE

The school nurse at Temple is present 2 days a week; she is at West Hampton High the remaining 3 days. A review of the daily clinic register for the preceding 6 weeks noted a clinic attendance of 141; the majority (72%) of those visiting suffered from stomachache or headache. Although none of the stomach ailments required early dismissal, 60% of the headaches were associated with fever and necessitated early dismissal from school. Remaining complaints were sore throats and minor cuts or falls. All children were screened biannually for vision and hearing problems. The nurse recognized the need for yearly screening but said she lacked the necessary time. She stated that if school policy would permit the recruitment and training of a parent volunteer(s), then yearly screening would be feasible. In addition to vision and hearing testing, all children are screened for head lice twice a year; children found to be infected are dismissed from school and are not readmitted until they have been successfully treated.

Some 62% of the youngsters participate in the free lunch program. The nurse expressed concern that several children who appear undernourished (displaying, for example, low weight for height and small arm circumference for age) do not qualify for the lunch program, whereas others who appear to be well nourished do qualify. Eligibility is based on family size and income.

Major health problems as described by the nurse include lack of hygiene (children frequently come to school dirty and inadequately clothed for cold weather); dental caries; high (30% to 40%) annual incidence head lice, especially in primary grades (kindergarten, first grade, and second grade); incomplete immunization status (92% of the youngsters have up-to-date immunizations); and lack of parent follow-through for needed medical care and treatment during illnesses.

To assess dental status, the nurse performed oral assessment of children who came to the clinic during one 4-week period. She found that 62% of the children have discolored areas or cavities in the pits of their teeth or between teeth. Most of the youngsters stated they had never been to a dentist, and many reported frequent tooth pain and difficulty chewing.

The nurse does not do any health teaching in the classroom because school policy mandates that the nurse be present in the clinic at all times. The ruling causes considerable frustration because the nurse's participation in the teaching and promotion of health habits is restricted to one-to-one clinic encounters (a time when the child is ill and not receptive to learning). When asked about staff and teacher usage of the clinic, the nurse discussed at length the need for health information expressed by both teachers and staff. Questions regarding exercise, stress, and diet modifications are common. The nurse would like to assess and identify specific health needs of staff and teachers.

COMMUNITY SERVICE

As a community service, Temple sponsors scout troops and basketball and softball teams and provides a meeting place for several newly formed church and community action groups. In addition, Monday through Thursday nights,

Temple houses extension courses from Hampton Community College. A full range of subjects is offered, including academic, vocational, and enrichment courses. Present enrollment exceeds 1200, an increase of 22% from the previous year.

All Rosemont residents were familiar with Temple Elementary; most had children who attended Temple, or else they themselves had attended Temple as youngsters. Residents felt that Temple was a community landmark and symbol of unity that links one generation to the next. The primary complaint, repeated by several families, was a perceived insensitivity of Temple's staff and teachers to ethnic and racial differences and needs. For example, all school notices are written in English, and all programs offered by the Parent Teachers Organization (PTO) are presented in English. Both Asian and Hispanic parents have brought specific concerns and needs to the staff and teachers at Temple but have repeatedly been told that all parental requests must come from appropriate PTO committees—an organization that seems alien to many Asian and Hispanic parents.

Day Care

One day care center is located in CT 402—the Busybee Nursery. There are no day care facilities in CT 403. Housed in a renovated building, Busybee accepts children aged 2 to 5 years. Some 60 youngsters are cared for by five staff members, and 43 children (primarily toddlers) are on the waiting list. The center is licensed by the state. Rosemont residents repeatedly lamented the lack of day care facilities. Many parents felt forced to leave their young children with other mothers or teenagers who have dropped out of school. Several mothers reported leaving their children daily with a babysitter who cares for from 8 to 10 youngsters.

Library

The Rosemont library is conveniently located adjacent to the main shopping district and offers a variety of adult, teen, and youth book programs, films, and special educational activities. Notices of all programs are published in the Rosemont Civic Association newsletter and posted on local bulletin boards.

Extracommunity

High school students from Rosemont attend Central Hampton High, a complex that houses 4800 students and is located 8 miles from Rosemont. Concerned about truancy and grade failure, Central Hampton began a "Failproof" program 2 years ago. Some 82% of students and their parents have participated. As a result, school scores on state and national proficiency tests have improved and truancy has decreased. The principal described numerous community outreach services offered by the school, including recreational programs in the evening and on the weekends, as well as a full complement of adult education courses.

The nurse at Central Hampton is present 5 days a week. The majority of visits to the clinic (an average of 30 daily) involve allergy-related complaints, gastrointestinal upsets, and minor sprains or strains that occur during physical exercise class. Because of HSD policies, the school nurse is also prohibited from offering health education in the classroom.

The nurse's major concern is the increased number of teenage pregnancies and the HSD Board's decision of 2 years ago not to permit sex education information in the classroom. Classes in sexuality, sexually transmitted disease, contraception, and decision making in the area of sexual activity had been offered at all high schools in Hampton before the new ruling. The nurse does not know the sequence of events that resulted in the sex education decision. A second major concern is the increased use of alcohol among students. A drug awareness curriculum was prepared by the state board of education and will be implemented during the next semester as part of the biology courses' content.

Numerous private preschool and grade schools are available in Hampton, and some are used by the residents of Rosemont, especially by people in CT 403. Some 20 colleges and universities are located in Hampton and Jefferson County; most offer a variety of general education and specialty training programs. One unique aspect of the area's educational resources is Hampton Community College, a junior college that provides classes in 21 public schools in Hampton and Jefferson County. (Temple Elementary is one of these campuses.) Numerous residents state that they prefer Hampton Community College to other area resources because of its convenient locations, low tuition, and employment-oriented approach to education.

RECREATION

The recreation facilities within and adjacent to Rosemont are listed in Table 9–34 and pictured in Figure 9–3. With the exception of the schoolyards, there is very little recreational area for children and almost none for adults and teenagers. Although there are funds in the budget of the Hampton Parks and Recreation Department for the acquisition of property, there are no plans for any development in the Rosemont area. However, the city has recently begun

TABLE 9–34 ■ Recreational Facilities in Rosemont and Adjacent Areas

	Acreage	Location	Facilities
San Juan	2.6	1650 Pleasant	Shelter building, playground equipment, softball field, and baseball field
Richards	1	1414 Redbud	Shelter building, playground equipment, picnic area, and basketball court (swimming pool recently filled in)
Applehurst	1.9	600 Water Oak	Recreation center, rest room, playground equipment, picnic area, tennis, basketball, and volleyball courts
Jeckle Park	0.08	1500 Maple	None
Buff's Bayou	?	"Greens" along the bayou	Park benches and jogging/bicycle trail

(Data from City of Hampton, Parks and Recreation Department, interview with JB [Director], May 1994.)

an improvement program along the banks of Buff's Bayou to create a "River Walk" similar to those in other cities with rivers. It will be several years before the project is completed.

The Rosemont Sports Association, according to its president, provides "quality organized recreation opportunities" for the local community. Programs consist of teams for winter bowling, spring bowling, summer bowling, softball, flag football, tennis, and so forth. The Rosemont Sports Association, however, is open only to members who pay a fee of $20 per year.

Churches of Rosemont (two were visited—see the Social Services section) offer a wide variety of activities for all ages. Exercise classes, craft classes, Mother's Day Out, preschool classes, senior citizens' groups, and many other programs are available to church members. Although other community residents are welcome to take advantage of these activities, the people interviewed at the churches reported that their participants are almost all church members.

Several residents spoke of an area along the northern bank of Buff's Bayou (just east of Way Drive) that is used as a gathering place by residents who live nearby. Families take their children there on summer evenings so parents can visit while the children play. The only facilities at this area are benches that have been placed along the grassy area.

A bicycle/jogging trail follows the bayou for several miles and is popular with the health-conscious residents who use it frequently, especially in the early morning and late evening hours. Some people have expressed fear of being mugged while using this trail, but there have been no official reports of crime in this area over the past year. The trail and all the land along the bayou are maintained by the city of Hampton.

The area residents of the east side tend to congregate for recreation on sidewalks and in neighborhood bars. The one playground in the area, other than the one at Temple Elementary, is located adjacent to the Audubon Parkway Village (the low-rent housing complex), and it is used exclusively by the residents of that complex. The playground equipment is in very poor repair, and there is virtually no grass left in the area. The Parks and Recreation Department has no plans to upgrade or replace the equipment or to replant the grass.

There is one movie theater and one theater for stage production in Rosemont, but movie theaters are accessible and near almost all areas surrounding the community. Other forms of evening entertainment are reflected in the numerous bars and restaurants that feature live music (as was mentioned in the physical examination of the community).

Extracommunity recreational facilities abound. A large city park that includes museums, a zoo, a bandshell, and picnic areas is less than a mile to the south of Rosemont. Another city park in downtown Hampton, called Serenity Park, is less than a mile to the northeast.

Virtually every major league sport has a team in Hampton. The sports arenas are some distance from the area, but there is adequate bus service to them.

An abundance of music and theater is available to those who can afford it. Hampton has a symphony orchestra, a ballet, both grand and light opera, and a legitimate stage company, to name a few options. In addition, water activities, such as boating and fishing, are as close as 30 miles away. According to several residents of Audubon Parkway Village, a special day out includes crabbing along the bay—which is often a successful endeavor to fill the dinner pot as well as provide fun for the whole family.

SUMMARY

The community assessment is never complete; however, we must pause at some point. Because we have addressed all parts of the model, this is where we will stop. A description of each community subsystem has been recorded. Note that at every step of the assessment, people in the community were included. Not only did we interview the "professionals" (for example, school nurses, principal, police chief, and so on), but clients of the subsystems were also included (parents, shoppers, patients, and people on the street). The assessment, like all steps in the process, is carried out in partnership with the community. The next step is analysis, a process that synthesizes the assessment information and derives from it diagnoses specific to the community.

Crucial to community assessment is a model, or map, to direct and guide that process. The model (community assessment wheel) shown in Figure 9–1 provided a framework, and the tool, "Learning About the Community on Foot" (see Table 9–1), guided the assessment of Rosemont. In the Suggested Readings list, several other approaches to community assessment are presented. As you are aware, there are other models you may wish to consider as you continue your practice of community health assessment.

SUGGESTED READINGS

Barton, J.A., Smith, M.C., Brown, N.J., & Supples, J.M. (1993). Methodological issues in a team approach to community health needs assessment. *Nursing Outlook, 41*(6), 253–261.

Bennett, E.J. (1993). Health needs assessment of a rural county: Impact evaluation of a student project. *Family & Community Health, 16*(1), 28–35.

Gerberich, S.S., Stearns, S.J., & Dowd, T. (1995). A critical skill for the future: Community assessment. *Journal of Community Health Nursing, 12*(4), 239–250.

Gregor, S. & Galazka, S.S. (1990). The use of key informant networks in assessment of community health. *Family Medicine, 22*(2), 118–121.

Hancock, T. & Minkler, M. (1997). Community health assessment or healthy community assessment: Whose community? Whose health? Whose assessment? In Minkler, M. (Ed.), *Community organizing and community building for health* (pp. 139–156). New Brunswick, NJ: Rutgers University Press.

Keppel, K.G. & Freedman, M.A. (1995). What is assessment? *Journal of Public Health Management, 1*(2), 1–7.

Kretzman, J.P. & McKnight, J.L. (1993). *Building communities from the inside out: A path toward finding and mobilizing a community's assets.* Chicago, IL: ACTA Publications.

Lindell, D.H. (1997). Community assessment for the home health nurse. *Home Healthcare Nurse, 15*(1), 618–626.

Palfrey, J.S. (1994). *Community child health: An action plan for today.* Westport, CT: Praeger.

Ruth, J., Eliason, K., & Schultz, P.R. (1992). Community assessment: A process of learning. *Journal of Nursing Education, 31*(4), 181–183.

Schultz, P.R. & Magilvy, J.K. (1988). Assessing community health needs of elderly populations: Comparisons of three strategies. *Journal of Advanced Nursing, 13,* 193–202.

Serafini, P. (1976). Nursing assessment in industry: A model. *American Journal of Public Health, 66*(8), 755–760.

Texas Department of Health. (1998). *Community assessment guidelines.* (Bureau of Community Oriented Primary Care). Austin, TX: Author.

———. (1998). *Community assessment resources.* (Bureau of Community Oriented Primary Care). Austin, TX: Author.

Urrutia-Rojas, X. & Aday, L.A. (1991). A framework for community assessment: Designing and conducting a survey in a Hispanic immigrant and refugee community. *Public Health Nursing, 8*(1), 20–26.

Walker, M. & Breuer, S. (1992). *Community assessment, health care and you.* Austin, TX: Health Care Options for Rural Communities (P.O. Box 15587, Austin, TX 78761-5587; Fax [512] 465-1090.)

White, J.E. & Valentine, V.L. (1993). Computer assisted video instruction & community assessment. *Nursing and Health Care, 14*(7), 349–353.

Women's Environment & Development Organization. (n.d.). *Women for a healthy planet—Community report card.* Available from the author at 845 Third Avenue, 15th Floor, New York, NY 10022; Fax (212) 759-8647. (Also available in Spanish.)

INTERNET RESOURCES

www.census.gov/
US Census

www.bca.doc.gov/
Bureau of Economic Analysis

www.cdc.gov/
Centers for Disease Control and Prevention

www.cdc.gov/nchswww/nchshome.htm
National Center for Health Statistics

www.cdc.gov/epo/mmwr.html
Morbidity and Mortality Weekly Report

www.nlm.nih.gov
National Library of Medicine

www.os.dhhs.gov/progorg/ophs/
Office of Public Health and Science

www.health.org/
National Clearinghouse for Alcohol and Drug Information

www.vote-smart.org/
State and national government and political information

Elizabeth T. Anderson **and** Judith McFarlane

CHAPTER

COMMUNITY ANALYSIS AND NURSING DIAGNOSIS

10

OBJECTIVES

This chapter is focused on the second phase of the nursing process, analysis, and the associated task of forming community nursing diagnoses.

After studying the chapter, you should be able to

- Critically analyze community assessment data.
- Formulate community nursing diagnoses.

INTRODUCTION

Analysis is the study and examination of data. These data may be quantitative (numerical) as well as qualitative. All aspects need to be considered. Analysis is necessary to determine community health needs and community strengths as well as to identify patterns of health responses and trends in health care use. During analysis, any need for further data collection is revealed as gaps and incongruities in the community assessment data. The end point of analysis is the community nursing diagnosis.

COMMUNITY ANALYSIS

Analysis, like so many procedures we carry out, may be viewed as a process with multiple steps. The phases we will use to help in the analysis are categorization, summarization, comparison, and inference elaboration. Each is described and illustrated below.

Categorize

To analyze community assessment data, it is helpful to first categorize the data. Data can be categorized in a variety of ways. Traditional categories of community assessment data include the following:

- Demographic characteristics (family size, age, sex, and ethnic and racial groupings)
- Geographic characteristics (area boundaries; number and size of neighborhoods, public spaces, and roads)
- Socioeconomic characteristics (occupation and income categories, educational attainment, and rental or home ownership patterns)
- Health resources and services (hospitals, clinics, mental health centers, and so forth)

However, models are being used increasingly in the organization and analysis of community health data because they provide a framework for data collection and a map to guide analysis. Because the community assessment wheel (see Figure 9–1) was used to direct the community assessment process in the Rosemont sample study, that same model can be used to guide analysis. Each of the community subsystems will be analyzed, and components within each subsystem specify the categories to be evaluated.

Summarize

Once a categorization method has been selected, the next task is to summarize the data within each category. Both summary statements and summary measures, such as rates, charts, and graphs, are required.

TAKE NOTE   Many health care agencies and educational institutions have access to computerized information systems—a system through which formatted data can be retrieved in a variety of forms—including summary health statistics. For example, data entered into a computer system as census figures can be configured into population pyramids, and census and vital statistics information can be programmed to calculate birth, death, and fertility rates. Calculations that previously required hours to complete are now computed in seconds. In your practice, make it a point to inquire as to the availability of computer systems and, if possible, use computer processes to complete quantitative data analysis. In addition, your local health department may be able to furnish the rates for you (for instance, the infant mortality rate [IMR]). Note, however, that the denominator used may not be the community as you have defined it.

Compare

Additional tasks of data analysis include the identification of data gaps, incongruencies, and omissions. Frequently, comparative data are needed to determine if a pattern or trend exists or if data do not seem correct and the need for revalidation of original information is required. Data gaps are inevitable, as are mistakes in recording data; the important task is to analyze data critically and be aware of the potential for gaps and omissions. To have professional colleagues as well as community residents review the analysis is helpful. Every person has a unique perspective; it is only through the sharing of views that a whole and comprehensive picture of community assessment data can evolve.

Using the data from your community, compare it with other similar data. For instance, you calculate (or discover) an infant mortality rate of 12 per 1000 live births—how does this compare with the city? the state? the nation? Is it for the entire infant population of your community? Is the IMR different based on race? (*Note:* This is a good time to review Chapter 2 to assist you with epidemiologic reasoning as you try to make sense of your data.)

Other resources for comparison are the documents dealing with objectives—for the nation and for individual states. *Healthy People 2010* presents national figures, such as incidence and prevalence when available, for our major health problems and proposes goals and objectives for each. *Healthy People 2010*—along with state and, if available, local health planning documents—can be invaluable to you both as you analyze your data and as you develop a plan based on those data.

Draw Inference

Having categorized, summarized, and compared the data you have collected, the final phase is to draw logical conclusions from the evidence; that is, to draw inferences that will lead to the statement of a community nursing diagnosis. This is where you synthesize what you know about the community; that is, what do these data *mean*? The remainder of this chapter will walk you through analysis of the data we collected in the community assessment of Rosemont.

ROSEMONT SAMPLE COMMUNITY ANALYSIS

After the analysis examples given below, information on how to form community nursing diagnoses is presented (see the Community Nursing Diagnosis section later in this chapter). The analysis of the Rosemont assessment data, as in the assessment process, begins with the community core, because it is the core (the people and their health) that is of interest to the community health nurse. Recall that the core is affected by (and affects) all of the subsystems depicted in the model surrounding it. Some subsystems will influence certain problems more than others, but it is important to assess the subsystems because of their contribution to the causes and alleviation of problems in the core.

Community Core

An analysis of Rosemont's core is presented in Table 10–1. Community core data include many demographic measures, a type of data that is especially amenable to graphs and charts. The adage "one picture is worth a thousand words" is particularly meaningful for demographic characteristics.

Perhaps the most representative illustration of the age and sex composition of a population is the population pyramid. Population pyramids for census tracts (CTs) 402 and 403 appear in Figure 10–1. A population pyramid for

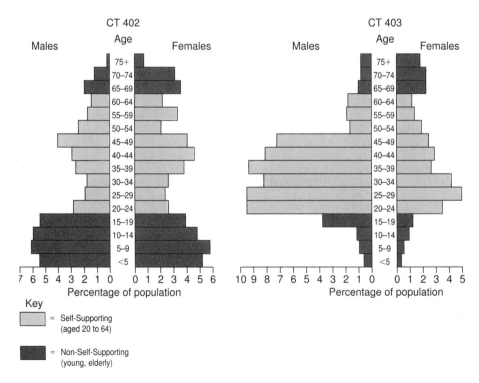

Figure 10–1. Population Pyramid: Age and sex structure of CT 402 and CT 403.

TABLE 10–1 ■ Analysis of Rosemont's Core

Categories of Data	Summary Statements/Measures	Inferences
History		
	Cultural and ethnic diversity	
	Renovation of business and homes	Community revitalization
	Pride and concern evident	Community pride
Demographics		
Age		
CT 402	42.5% of population ≤ 19 years	Large % of children and
	53% of population ≤ 19 years or ≥ 65 years	adolescents
		High dependency ratio*
	10% of population ≥ 65 years	Large % of elderly compared to Hampton and Jefferson County
Data gap: Need prior census data to determine if demographics are consistent or changing.		
CT 403	7.5% of population ≤ 19 years	Small % of children and
	15.2% of population ≤ 19 years or ≥ 65 years	adolescents
		Low dependency ratio
	7.7% of population ≥ 65 years	
Data gap: Need census data on 5-year increments to construct population pyramids.		
Sex		
CT 402	48% of population is male.	Equal % of males and females
	45% of population aged 20–64 is male.	
CT 403	65% of population is male.	High % of males
	69% of population aged 20–64 is male.	
Data gap: Need prior census data to determine if demographics are consistent or changing.		
Racial/ethnic		
CT 402	Diversity: black 54%, Asian 19%, white 12%, Hispanic 9%	Racial and ethnic diversity
CT 403	Homogeneity: white 89%	Racial and ethnic homogeneity
Data gap: Need census data from 1970 to determine if demographics are consistent or changing.		
Household types		
CT 402	83% of households are family.	Family households dominate
CT 403	36% of households are family.	Nonfamily households dominate
Marital status		
CT 402	15% single, 60% married, 14% divorced	Small % of single adults
		Majority of adults married
CT 403	53% single, 24% married, 15% divorced	Large % of single adults
		Small % married
Data gap: Need prior census data to determine if demographics are consistent or changing.		

Continued

TABLE 10–1 ■ Analysis of Rosemont's Core (Continued)

Categories of Data	Summary Statements/Measures	Inferences
Vital Statistics (Refer to Chapter 2 for rate calculation)		
		(When Compared to Hampton and Jefferson County Data)
Births CT 402	*Rate per 1000* 30.5	A higher birth rate
CT 403	17.3	A lower birth rate
Hampton	19.4	
Jefferson County	25.2	
Data gap: Need general fertility rate and age-specific birth rate.		
		(When Compared to Hampton and Jefferson County Data)
Deaths	*Rate per 1000*	
CT 402 Infant Neonatal Fetal Crude	 33.3 23.8 76.2 10.4	A higher death rate for all ages
CT 403 Infant Neonatal Fetal Crude	 17.1 17.1 8.5 6.2	A higher infant and neonatal rate
Data gap: Need vital statistics from previous 3 to 5 years to determine if rates are consistent or changing.		
Hampton Infant Neonatal Fetal Crude	 12.1 7.9 12.6 6.0	
Jefferson County Infant Neonatal Fetal Crude	 12.3 8.3 15.3 7.3	
		(When Compared to Hampton and Jefferson County Data)
Causes of Death CT 402	Heart disease 22.2%; malignant neoplasms 23.6%; cerebrovascular 8.3%; accidents 5.6%; diseases of early infancy 9.7%; homicides 8.3%; pneumonia 2.8%; suicides 4.2%; tuberculosis 1.4%; all other causes 13.9%	A much higher % of deaths due to Diseases of infancy Homicides Suicides Tuberculosis A higher % of deaths due to cerebrovascular disease A lower % of deaths due to heart disease

TABLE 10-1 ■ Analysis of Rosemont's Core *(Continued)*

Categories of Data	Summary Statements/Measures	Inferences
Vital Statistics *Causes of Death*		*(When Compared to Hampton and Jefferson County Data)*

CT 403	Heart disease 23.8%; malignant neoplasms 26.1%; cerebrovascular 4.7%; accidents 9.5%; diseases of early infancy 2.4%; homicides 2.4%; cirrhosis of liver 2.4%; pneumonia 2.4%; suicides 2.4%; diabetes mellitus 4.8%; congenital anomalies 4.8%; all other causes 14.3%	A higher % of deaths due to
		  Accidents
		  Diabetes mellitus
		  Congenital anomalies
		A lower % of deaths due to heart disease

Data gap: Need comparative data for past 3 to 5 years.		
Hampton	Disease of heart 33.4%; malignant neoplasms 21.8%; cerebrovascular 7.3%; accidents 6.2%; emphysema, asthma, bronchitis 0.8%; diseases of early infancy 2.6%; homicides 6.2%; cirrhosis of liver 1.7%; pneumonia 2.2%; suicides 2%; diabetes mellitus 1.4%; congenital anomalies 1%; nephritis and nephrosis 0.1%; tuberculosis 0.2%; all other causes 13%	
Jefferson County	Disease of heart 36%; malignant neoplasms 24.2%; cerebrovascular 7.4%; accidents 5.7%; emphysema, asthma, bronchitis 0.7%; diseases of early infancy 3%; homicides 1.5%; pneumonia 2.2%; suicides 1.4%; diabetes mellitus 1.8%; congenital anomalies 1.5%; nephritis and nephrosis 0.2%; tuberculosis 0.2%; all other causes 9.1%	

*Dependency ratio describes the potentially self-supporting portion of the population and the dependent portions at the extremes of age. The dependency ratio is usually computed as follows:

$$\frac{\text{population under 20} + \text{population 65 and over}}{\text{population 20 to 64 years of age}} \times 100$$

The dependency ratio for CT 402 is 91, meaning for every 100 persons aged 20 to 65 (supposedly self-supporting because of age), there are 91 persons under age 20 or over age 65 needing support (because of age). In contrast, the dependency ratio for CT 403 is 19.

Rosemont is included as Figure 10–2. Several other graphic display methods (pie chart, frequency graph, bar chart, and map) may be used. An example of each is included in Figure 10–3.

TAKE NOTE

The population pyramid is formed of bars; each bar represents an age group. Usually 5- or 10-year age groups are used, although adaptations can be made for smaller or larger age ranges. Bars are stacked horizontally, one on another, with bars for males on the left of a central axis and those for females on the right. The percentage of males and females in a particular age group is indicated by the length of the bars, as measured from the central axis. All age groups in a pyramid should be the same interval.

To construct a population pyramid, use Table 10–2 to calculate the percentage contribution of each age and sex class and Table 10–3 for actual pyramid construction. Note that parts of the population pyramids in Figure 10–1, those depicting people younger than 20 years and older than 65, are shaded; this was done to denote the dependent portions of the population.

Studying the population pyramids for CT 402 and CT 403 reveals striking age and sex differences, and this illustrates an important lesson. If the demographics of Rosemont had been presented as one population pyramid (see

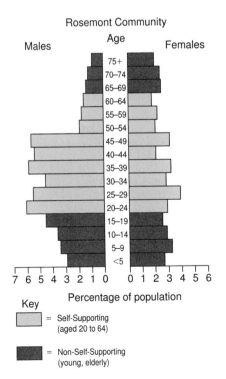

Figure 10–2. Population Pyramid of Rosemont: Age and sex structure.

Position of Infant in Sudden Infant Death Syndrome

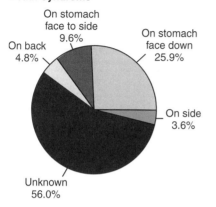

Suicide by Race and Age Group, 1994–1996

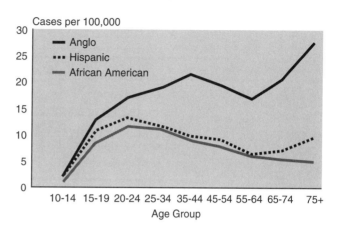

Reported Cases of Hepatitis C by Sex, Race/Ethnicity, and Age

E. coli 0157:H7 incidence Rates by Public Health Region

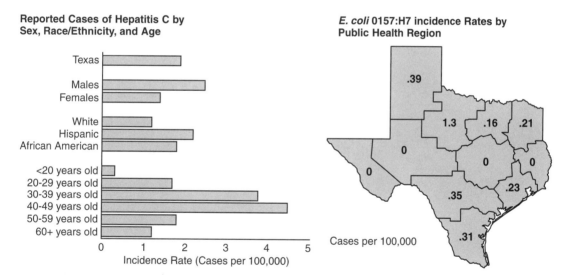

Figure 10–3. Graphic models to display assessment data. Source: Texas Department of Health (1998). _Epidemiology in Texas 1997 Annual Report._ Austin, TX: Author.

Figure 10–3), important age and sex differences might have been minimized or have gone unrecognized, and their associated age- and sex-related health needs would be left unmet. This hazard in data analysis is referred to as aggregating or pooling the data. It is important to divide data along all possibly meaningful lines so important information is not overlooked. Be alert to this problem as you proceed with your analysis.

TABLE 10–2 ■ Calculations for a Population Pyramid

Community Name, Census Tract, or Geographic Boundaries: _____

Total Population: _____

Ages (Years)	Males		Females	
	Number	% of Total Population	Number	% of Total Population
Total				
Younger than 5				
5–9				
10–14				
15–19				
20–24				
25–29				
30–34				
35–39				
40–44				
45–49				
50–54				
55–59				
60–64				
65–69				
70–74				
75 and over				

Studying the inferences presented in Table 10–1, in conjunction with the population pyramids, Figures 10–1 and 10–2, the following statements can be made about Rosemont's core. In CT 402, there exists the following:

- A large percentage (42.5%) of children and adolescents
- A high dependency ratio
- An equal percentage of adult men and women aged 20 to 64 years
- A larger percentage (10%) of elderly than Hampton or Jefferson County
- A small percentage (15.2%) of single adults
- A moderate percentage (60.7%) of married adults
- A predominance (83%) of family households

TABLE 10–3 ■ Constructing a Population Pyramid

Population Pyramid For _____ : 20_____

Males													Females
						75 & Over							
						70–74							
						65–69							
						60–64							
						55–59							
						50–54							
						45–49							
						40–44							
						35–39							
						30–34							
						25–29							
						20–24							
						15–19							
						10–14							
						5–9							
						Younger than 5							

8   6   4   2   0   2   4   6   8

Percentage of Population

- A mixed racial/ethnic composition with 54% black, 19% Asian, 12% white, and 9% Hispanic
- An extremely high infant and fetal death rate
  - Infant mortality rate (33 per 1000 live births)
  - Neonatal mortality rate (24 per 1000 live births)
  - Fetal mortality rate (76 per 1000 live births)
- A higher birth rate (31 per 1000 population) than Hampton (19 per 1000 population) or Jefferson County (25 per 1000 population)
- A higher crude death rate (10 per 1000 population) than Hampton (6 per 1000 population) or Jefferson County (7 per 1000 population)
- A much higher percentage of deaths owing to diseases of early infancy, homicides, suicides, and tuberculosis than Hampton or Jefferson County

- A slightly higher percentage of deaths owing to cerebrovascular disorders than Hampton or Jefferson County

  In contrast, it can be seen that CT 403 has the following factors:

- A small percentage (7.5%) of children and adolescents
- A low dependency ratio
- A larger percentage (7.7%) of elderly than Hampton or Jefferson County
- A high percentage (69%) of adult males aged 20 to 64 years
- Racial and ethnic homogeneity, with 89% of the population white
- A predominance (64%) of nonfamily households
- A large percentage (53%) of single adults
- A small percentage (24%) of married adults
- A lower birth rate (17 per 1000 population) than Hampton or Jefferson County
- A higher infant mortality (17 per 1000 live births) and a higher neonatal mortality (17 per 1000 live births) than Hampton or Jefferson County
- A lower crude death rate (6.2 per 1000 population) than Hampton or Jefferson County
- A higher percentage of deaths owing to accidents, diabetes mellitus, and congenital anomalies than Hampton or Jefferson County
- A lower percentage of deaths due to heart disease than Hampton or Jefferson County

Having analyzed the core characteristics of Rosemont, it is evident that major differences exist between CT 402 and CT 403, although both are part of Rosemont. In the following sections, this finding will be given more detail as each subsystem in our community assessment wheel model is analyzed.

Physical Environment

To study the physical components of Rosemont, data were collected that began with community inspection (that is, the "Learning About the Community on Foot" survey) and concluded with a systems review and laboratory studies (in other words, census and chamber of commerce data). Table 10–4 presents an analysis of the physical examination data.

Studying the inferences in Table 10–4, the following statements about Rosemont's physical components can be made:

- Rosemont is a community of contrasts and diversity.
- Densely populated residential areas, composed mainly of older homes, abut businesses of various types.

TABLE 10–4 ■ Analysis of Rosemont's Physical Examination Data		
Categories of Data	**Summary Statements/Measures**	**Inferences**
Inspection		
Windshield survey "Learning About the Community on Foot"	A community of contrast: bustling business areas and quiet neighborhoods	Ethnic and business diversity Congested streets lined with homes or businesses
	Ethnic diversity evident in foods	Minimal industry
		Little "open" space
Vital Signs		
	Flat terrain and mild climate	Mild climate, abundant flora
	Densely populated (14 persons per acre)	Densely populated (14 persons per acre)
	Posters abound, sharing information and heralding forthcoming events	Note: in CT 402, there are 221 persons per acre at one housing development.
Systems Review *Land Usage*		
CT 402	37% of land in commercial usage, 28% single family, 8% multifamily, and 9% open	CT 402 has almost twice the commercial usage of land (37%) compared to CT 403 (20%).
CT 403	20% of land in commercial usage, 32% single family, 15% multifamily, and 18% open	CT 403 has twice the percentage of open space (18%) compared to CT 402 (9%).
Housing Values CT 402	From 1980 to 1990, average home values increased 6.8% and average rents increased 16.9%.	Sharp contrast between average home values; in CT 402, average home value is $43,300, compared to $62,400 in CT 403.
CT 403	From 1980 to 1990, average home values increased 6.8% and average rents increased 16.9%.	Average rent is similar for both census tracts and comparable to Hampton.

(Note: No data gaps identified; data for this area are complete.)

- Industry is minimal and is concentrated entirely in CT 402.
- Housing values increased greatly in CT 402; in both CT 402 and CT 403, only rents rose at the same rate.

Health and Social Services

An analysis of the health and social services in Rosemont is presented in Table 10–5. Because the data were categorized initially as extra- and intracommunity health and social services, the same format has been used in the analysis.

TABLE 10–5 ■ Analysis of Health and Social Services in Rosemont

Categories of Data	Summary Statements/Measures	Inferences
Health Facilities		
Extracommunity		
Hospitals	Most are referral or private. One public hospital, Jefferson Memorial, has problems of Long waits (≥ 8 hr) Fragmented care Inaccessibility	Only one public hospital; users complain of lengthy waits and fragmented care.
Private care Health department (Sunvalley Clinic)	Numerous options, including HMOs Health providers feel Sunvalley Clinic has Inadequate antepartal services; women wait 8–10 weeks for an initial appointment that is often after their expected date of confinement Inadequate nursing services to meet elderly's needs Rosemont residents feel the clinic is Inaccessible (no direct bus connection) Impersonal (no primary care providers)	Variety of private care options Inadequate antepartal services Many women deliver at Jefferson Memorial with no antepartal care. Many women are forced to self-deliver at home because they do not meet eligibility requirements at Jefferson Memorial. Inaccessibility and unacceptability of Sunvalley services

Data gap:
Number of Rosemont residents using
  Well and ill infant, child, adolescent, adult services
  Mental health counseling and referral services
User's perception of adequacy, accessibility, and acceptability of the above services

| Home health | One large Visiting Nurse Association (VNA) Numerous home health agencies; most require fee-for-service or third-party reimbursement. | Numerous options for home health care |

Data gap: Frequency and type of VNA services used by Rosemont residents

| Continuing care | Two long-term licensed facilities close (eight miles) from Rosemont | Two long-term licensed facilities |

Data gap: Adequacy of facilities as perceived by health administrators, staff, and patients

| Emergency services: Medical emergency ambulance service (MEAS) | Cardiac and cerebrovascular accident (CVA) are major reasons for MEAS visits to Rosemont. | Cardiac and CVA are major reasons for MEAS visits, followed by accidents and home falls. |

Data gap: Number of persons using MEAS and their age, sex, race, and ethnic characteristics

| *Intracommunity Health Services* | | |
| Health care practitioners | Rosemont has no Obstetric, gynecologic, or family practitioners Bilingual health practitioners | Lack of OB/GYN and family practitioners No bilingual health practitioners |

TABLE 10–5 ■ Analysis of Health and Social Services in Rosemont *(Continued)*		
Categories of Data	**Summary Statements/Measures**	**Inferences**
Clinics		

Third Street Clinic	Health care providers feel immediate health needs include
	    Ill infant, child, adolescent, and adult assessment, treatment, and follow-up
	    Dental assessment and restoration
	    Counseling, referral, and treatment for substance abuse
	    Group health teaching
	    Support groups for single parents and senior citizens
	Additional needs of the clinic include recruitment and retainment of health care providers.
		Inadequate health services for
		    Ill persons (all ages)
		    Dental assessment and restoration
		    Counseling and treatment for substance abuse
		    Health education
		    Self-help/support groups

	Many Rosemont residents use the clinic routinely; people feel welcomed and comply with medical care. Residents agree that additional services are needed.	Rosemont residents state that care at Third Street Clinic is acceptable and accessible.

Data gap:

Number of persons requesting services that health care providers feel are needed

Characteristics of people requesting medical care services

Rosemont Health Center	Director of clinic feels immediate needs are
	    Formation of counseling and support groups
	    Orientation program and inservice for staff (all are volunteers)
		Highly acceptable, accessible, and affordable care for sexually transmitted diseases
		Inadequate counseling and support groups
		Lack of orientation and inservice for the staff
		Lack of procedure manuals and posted protocols for emergency care
		Lack of safety procedures including visible emergency cart and proper syringe disposal

Data gap:

What do staff perceive as needs?

What do residents perceive as needs?

Social Facilities		
Extracommunity		
Hampton Community Counseling Center (HCCC)	HCCC offers counseling to adolescent drug users. Most patients are middle- or upper-class males; all are white.	HCCC is close to Rosemont and offers needed counseling for substance abuse, yet HCCC is not used by Rosemont residents.

Continued

TABLE 10–5 ■ Analysis of Health and Social Services in Rosemont *(Continued)*

Categories of Data	Summary Statements/Measures	Inferences
Social Facilities		
Extracommunity		
	Staff feels that they are meeting community needs. Rosemont residents are not aware that the center exists.	
YMCA Indo–Chinese Refugee Program	Cultural-orientation programs for Asian immigrants; staff perceive immediate needs are for programs on the following: Substance abuse Basic life survival skills (for example, employment, self-health care) Many Rosemont residents use the YMCA services; all agree the programs are excellent but state the waiting period for classes is long and frustrating.	Insufficient number of cultural programs resulting in long waiting periods and frustration
Intracommunity Churches		
South Main	Extensive social service programs; social program for gay men despite resistance from older members	Social outreach programs offered by both churches Only South Main offers program for gay men although older members of South Main resent the program.
Westpark	Extensive social service program No social programs for gay men	
Lambda Alcoholic Anonymous (AA)	Active AA program for gay men: membership exceeds 120.	Active chapter of Lambda AA

Notice that statements from health care providers have been reported separately from those of health care recipients. This is because health care providers frequently have a different concept of the adequacy, accessibility, and acceptability of health services than that held by health care recipients. Be sure to collect and analyze data from both perspectives.

After reviewing Table 10–5, the following statements can be made about Rosemont's health services:

- The Sunvalley Clinic, operated by the city health department, has inadequate antepartum services for Rosemont women; this results in
  - Many women delivering at Jefferson Memorial with no antepartum care

- Women forced to self-deliver at home because they do not meet eligibility requirements at Jefferson Memorial
- There are no practicing private obstetric, gynecologic, or family practitioners nor are there any nurse-midwives in Rosemont.
- The Third Street Clinic has inadequate health services, specifically a lack of
  - Assessment and treatment of people who are ill
  - Dental assessment and restoration
  - Counseling and treatment programs for substance abuse
  - Health education programs responsive to residents' needs
  - Support and self-help groups as needed and requested by residents
- The Rosemont Health Center offers acceptable, accessible, and affordable services for sexually transmitted diseases (STD); however, there is a lack of
  - Orientation and education for the staff
  - Procedure manuals and posted protocols for emergency care
  - Safe disposal methods for syringes
  - A visible emergency cart

The following deductions can be made about Rosemont's social services:

- Hampton Community Counseling Center (HCCC) is located close to Rosemont but is not used by Rosemont residents, although residents repeatedly expressed a wish for substance-abuse counseling programs.
- The YMCA Indo–Chinese Refugee Program is heavily used by Asians in Rosemont; however, present programs of cultural orientation are inadequate to meet the demand. Both the YMCA staff and Rosemont residents see a need for additional programs.
- South Main and Westpark churches offer numerous social service programs; however, only South Main offers a social program especially for the gay male population—a program that is resisted by older parishioners.
- An active chapter of Lambda AA is located in Rosemont.

Economics

An analysis of the economic and financial characteristics of Rosemont is presented in Table 10–6. The analysis begins with individual wealth indices (such as income), proceeds to indicators of business and industrial wealth, and concludes with employment status of community residents. As with other subsystems, the categories for data assessment have become categories for data analysis.

After studying Table 10–6, the following statements can be made about the economic status of Rosemont. Striking differences exist in the financial characteristics between households in CT 402 and CT 403.

TABLE 10–6 ■ Analysis of Economic Indicators of Rosemont

Categories of Data	Summary Statements/ Measures	Inferences
Financial Characteristics of Households		
Median household income (1990)		
CT 402 $10,693		Medial household income in CT
CT 403 $31,273		403 is considerably higher than in
Hampton $30,483		CT 402.
% of families with incomes below poverty level (1990)		
CT 402 53.7%		In CT 402, over half of all families
CT 403 5.4%		have incomes below the poverty
Hampton 7.1%		level.
% of families on public assistance/welfare		
CT 402 36.4%		In CT 402, 36.4% of all families are
CT 403 4.3%		on public assistance/welfare
Hampton 3.4%		compared to 4.3% in CT 403 and
		3.4% in Hampton.
% of female head of households (1990)		
CT 402 49.2%		In CT 402, half of the households
CT 403 11.1%		are headed by females.
Hampton 15.4%		
Business/industry characteristics (1990)		
CT 402	Nearly equal percentage of wholesale/retail (48%) and professional (42%)	In CT 402, equal percentage of wholesale and professional businesses
CT 403	Predominance of professional (48%) over wholesale/retail (37%)	In CT 403, predominance of professional businesses
Labor force characteristics (1990): age (% of persons ≥ 16 years)		
CT 402 39.8%		Only 40% of persons in CT 402
CT 403 85.4%		are of employable age (≥ 16)
Hampton 71.5%		compared to 85% in CT 403 and
		71% in Hampton.
Wage class: % private, % government, % self-employed		
CT 402 67%, 18%, 2%		Wage class data similar for CT
CT 403 76%, 12%, 6%		402 and CT 403, with the majority of all wages derived from private businesses

	Summary Statements/	
Categories of Data	**Measures**	**Inferences**
Financial Characteristics *of Households*		
Occupational groups		
Managerial/professional		
CT 402 7.1%		Striking differences between
CT 403 42.1%		occupational categories
Technical/sales		
CT 402 12.1%		In CT 402, 67% of workers are in
CT 403 34.1%		service or operator occupations,
		compared to 14.8% in CT 403.
Service		
CT 402 44.2%		In CT 403, 76% of workers are in
CT 403 10.5%		managerial or technical
		occupations, compared to 19% in
		CT 402.
Operators/laborers		
CT 402 23.6%		
CT 403 4.3%		

TABLE 10–6 ■ Analysis of Economic Indicators of Rosemont *(Continued)*

(Note: No data gaps identified; data in this area are complete.)

In CT 402, it was found that

- The median household income of $10,693 is only 34% of the median income in CT 403 and Hampton.
- The majority of families (53.7%) have incomes below the poverty level.
- Half of all households are headed by females.
- One third of all families receive public assistance/welfare.

In CT 403, the following factors exist:

- The median household income of $31,273 is much greater than that of CT 402, as well as that of Hampton.
- Only 5.4% of families have incomes below the poverty line.
- Only 11.1% of all households are headed by females.
- Only 4.3% of families receive public assistance/welfare.

Striking differences also exist between the labor force characteristics of CT 402 and CT 403.

In CT 402, it was found that

- Only 39.8% of the population is of employable age (16 years or older).
- Most people (67.8%) work in service or operator/labor occupations.

CT 403 presented a contrasting picture:

- Of the population, 85.4% is of employable age (16 years or older).
- Most people (76.2%) work in managerial or professional positions.

Safety and Transportation

An analysis of the safety and transportation services in Rosemont is set forth in Table 10–7.

Reviewing the data, the following statements can be made about Rosemont's safety (protection) services and associated concerns:

- Grease fires are the major cause of house fires.
- Thefts and burglaries are the major reported crimes, followed by robbery and vehicle theft; elderly people and gay men feel especially victimized. Both groups related numerous stories of harassment and violence.
- There is no fluoride in Rosemont's drinking water, and neither is there routine testing for arsenic or heavy metals, substances that residents fear are contaminating the water.
- Owing to abandoned vehicles and dumping of machinery and appliances, residents, especially children, are at increased risk of accidental injury.
- Air pollution has increased; the Air Control Board believes that citizens are inadequately informed about air pollution advisories as well as personal actions that can be taken to decrease pollution.

Regarding Rosemont's transportation services, the following deductions are made:

- A large percentage of residents in CT 403 drive to work alone (64%) compared to those in CT 402 (43%); however, 48% of the residents in CT 402 use carpools or public transportation to get to work, compared to 26% in CT 403.
- When compared to CT 403, a substantially larger percentage of the population in CT 402 have a transportation disability, especially among those over age 65.

Politics and Government

A rich diversity of political organizations exists in Rosemont. However, at this point in the nursing process—analysis—it is sufficient to describe the organizations and identify key persons. Consider your information about the political

TABLE 10-7 ■ Analysis of Safety and Transportation Services in Rosemont		
Categories of Data	**Summary Statements/Measures**	**Inferences**

Safety
Protection Services

Fire	45 fires during past 90 days; of these, 40 occurred in homes (usually a grease fire).	Major cause of fires within last 90 days was grease.

Data gap:
Obtain additional data (12 months) and determine if grease fires are major cause.
Document age, sex, and racial characteristics, as well as time of day and associated circumstances.

Police	Crime statistics for past four years show thefts as the leading crime, followed by burglary. Frequency of occurrence is high for both census tracts. Robbery is twice as prevalent in CT 402 compared to CT 403, and vehicle theft is three times more common in CT 403. Residents expressed fear and related stories of muggings and violence directed especially toward the elderly and gay male populations.	Thefts and burglaries are the major crimes; the elderly and gay men feel especially victimized.

Data gap:
Assess residents' knowledge about self-protection measures against crime.
Assess residents' interest and past participation in crime prevention programs.
Assess available crime prevention programs.

Sanitation

Sewage	Sewage moratorium exists owing to overcapacity of present facility.	Inadequate sewage treatment facilities resulting in building restrictions
Potable water	No fluoride in drinking water No routine testing of drinking water for arsenic or heavy metals (elements that residents believe may be contaminating the water)	Lack of fluoride in drinking water No routine tests of drinking water for arsenic or heavy metals

Data gap:
Assess history of fluoride issue. Has fluoride been proposed, voted on? What is the present position of the health department, city council, civic associations, and the general public?

Regarding arsenic and heavy metals: Is Lake Hampton tested for arsenic or heavy metals? What is the position and plan of the health department, city council, and civic associations?

Solid waste	Increased illegal dumping of machinery and appliances; unoperable autos are parked on the streets for months before removal by the City of Hampton.	Potential for accidents (with consequences such as trauma and suffocation) as people explore abandoned objects and automobiles

TABLE 10–7 ■ Analysis of Safety and Transportation Services in Rosemont *(Continued)*

Categories of Data	Summary Statements/Measures	Inferences
Sanitation		
Data gap: Document laws and fees for illegal dumping. Are signs posted to notify persons of law and associated fines? What actions have been taken by residents, civic associations, businesses?		
Air	Rise in air population attributed to increase in industrial growth and population density. Residents complain of eye irritation and increased number of respiratory conditions.	Increased air pollution
	Air Board feels citizens are inadequately informed regarding actions needed during an air stagnation advisory and individual responsibility to decrease pollution.	Citizens may be inadequately informed regarding personal actions needed during an air stagnation advisory to decrease air pollution.
Data gap: Assess if public awareness programs have occurred. If so, when, and what was the response? What do residents understand about air pollution, air advisories, and their role in decreasing air pollution? Do residents desire more information about air pollution?		
Transportation		
Private (to work)		
CT 402	43% of people drive alone, 24% carpool, and 23% use public transportation.	Almost half (43%) drive alone to work, with equal percentages (24%) carpooling or using public transportation.
CT 403	64% of people drive alone, 16% carpool, and 11% use public transportation.	Most people (64%) drive alone to work, some carpool (16%), and only a few use public transportation (11%).
Transportation Disability		
CT 402	6% of persons aged 16 to 64 and 21% of over age 65 have a disability.	When compared to CT 403, a large percentage of residents in CT 402 have a transportation disability, especially those over age 65.
CT 403	0.3% of persons aged 16 to 64 and 11% of those over age 65 have a disability.	

system and form of government to be reference material that will be useful at the next stage of the nursing process—program planning with the community.

Communication

Ample formal and informal communication sources exist in Rosemont. No analysis is required of the data. Consider the communication data to be reference material that will be useful at the next stage of the nursing process— program planning with the community.

TAKE NOTE

If sufficient information is collected regarding a community's communication system (refer to Table 9–29 in Chapter 9 for components to assess), then there is no need to further analyze the data.

Education

An analysis of Rosemont's general educational status (characteristics of school enrollment, years of schooling completed, and language spoken) and specific educational sources (for example, public and private schools, both intra- and extracommunity) is presented in Table 10–8.

Major differences exist between the general educational status of CT 402 and CT 403. The status in CT 402 is as follows:

- A small percentage of residents are high school graduates (28%), with the majority of persons enrolled in school attending elementary grades. Some 75% of the population has poor English proficiency.

 In contrast, the CT 403 data show that

- A large percentage of residents are high school graduates (89%), and the majority of the persons who attend school are in college. Only 19% of the residents have poor English proficiency.

 With regard to specific educational sources, Temple Elementary is the primary educational resource in Rosemont. Temple has an enrollment of 924 youngsters. The principal, teachers, nurse, and parents were interviewed during the assessment process. To summarize the situation at Temple, it has been concluded that

TABLE 10–8 ■ Analysis of Educational Sources in Rosemont

Categories of Data	Summary Statements/ Measures	Inferences
Educational Status		
Years of schooling completed: % high school graduates		
CT 402 28%		In CT 402, only 28% of persons
CT 403 89%		over age 25 are high school
Hampton 68%		graduates, compared to 89% in CT 403 and 68% in Hampton.
School enrollment: % elementary, % high school, % college		
CT 402 59%, 23%, 4%		The majority of persons attending school in CT 402 are
CT 403 15%, 7%, 73%		elementary grade students; in
Hampton 48%, 23%, 19%		CT 403, the majority of those attending school are in college.
Language spoken: % of population with poor English proficiency		
Age 5–17 Age 18+		In CT 402, some 75% of the
CT 402 76% 74%		population has poor English
CT 403 11% 19%		proficiency, compared to small
Hampton 21% 26%		percentages in CT 403.
Educational Sources		
Intracommunity		
Temple Elementary	Grades K to eighth Enrollment 924 Ethnicity 42% black 33% Asian 18% Hispanic 5% white	Mixed ethnicity, predominance of black children
	Principal feels major problems are Truancy Academic failure Principal wants to stop bilingual classes.	According to staff, major problems are Truancy Academic failure (22%) Inadequate parent–teacher relationships English insufficiencies Stressed home environments with inadequate adult supervision

Data gap:
Explore the principal's statement about bilingual education. Why the opposition? What is the position and policy on bilingual education in Hampton Independent School District (HISD)?
What is the principal's perception of parental concerns?

TABLE 10–8 ■ Analysis of Educational Sources in Rosemont *(Continued)*

Categories of Data	Summary Statements/ Measures	Inferences
Educational Sources *Intracommunity*	*Teachers feel* major impediments to student learning are Inadequate parent–teacher communication Poor English proficiency Stressed home environment Inadequate adult supervision	Same as above

Data gap:
Explore teachers' perceptions of bilingual education.
What are teachers' perceptions of parental concerns?

Temple Elementary	*Nurse feels* major health problems of youngsters are Poor hygiene Dental caries Prevalence of head lice Incomplete immunizations Lack of parent follow- through for needed medical care	Major student health problems are Inadequate hygiene Control of dental caries Control of head lice Parent follow-through with needed medical care Health education

Data gap:
Document age, sex, ethnicity, and racial characteristics of children with specific health problems.

	Nurse feels more health teaching and screening would be possible with parent volunteers. Present policy restricts nurse to clinic, permitting no classroom teaching.	Same as above

Data gap:
Document school policy regarding
   Recruitment and training of parent volunteers
   The nurse's presence and role in the clinic

Explore nurse's attitude toward health education.
   Discuss options for health programs for students, staff, and parents.

Temple Elementary	*Parents feel* Temple is a community strength *but* the present staff members are insensitive to ethnic and racial needs; attempts to discuss these concerns with Temple's staff have been frustrating.	Parental concern and involvement are evident; however, attempts to discuss concerns with staff have been frustrating.

Continued

TABLE 10–8 ■ Analysis of Educational Sources in Rosemont *(Continued)*

Categories of Data	Summary Statements/ Measures	Inferences
Educational Sources		
Intracommunity		
Data gap:		
Identify officers and key people (committee chairs) of Temple's PTO. Are these officers/key people aware of ethnic and racial needs?		
Identify students' perceptions of their school. What activities do they enjoy? Are there afterschool activities? Who participates? What activities are needed?		
Busybee Day Care	One day care center in CT 402; no facility in CT 403	Inadequate day care facilities Parents leave children in crowded homes
Extracommunity Central Hampton High	Truancy and grade failure reversed with "Failproof" program Increased number of teenage pregnancies Decision by school board not to permit sex education classes Increased use of alcohol	Increased number of teenage pregnancies Increased use of alcohol among high school students Sex education classes not permitted in high school

Data gap:
Number of pregnancies last 3 to 5 years (for comparison) and age, grade level, racial, and ethnic characteristics of girls.

History and reason for HISD Board decision to stop sex education.

Document scope of alcohol use and characteristics of users.

- Problems of truancy exist, especially among Hispanic boys. There are large numbers of academic failures (22% of students last year).
- Large numbers of students have English-skills insufficiencies, further documented by general educational data.
- Inadequate working relationships exist between parents and teachers, compounded by the language barrier.
- Student health problems consist of
  - Dental caries (62% of youngsters)
  - Head lice, especially in grades kindergarten to second
  - Incomplete immunizations
  - Poor hygiene
  - Inadequate parent follow-through of needed medical care
  - Inadequate health education program
- There is parental concern and involvement and a desire to communicate needs to staff.

One day care facility exists in Rosemont—the Busybee. This facility is extremely inadequate. As a result, parents are forced to leave children in conditions that may be crowded and undersupervised.

The major extracommunity educational facility is Central Hampton High. The major problems of Central Hampton High, according to the school nurse, include

- Increased number of teenage pregnancies
- Lack of sex education classes
- Increased use of alcohol

Central Hampton has succeeded in reducing truancy and grade failure through a program called "Failproof."

Recreation

Recreational space and facilities are minimal. A sum of 5.6 acres of public recreational space is available for a population of 13,631 (combined populations of CT 402 and CT 403). The organized sports and recreational programs that are available through churches and associations require membership and usually charge a fee. There are no public recreational programs, and the few pieces of public recreational equipment that exist are in need of repair.

Community Nursing Diagnosis

In the preceding pages, each subsystem of the Rosemont sample has been analyzed in relation to its effect on the core (the people), and inferences have been drawn. The final task of analysis is the synthesis of the inference statements into community nursing diagnoses.

A *diagnosis* is a statement that synthesizes assessment data. A diagnosis is a label that both *describes a situation* (or state) and *implies an etiology* (reason).

A *nursing diagnosis* limits the diagnostic process to those diagnoses that represent *human responses to actual or potential health problems that nurses are licensed to treat*. This stipulation is based on the American Nurses Association (ANA) Social Policy Statement (see the Suggested Readings list). Although no standard format exists, most nursing diagnoses have three parts:

1. A *description* of the problem, response, or state
2. Identification of factors *etiologically* related to the problem
3. *Signs and symptoms* that are characteristic of the problem

A *community nursing diagnosis* focuses the diagnosis on a *community*—usually defined as a *group, population, or cluster of people with at least one common characteristic* (such as geographic location, occupation, ethnicity, or housing condition). To derive a community nursing diagnosis, community assessment data are analyzed and inferences are presented. Inference statements shape nursing diagnoses. Some inference statements form the *descriptive* part of the nursing diagnosis; that is, they testify to a *potential or actual community health problem* or concern—for example

- High infant mortality rate in Rosemont
- High prevalence of dental caries among youngsters at Temple Elementary School in Rosemont

Other inference statements are *etiologic* and document the possible reasons for the health problem or concern. Etiologic statements are linked to the descriptive statements with a *"related to"* clause—for example

- High infant mortality in Rosemont is related to
  - Inadequate resources at the health department's Sunvalley Clinic to meet antepartum care needs
  - Inaccessibility and unacceptability of present antepartum services at the Sunvalley Clinic
  - Lack of obstetric and family practitioners in Rosemont
- High prevalence of dental caries among youngsters at Temple Elementary School in Rosemont is related to
  - Lack of dental assessment and treatment at the Third Street Clinic
  - Lack of fluoride in Rosemont's drinking water
  - Low median household income in CT 402 and associated limited economic resources for purchasing dental care
  - No dental hygiene education offered at Temple Elementary

Finally, the *signs and symptoms* of the community nursing diagnosis are the inference statements that *document the duration or magnitude of the problem*. Examples of documentation include record accounts, census reports, and vital statistics. This final piece of the community nursing diagnosis is linked to the first two parts with an *"as manifested by"* clause—for example

- High infant mortality rate in Rosemont is related to
  - Inadequate resources at the health department's Sunvalley Clinic to meet antepartum care needs
  - Inaccessibility and unacceptability of present antepartum services at the Sunvalley Clinic

- Lack of obstetric and family practitioners in Rosemont
- *As manifested by* many Rosemont women who deliver at Jefferson Memorial with no antepartum care, many Rosemont women who self-deliver at home, and an IMR of 17 per 1000 live births.
- High prevalence of dental caries among youngsters at Temple Elementary School in Rosemont is related to
  - Lack of dental assessment and treatment at the Third Street Clinic
  - Lack of fluoride in Rosemont's drinking water
  - Low median household income in CT 402 and associated limited economic resources for purchasing dental care
  - No dental hygiene education offered at Temple Elementary
  - *As manifested by* 62% of youngsters at Temple Elementary who have dental caries on inspection

Although a single problem is stated, the etiology and signs and symptoms may be multiple. Also notice that, although the health problem inference is drawn from the analysis of one subsystem (such as the health and social services subsystem or the educational subsystem), the etiologies may be, and usually are, drawn from several subsystems. For example, regarding the health problem of dental caries among youngsters at Temple Elementary, etiologic inferences were derived from four subsystems—educational, health and social services, safety and transportation, and economic. This example sums up the most important lesson of community health nursing: *All community factors (subsystems) join to determine the health status of a community. No one subsystem is more important or crucial than any other in determining a community's health.*

The process of deriving community nursing diagnoses always remains the same. First, assessment data are categorized and studied for inferences that are descriptive of potential or actual health problems amenable to nursing interventions; next, associated inferences are identified that explain the derivation or continuation of the problem; and last, documentation is presented. Additional community nursing diagnoses for Rosemont are presented in Table 10–9. There is no particular order to the list, and neither is the list conclusive. Determining the order of priority among community nursing diagnoses is part of program planning and depends on existing community goals and resources. This important skill is discussed in the next chapter.

Deriving community nursing diagnoses requires critical decision making and astute study; it is a challenging and vital task. The completeness and validity of the diagnoses that have been derived will be tested during the next stage of the nursing process and will form the foundation of that stage—the planning of a health program.

TABLE 10–9 ■ Community Nursing Diagnoses

Community Response/ Concern/Problem (Actual or Potential)	Etiology Related to . . .	Documentation Signs and Symptoms as Manifested by . . .
Stress and anxiety of being criminally victimized	Increased episodes of thefts and burglaries Inadequate knowledge on the part of residents regarding self-protection measures	Police crime statistics of past four years Personal testimony of residents, especially gay men and the elderly
Potential for accidents (such as trauma and suffocation) as children and adults explore abandoned goods	Illegal dumping of machinery and appliances Abandonment of automobiles Nonenforcement of city ordinances	Parental concern for safety Observation of persons exploring abandoned goods
Potential for health problems associated with air pollution (such as initiation and exacerbation of respiratory conditions)	Increased air pollution Lack of knowledge regarding personal action required during an air stagnation advisory to decrease air pollution	Air Board reports of current air pollution levels Residents' complaints of eye irritation and increased number of respiratory conditions
Truancy and academic failure at Temple Elementary	Large number of students with poor English proficiency Stressed home environment in CT 402, where 50% of homes are headed by females and 54% of families are below poverty level Inadequate communication links between parents and school personnel	Records at Temple Elementary
Stress within Rosemont between the gay and heterosexual populations	Differing lifestyles of gay men Lack of acceptance of gay male lifestyle	Lack of social programs for gay men in Westpark Church Resistance of older church members in South Main to existing program for gay men Large percentage of single males in CT 403
Potential for inadequate coping of single parents, the elderly, and persons with sexually transmitted diseases (STDs)	Lack of support groups and programs for single parents, the elderly, and persons with STDs Inadequate resources at Third Street Clinic to offer programs although the need is recognized Inadequate resources at Hampton Health Center to offer programs although the need is recognized	Health providers' perceptions of the Third Street Clinic Health providers' perceptions of the Rosemont Health Center High percentage of deaths owing to homicides and suicides in CT 402

TABLE 10–9 ■ Community Nursing Diagnoses (Continued)

Community Response/ Concern/Problem (Actual or Potential)	Etiology Related to . . .	Documentation Signs and Symptoms as Manifested by . . .
Unsafe working environment at Rosemont Health Center	Lack of orientation and inservice programs for staff Lack of procedure manuals and posted protocols for emergency care Lack of safety procedures	Visual assessment Perceptions of administration Perception of volunteer nurse
Potential for inadequate cultural assimilation of Asian immigrants	Lack of programs to meet present needs Lack of staff at Indo–Chinese Refugee Program Increased need for programs Large Asian population in CT 402 (19%) Large percentage of population in CT 402 (75%) with poor English proficiency	Perceived needs of Asians in Rosemont
Incomplete immunization status of children at Temple Elementary	Inadequate communication between parents and school's staff Inaccessibility and unacceptability of Health Department's Sunvalley Clinic Inadequate income in CT 402 to purchase immunizations	School health records at Temple Elementary
High infant, neonatal, and fetal mortality rate	Inadequate antepartum care at Sunvalley Clinic Lack of obstetric and family practitioners in Rosemont Lack of bilingual practitioners in Rosemont Inadequate income in CT 402 to purchase essential medical care	Vital statistics
Potential for boredom and associated consequences (violence, vandalism)	Lack of public, no-fee recreational programs Minimal public recreational areas and equipment	A total of 5.6 acres of public recreational space in Rosemont Visual inspection of available land and equipment
High prevalence of pediculosis capitis among children at Temple Elementary	Crowded living conditions Knowledge deficit regarding transmission and treatment	Cases reported by school nurse at Temple Elementary

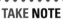

TAKE NOTE

This is an excellent time to share your assessment data with colleagues and people in the community to solicit their analysis. Because we all have opinions and values that color our perceptions, group critiquing and analysis of assessment data are ways to foster objectivity.

SUMMARY

Critical analysis of the Rosemont community has been completed using the community assessment wheel as a guide. Subsequently, community nursing diagnoses were formulated, based on the inferences of the analyses. Although community nursing diagnoses are relatively new to practice, community health nurses have, since the profession's inception, derived inferences from assessment data and have acted on those data. However, the terminology and format that have surrounded these informally produced inferences (diagnoses) have been inconsistent. There is considerable discussion, and some controversy, regarding the structure and terminology that would be optimal for community-focused nursing diagnoses. In your practice, you will be exposed to various formats for making community nursing diagnoses—evaluate and test the usefulness of each. It is only through collaboration and vigorous testing that a standard format will evolve. In the Suggested Readings list, there are additional sources to help you as you develop community nursing diagnoses.

SUGGESTED READINGS

Allor, M.T. (1983). The "community profile." *Journal of Nursing Education, 22*, 12–16.
American Nurses Association. (1980). *Nursing: A social policy statement*. Kansas City, MO: Author.
Anderson, E.T. (1990, Fall). Community diagnosis: A guide for planning. *Visions* (A publication of Population-Focused Community Health Nursing Education at Pacific Lutheran University, Tacoma, WA), 8–10.
Bjaras, G. (1993). The potential of community diagnosis as a tool in planning an intervention programme aimed at preventing injuries. *Accident Analysis & Prevention, 25*, 3–10.
Stoner, M.H., Magilvy, J.K., & Schultz, P.R. (1992). Community analysis in community health nursing practice: The GENESIS Model. *Public Health Nursing, 9*, 223–227.
US Department of Health and Human Services. Public Health Service. (1990). *Healthy People 2000: National health promotion and disease prevention objectives*. Washington, DC: US Government Printing Office.
US Department of Health and Human Services. Office of Disease Prevention and Health Promotion. (1997). *Developing objectives for Healthy People 2010*. Washington, DC: US Government Printing Office.

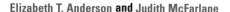

Elizabeth T. Anderson **and** Judith McFarlane

C H A P T E R

PLANNING A COMMUNITY HEALTH PROGRAM

11

OBJECTIVES

This chapter covers the planning of nursing actions to promote the health of a community.

After studying this chapter, you should be able to

- Validate your community nursing diagnoses with your community.
- Use principles of change theory to direct the planning process.
- In partnership with the community, plan a community-focused health program that includes
  - Measurable goals and behavioral objectives
  - A sequence of actions and a time schedule for achieving goals
  - Resources needed to accomplish the plan
  - Potential obstacles to planned actions and revised actions
  - Revisions to the plan as goals and objectives are achieved or changed
  - A recording of the plan in a concise, standardized, and retrievable form.

INTRODUCTION

Once a community's health has been assessed, the data analyzed, and community nursing diagnoses derived, it is time to consider nursing interventions that will promote the community's health—to formulate a community-focused plan. Each of the three parts of the diagnosis statement—the descriptions of the actual or potential problem, its causes, and its signs and symptoms—directs planning efforts for the nurse. All three provide equally important information from which to plan. Figure 11–1 displays the process for deriving a community nursing diagnosis and summarizes how the parts of the diagnosis both describe the community assessment and give direction for program planning, intervention, and evaluation. Community-focused plans are based on the nursing diagnoses and contain specific goals and interventions for achieving

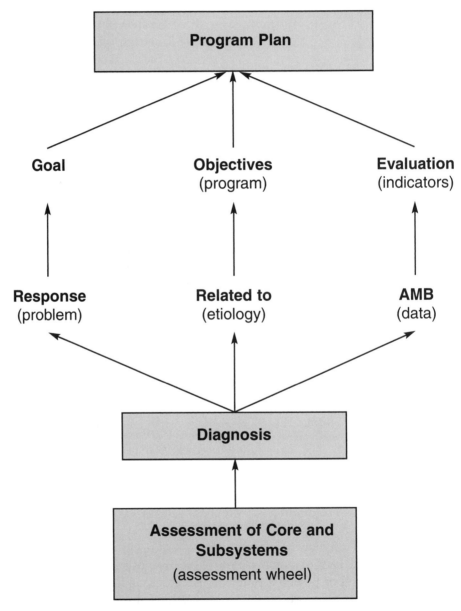

Figure 11–1. Basis for program planning.

desired outcomes. Planning, like assessment and analysis, is a systematic process completed in partnership with the community.

TAKE NOTE

Before proceeding, let's stop and consider the word *partnership* and its implications for community health nursing. Recall that a community is a social group determined by geographic boundaries and common values and interests. Community members function and interact within a particular social structure that both creates and exhibits behaviors and values. The normative behaviors and value systems of individuals, families, and the community that you have assessed may be very different from your own individual and family behaviors and values as well as the shared values of the community in which you reside. This creates a potential conflict. What may appear to you as a primary health problem of the community (for example, the incomplete immunization status at Temple Elementary in Rosemont) may not hold the same importance for the community's residents. They may be far more concerned about the possibility of being criminally victimized. Hence, there is a real need to validate community nursing diagnoses with the community. There is one question to ask: Are the community nursing diagnoses of importance to community residents? Methods of validating community nursing diagnoses will be presented in this chapter.

Validating your community nursing diagnoses with the community residents is an important step for establishing and maintaining the partnership. Equally important is the right of community leaders, organizations, and residents to confidentiality of privileged information and their right to choose not to participate in health planning. Communities have the right to identify their own health needs and to negotiate with the community health nurse with regard to interventions and specific programs. In turn, the community health nurse has the responsibility to provide or assist with the development of information needed for this process. The American Nurses Association's *Code for Nurses With Interpretive Standards* (1985) provides a guide for the many human rights issues that the community health nurse encounters.

In addition to forming a partnership with the community, the community health nurse must consider the influences of social, economic, ecologic, and political issues. Many (if not all) community health issues are directly and profoundly affected by larger policy issues. The high prevalence of dental caries among youngsters at Temple Elementary is related as much to the lack of fluoride in Rosemont's drinking water as it is to the lack of dental hygiene education at the school. In turn, each etiologic antecedent is influenced by city, county, state, and national legislative actions and policies. None of the nursing diagnoses for Rosemont can be considered to be separate from the remaining diagnoses; all diagnoses document the health status of Rosemont and must be considered as a whole during the community-focused planning.

Additional considerations of the nurse who is involved in community-focused health planning are the health needs of populations at risk. Special at-risk groups reside in all communities—the homeless, the poor, people who are infected with HIV, pregnant women, infants, children, and the elderly are groups at increased risk for decreased health status. The health needs of at-risk groups must be considered as part of all community health plans.

Last, community-focused planning involves an awareness and application of planned change—a process of well-thought-out actions to make something happen. Planned change is discussed in detail later in this chapter.

VALIDATING COMMUNITY NURSING DIAGNOSES

In reviewing the community nursing diagnoses for Rosemont (see Table 10–9), it can be seen that several diagnoses focus on the health status of children and others focus on the health of special groups such as the Asian and gay male populations. Many diagnoses seem to affect all residents, such as the stress and anxiety of being criminally victimized. It may be helpful to stop and review your community nursing diagnoses and categorize them according to the population most affected. A categorization of Rosemont's diagnoses appears in the displayed material, Community Nursing Diagnoses for Rosemont by Population Group.

Because several diagnoses focus on children and because the age and dependency status of children place them at increased risk of decreased health status, a decision was made to begin the planning process by validating the diagnoses that focused on children.

PLANNED CHANGE

We all experience change. As you read these words, your knowledge level is changing. Yet planned change differs from change in that actions occur in a definite sequence, with each one serving as preparation for the next. Planned change is a well-thought-out effort designed to make something happen; all efforts are directed and targeted to produce change. (Many theorists have written about planned change; several works are listed at the end of this chapter.) Reinkemeyer's stages of planned change are presented in the displayed material. The stages are like a recipe in that to produce the intended outcome, it is helpful to follow them strictly and completely to reach the intended outcomes.

One theorist, Kurt Lewin (1958), described three stages of planned change: unfreezing, moving, and refreezing, as shown in the displayed material on

Community Nursing Diagnosis for Rosemont by Population Group

Children

■ Potential for accidents (for example, trauma or suffocation as children explore abandoned machinery)

Specific to children at Temple elementary:

■ Truancy and academic failure
■ Incomplete immunization status
■ High prevalence of pediculosis capitus
■ High prevalence of dental caries
■ Lack of health promotion information, including nutrition, exercise, and safety

Infants

■ High infant, neonatal, and fetal mortality rate

Gay Men

■ Stress within Rosemont between the gay and heterosexual populations (especially the older heterosexuals)
■ Potential for inadequate coping of people with sexually transmitted diseases

All Rosemont Residents

■ Stress and anxiety of being criminally victimized
■ Potential for health problems associated with air pollution
■ At Rosemont Health Center, unsafe working environment

Lewin. It is during the unfreezing stage that the client system (in other words, the organization, community, or at-risk population) becomes aware of a problem and the need for change. Then the problem is diagnosed, and solutions to the problem are identified. From these alternative solutions, one is chosen that seems most appropriate for the situation. In the moving stage, the change actually occurs. The problem is clarified, and the program for solving the problem is planned in detail and begun. Finally, the refreezing stage consists of the accomplished changes becoming integrated into the values of the client system. In this stage, the idea is established and continues to be influential. Lewin also addressed forces that help or hinder change to occur, labeling them the driving forces and the restraining forces, respectively.

Reinkemeyer's Stages of Planned Change

Stage 1   Development of a felt need and desire for the change
Stage 2   Development of a change relationship between the agent and the client system
Stage 3   Clarification or diagnosis of the client system's problem, need, or objective
Stage 4   Examination of alternative routes and tentative goals and intentions of actions
Stage 5   Transformation of intentions into actual change
Stage 6   Stabilization
Stage 7   Termination of the relationship between the change agent and the client system

Reinkemeyer, A. (1970). Nursing's need: Commitment to an ideology & change. *Nursing Forum, 9*(4), 340–355.

Lewin's Stages of Planned Change and Their Application to the Planning Process

Lewin's Stages of Planned Change	Application to the Planning Process
>> ♦ Unfreezing	♦ Unfreezing ● Identification of a need for change
>> >> ♦ Moving process	♦ Moving process ● Presence of a change agent ● Identification of problems ● Consideration of alternatives ● Adaptation of plan to circumstances
>> >> >> ♦ Refreezing	♦ Refreezing ● Implementation of the plan ● Stabilization of the situation

Lewin, K. (1958). Group decision and social change. In E. Maccoby (Ed.), *Readings in social psychology* (3rd ed.). New York, NY: Holt, Rinehart and Winston.

Theories of planned change are important because they can be used to guide and direct the planning process.

APPLYING CHANGE THEORY TO COMMUNITY HEALTH PLANNING

To validate our nursing diagnoses and initiate the planning process, Reinkemeyer's stages of planned change have been chosen as a guide.

Stage 1: Development of a Felt Need and Desire for the Change

To initiate a felt need and desire for change within the Rosemont community, those organizations that reported actual or potential health concerns of youngsters were contacted, and a meeting was suggested in order to report the findings of the Rosemont community assessment. Meetings were arranged with the staffs of Temple Elementary, the Third Street Clinic, and the YMCA Indo–Chinese Refugee Program. During the meetings, input from all staff members was sought regarding their observations and perceptions of child health needs as well as their desire to become involved in a planned program of health promotion.

Temple Elementary requested that the assessment data be shared with representatives of the Parent Teacher Organization (PTO) as well as with the school's newly formed parent–teacher liaison group. Both the Third Street Clinic and the YMCA Indo–Chinese Refugee Program requested a presentation to their community advisory boards.

Stage 2: Development of a Change Relationship Between the Agent and the Client (Partner) System

Both Stages 1 and 2 were completed during the assessment presentations. All staff members were keenly aware of child health needs, and each organization desired to become involved in the planning process. To expedite planning, the Rosemont Health Promotion Council was formed. Each of the three organizations, Temple Elementary, the Third Street Clinic, and the YMCA Indo–Chinese Refugee Program, decided to send one staff member and one interested parent to the planning meetings. At this point, the community health nurse functioned as a change agent to guide and facilitate but not to direct the planning process. The council elected a chairperson and agreed on meeting dates. The purpose of the council was to coordinate interagency planning for a community-focused health-promotion program.

Stage 3: Clarification or Diagnosis of the Client System's Problem, Need, or Objective

Now the time has arrived to validate the community nursing diagnoses. At the conclusion of each presentation, the community health nurse proposed a survey questionnaire to assess the target population's perception of their health concerns. Revisions were solicited from staff and community groups, and the final, agreed-on questionnaire is presented here. Notice that the questionnaire is directed to parents, yet the nursing diagnoses are focused on children. Why not ask the children? This suggestion was made by several council participants. Some members felt two questionnaires were necessary—one for the parents and one for the youngsters. What do you think? Because of the age of the youngsters (some had not learned how to read) and the associated time and costs of two questionnaires, it was decided to use one questionnaire directed at the parents. The questionnaire is presented in Figure 11-2.

Although the Rosemont questionnaire is focused on child health, the same format could be used to validate assessed health concerns of the elderly, well adults, teenagers, or pregnant women. The process of checking your assessed community data against the perceptions of the target population can be completed by a survey questionnaire (such as the one in the displayed material) that can be mailed or given as an interview. Or you may choose to validate assessed data by interviewing community leaders and civic groups that are representative of the target population. The word *representative* is very important. For example, the Temple Elementary PTO would not be representative of parents in Rosemont because, as was noted during the assessment, most parents are not active in the organization.

Before we continue, a few words are needed about composing questionnaires. Everyone is confronted daily with people who are asking questions. Questionnaires arrive in the mail, and people call on the phone. Frequently, the interviewees neither learn the purpose of the questionnaire nor how the information will be used. When you draft a questionnaire, begin with introductory information that states who you are and what the purpose of the questionnaire is. Emphasize that participation is voluntary and that the information given will be confidential. Sign your name and, if the questionnaire is to be mailed,

Dear Parent:

We are nursing students who are interested in learning more about what you think are the most important health needs of your family. Answering a few short questions will help us plan some information sessions for you about how to keep your family healthy. Please either place a √ in the appropriate box or fill in the line. Your participation is voluntary. All information is confidential, and you will not be identified in any way. If you have questions, please feel free to call us. Thank you.

Virginia Brown
Ricardo Guerrero
Ann Nguyen
Alice Washington

1. How many children do you have?
2. What are their ages?
3. If you have a baby, do you breast-feed? Yes [ ] No [ ]
4. If you have a baby, do you bottle-feed? Yes [ ] No [ ]
5. What other foods do you feed your baby?
6. What foods do you usually feed your children?
7. Would you like to know more about what to feed your baby and children to keep them healthy? Yes [ ] No [ ]
8. Would you like to know where you can take your children for health care, both when they are well and sick? Yes [ ] No [ ]
9. Check (√) the following common problems you would like to know more about.
   [ ] Vomiting
   [ ] Diarrhea
   [ ] Colds and allergies
   [ ] Skin rashes
   [ ] Cuts and falls
   [ ] Head lice
   [ ] Worms
   [ ] Fever
   [ ] Temper tantrums and angry behaviors
   [ ] Refusal to do homework or go to school
   [ ] Poor school grades
10. Other concerns that you would like information about (this can include information for yourself, a friend, or a child):
   _____
   _____

11. Have you ever felt that you, a sibling, or another adult hurt your child when the child was punished? Yes [ ] No [ ]
12. Would you like to learn about ways to keep from hurting children when adults are angry? Yes [ ] No [ ]   *Continued*

Figure 11–2. Questionnaire to Validate Community Nursing Diagnosis.

13. Circle the best days and times for you to attend information sessions.

Monday	am	pm
Tuesday	am	pm
Wednesday	am	pm
Thursday	am	pm
Friday	am	pm
Saturday	am	pm
Sunday	am	pm

14. Circle the best place for you to attend information sessions:

Temple Elementary
Third Street Clinic
YMCA
Other (specify where)

Figure 11–2 *(Continued).*

include a phone number where you can be contacted. Write questions that can be answered quickly (the whole questionnaire should not take longer than 10 minutes to complete). Ideally, place all questions on one side of a standard 8½-inch by 11-inch piece of paper that, if it is to be mailed, can be refolded so that a return address shows. Before sharing the questionnaire with agencies or community residents, administer it informally to friends and family; any comments made (such as "What do you mean by . . .?" or "I don't understand. . . .") signal the need for further rewriting and clarification.

Because Rosemont has a large population of Spanish- and Vietnamese-speaking residents, staff at Temple Elementary and the YMCA Indo–Chinese Refugee Program volunteered to translate the questionnaire into these languages. The questionnaire was then ready for distribution.

TAKE NOTE

How should the questionnaire be administered? Should the questionnaire be mailed to all households of children at Temple Elementary? Should the questionnaire be given to all adults who bring their children to the Third Street Clinic? Or should the questionnaire be used as an interview and given to a selected number of parents at Temple Elementary or to clients at the Third Street Clinic or to adults attending the YMCA Indo–Chinese Refugee Program? (Recall from research that people who have been randomly selected can be considered representative of the total population.) What would you recommend? Before making a decision, list each option and consider the benefits and drawbacks of each. Here is some information for your decision making: Mailed questionnaires have about a 50% return rate that can be increased somewhat with a reminder postcard or telephone call, whereas questionnaires administered as an interview potentially have a 100% return rate. However, interviews require interviewers and about 5 minutes per person per page of questionnaire, whereas mailed questionnaires require less labor but have the financial cost of postage. Decisions . . . decisions. . . .

After several discussions of the Rosemont Health Promotion Council, it was decided to distribute the questionnaire from Temple Elementary by sending one form home with each child. The questionnaires were color-coded by language, and each child was given a questionnaire in the language that was spoken commonly at home.

Within 2 weeks, 410 of the 736 questionnaires had been returned. The results were tabulated and summarized by the community health nurse and the student nurses from the local university who were helping her. The summaries were then presented to the Rosemont Health Promotion Council. Examples of the summarized data are presented in Tables 11–1 through 11–4. Why do you think the information was presented by ethnicity? What differences do you notice between family composition and ethnicity, health information desired and ethnicity, and further concerns and ethnicity? Of what importance are these ethnic differences for community health planning?

TAKE NOTE

The Rosemont questionnaires were categorized by ethnicity (surmised from the language commonly spoken in the home). However, depending on the community, responses may be categorized by urban versus rural residence, age of respondents, or other meaningful variables. Once summarized, no preferred day and time emerged for the classes. However, a definite preference was shown for location, with all Vietnamese-speaking families preferring the YMCA location and Spanish-speaking clients preferring the Third Street Clinic.

Stage 4: Examination of Alternative Routes and Tentative Goals and Intention of Actions

Having validated the community nursing diagnoses, the Rosemont Health Promotion Council was anxious to establish a plan. Much discussion followed the presentation of the questionnaire results. Representatives from Temple

TABLE 11–1 ■ Family Composition by Ethnicity						
	Hispanic		Vietnamese		Other*	
Number of Children	**N**	**%**	**N**	**%**	**N**	**%**
One only	82	57	44	61	31	16
Two children	12	8	3	4	112	58
Three children	24	17	10	14	34	18
Four or more children	26	18	15	21	17	8
Total	144	100	72	100	194	100

*Primarily white and black.

TABLE 11-2 ■ Health Information Desired by Ethnicity

	Hispanic		Vietnamese		Other*	
	N	%	N	%	N	%
Vomiting	124	86	65	90	22	11
Diarrhea	134	93	71	98	34	18
Skin rashes	114	79	11	15	52	29
Cuts/falls	45	31	60	83	5	3
Colds/allergies	46	32	5	7	62	32
Head lice	24	17	10	14	74	38
Worms	85	59	70	97	10	5
Fever	132	92	69	96	93	48
Tantrums/angry behavior	10	7	4	5	175	90
School refusal	5	3	6	8	165	85
Poor grades	4	3	2	3	132	68
Total respondents	144		72		194	

*Primarily white and black.

Elementary focused on questions 9 and 10 and were anxious to present a series of effective parenting seminars on discipline. Temple also felt the high percentage of white and black families who requested information about school phobias and poor grades merited sessions on that topic. Temple's staff discussed how programs to meet the questionnaire needs were consistent with the school's goal of improved communication between teachers and parents as well as with the goals of their Failproof program. In addition, recent state programs developed to prevent child abuse were proposed for presentation.

TABLE 11-3 ■ Percentage of Respondents Noting Other Concerns by Ethnicity

	Hispanic (%)	Vietnamese (%)	Other (%)*
Legal issues (child support, custody rights)	32	15	64
Finances/budgeting	23	26	51
Child-care programs	82	12	75
Adult health (weight reduction, birth control)	75	11	68
Employment	82	95	75
Crime prevention, especially prevention of rape and child molestation	88	84	89

*Primarily white and black.

TABLE 11–4 ■ Percentage of Respondents Answering Yes to Questions 11 and 12 by Ethnicity

	Answered Yes		
	Hispanic (%)	Vietnamese (%)	Other (%)*
Question 11: Have you ever felt that you, a sibling, or another adult hurt your child when the child was punished?	89	92	94
Question 12: Would you like to learn about ways to keep from hurting children when adults are angry?	94	95	98

*Primarily white and black.

The staff of the Third Street Clinic focused on the families with infants and the associated desire for information on nutrition and the care of common health conditions. The Third Street Clinic had recently initiated a Healthy Baby Program, consisting of evening and Saturday well-child and prenatal clinics as well as a total service day on Friday when clients could drop in without appointments for immunizations and screening tests for blood pressure, vision, and hearing. Informal counseling was also offered on Friday. The goal for the next 6 months was to invite various service providers, such as optometry and dental hygiene students as well as Medicare and State Unemployment Commission representatives, to jointly use the clinic space for information sessions and services. After considering the results of the questionnaire, the staff began to discuss the possibility of offering health promotion classes on Fridays that would focus on weight reduction, exercise fitness, and information about common conditions. The idea of inviting the police department to make presentations on crime prevention and legal rights was proposed and agreed on by everyone.

Representatives from the YMCA Indo–Chinese Refugee Program believed that, because of cultural taboos against discussing topics such as birth control in public, the information would be best accepted if offered at the YMCA by a respected member of the Vietnamese community. The YMCA was beginning a day care service for mothers of preschoolers, and staff members believed that some of the information on child care could become part of the new program, as well as basic child health screening services of development, vision, and hearing. The YMCA representatives were equally concerned that Vietnamese refugees be culturally assimilated into the Rosemont community, and they wanted to plan interagency programs about crime prevention and legal rights that would bring the Vietnamese into more contact with other Rosemont residents. The suggestion was made that a program on crime prevention would bring not only residents of different cultures together but also residents of different lifestyles. Keenly aware of the tension and stress between the homosexual and heterosexual populations, a community awareness program on crime prevention was suggested that would involve all three agencies and all residents of Rosemont. The idea was agreed on by all council members.

TAKE NOTE

Notice that each agency is considering how information learned from the questionnaire can be assimilated into existing or planned programs. All agencies have budgets and a set number of staff members to deliver services. Agencies must be as cost-efficient as possible and will want to consider how to include new services (such as information desired by parents) into an existing program. Community health nurses can facilitate this process by becoming familiar with the organizational structure and purpose of each agency. When you establish a planned-change relationship with an agency, ask about their organizational structure (most agencies have an organizational chart with positions arranged according to authority). Decision making usually follows the organizational chart, with consent from all levels being required before major changes can be made or a new program can be begun. Learn the names of the staff members and their position on the organizational chart. (An organizational chart for the Third Street Clinic appears in Figure 11–3.) Ask for a statement of the agency's mission and goals. Ask if you can attend a board meeting and pertinent committee meetings. Your purpose is to learn as much as possible about the services and decision-making process of the agency to facilitate the planned-change nursing interventions.

COMMUNITY HEALTH GOAL

Now is the time to transform the ideas and proposals of each agency into a community-focused goal and concrete intentions of action. After validating the nursing diagnoses with the community, the community-focused goal was this: to provide health-promotion programs on issues desired by the community residents, using methods acceptable to cultural norms and offered in an accessible location at a cost the community can afford.

This is a very comprehensive statement and can be considered to be an umbrella goal for the Rosemont community under which each agency will have goals. Goals specific to Temple Elementary included

- Reduce truancy 20% by the end of one school year
- Reduce grade failures 20% by the end of one school year

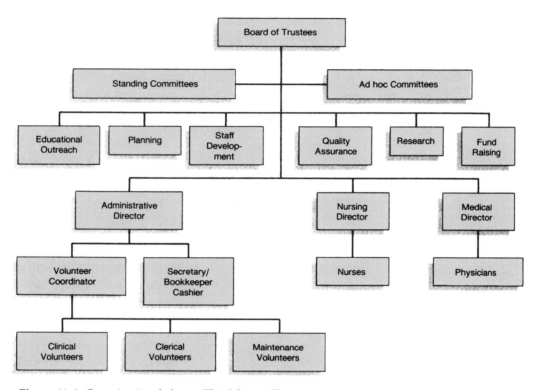

Figure 11–3. Organizational chart—Third Street Clinic.

- Increase immunization levels to 95% within one year
- Improve communication between parents and teachers
- Increase parental knowledge on how to protect children from molestation

Goals for the Third Street Clinic that were congruent with the community goal included

- Increased knowledge of community residents regarding crime prevention and legal rights
- Increased knowledge of parents regarding common health problems of children
- Increased knowledge and practice of effective parenting skills
- Increased percentage of adults who practice healthy lifestyle practices, including
  - Exercise fitness
  - Weight control
  - Stress management

Goals for the YMCA Indo–Chinese Refugee Program included

- 100% of children in the day care program screened for vision and hearing problems
- Increased knowledge and correct use of contraceptives
- Increased knowledge of parents regarding common health problems of children
- Increased rate of employed adults by 50%
- Increased rate of employed teenagers by 20%
- Increased knowledge of community residents regarding crime prevention and legal rights

PROGRAM ACTIVITIES

After formulation of goals, the next step is specifying the program activities. Program activities map out the actions necessary to deliver the program and thereby reach the goal(s). For example, one goal of the Third Street Clinic was increased knowledge of parents regarding health problems of children. Program activities for the goal might include

- Third Street Clinic staff and the community health nurse will select topics that are congruent with the questionnaire results to be included in classes for parents on common health problems of children.
- Third Street Clinic staff and the community health nurse will select resources (such as audiovisual aids and pamphlets) for presentation on the selected topics.
- Third Street Clinic staff and the community health nurse will decide on a day, time, and presentation schedule that are congruent with the questionnaire results.

Each program activity deals with planning the program and is written as sequential steps, each step being required to reach the goal. In addition, each program activity needs a date of accomplishment (for example: "By June 15th, the Third Street Clinic staff and the community health nurse will...").

LEARNING OBJECTIVES

Once program activities have been established, learning objectives are written. Learning objectives are derived from a goal and describe the precise behavior or changes that will be required to achieve the goal. Whereas program activities map out the actions necessary to deliver the program, learning objectives specify what changes in knowledge, behaviors, or attitudes are expected as a result of program activities.

Learning objectives focus on the learner and state what changes the learner can expect as a result of participating in the program. For example, one topic selected for presentation during the classes on common health problems of children was fever assessment and home management. The learning objectives were as follows:

- After the class and practice session on fever assessment and management of the fever at home, each participant will be able to
  - Demonstrate how to take a rectal and axillary temperature
  - Discuss common causes and dangers of fever during childhood
  - State what constitutes a fever
  - Explain at least three methods to reduce a fever
  - Describe danger signs that require a medical assessment

Both program and learning objectives can be written in sequential steps that are required to reach the goal, or each objective may have different aspects that, when combined, achieve the goal. Goals and objectives need to be measurable. To make statements measurable, use precise words. Examples of precise terms and less precise terms appear below:

Less Precise Terms (many interpretations)

To know
To understand
To realize
To appreciate
To be aware
To lower

More Precise Terms (fewer interpretations)

To identify
To discuss
To list
To compare and contrast
To state
To decrease by 20%

In addition, strive for each goal and objective to include

- A time frame for attaining the change (for example, "By June 15th . . .")
- The direction and magnitude of the change (for example, "Increase immunization levels to 95%")

• The method of measuring the change (for example, "After the session, each participant will demonstrate . . .")

Goals and subparts of the goals (objectives) help to clarify a program and establish the expected changes that will result from the program. Although much has been written on the mechanics of writing goals and objectives (several such texts are listed at the conclusion of this chapter), little information exists on the collaborative relationship that must exist between the community health nurse and community agency(ies) before meaningful goals and objectives can result.

COLLABORATION

What is meant by a collaborative relationship? Recall from the initial community assessment data that the staff of Temple Elementary had voiced concerns about truancy and grade failure; these same concerns are their first two goals. However, when the nursing diagnoses were validated with the community, parents were more concerned about ways in which they could protect their children from molestation. Could the concerns of the parents and those of the Temple Elementary staff be addressed in the same program? If they could, what would be the program goal? the objectives? This process is an example of collaborative planning and is the essence of community health nursing. You may be wondering how to establish collaborative planning and inform agencies about the usefulness of goals and objectives. Although you may be convinced of the value of planned change, how do you convince others to agree, especially because planned change is not commonly practiced in agencies? Role modeling is probably the best strategy. After reviewing the community nursing diagnoses and validating data with an agency, propose goals and objectives that are congruent with the agency's purpose and organizational structure. Solicit input from the group and continue to revise the goals and objectives until a group consensus is reached.

RESOURCES, CONSTRAINTS, AND REVISED PLANS

Once goals and objectives are written, the next step is to identify available resources and any constraints to the plan. These are analogous to Lewin's driving and restraining forces. Last, revised plans are proposed to the planning group. Resources are all the available means for accomplishing a task, including staff and budget as well as physical space and equipment. Recall that part of your community assessment included the identification of strengths. As you consider resources, include those strengths that may facilitate meeting program goals and objectives. For program planning, it is important to identify the resources needed as well as the resources available. Constraints are obstacles that restrict or limit actions and can include a lack of staff, budget, physical space, and equipment. Constraints may be thought of as the difference between needs and resources. Revised plans are actions that are proposed based on the knowledge of resources and constraints.

Following much discussion and self-examination, each agency of the Rosemont Health Promotion Council formed program goals and objectives. Then, alongside each goal and objective, necessary resources were listed. For example, at the Third Street Clinic, the following resources were identified as crucial to the goal:

 To increase the knowledge of parents regarding common health problems of children

Resources Needed

- Staff member to develop and assemble existing information on common health problems of children
- Staff member to present the information materials in English, Spanish, and Vietnamese
- Physical space and necessary equipment (eg, thermometers, basins) to teach assessment and home care skills

Resources Available

- Staff members who speak English and Spanish
- Staff nurse knowledgeable about the care of children
- Physical space and some necessary equipment
- Staff interest and desire to offer information requested by parents

Constraints

It may be helpful to consider constraints as the mismatch between resources needed and resources available. Constraints at the Third Street Clinic include:

- No staff member who speaks Vietnamese
- Discomfort of staff because of inexperience in developing and adapting learning materials

- Time limitations
- Staff members' insecurity about their ability to perform group teaching (all previous teaching was one on one)
- Lack of resource material (for example, audiovisuals and brochures on care of common childhood problems)

TAKE NOTE

Universal constraints are staff and money—agencies never have enough. An additional constraint is resistance to change. All people are reluctant to change existing routines and patterns of behavior. Initially, change is uncomfortable, and until new roles are learned, there is anxiety. Making people aware of the natural discomfort associated with change can build rapport and establish a collaborative relationship.

When each agency had listed its program goals, objectives, and activities, along with resources and constraints, several alternative actions became apparent. For example, a constraint of the Third Street Clinic was lack of staff members who spoke Vietnamese. A similar constraint of the YMCA Indo–Chinese Refugee Program was lack of a staff with necessary knowledge to offer classes on contraception or the care of children with common health problems. Therefore, the following revised plan was proposed:

R E V I S E D   P L A N

A bilingual (English–Vietnamese) staff member from the YMCA would attend the classes offered in English at the Third Street Clinic and then offer the classes in Vietnamese at the YMCA.

Both the Third Street Clinic and the YMCA noted a lack of resource materials as a constraint to program implementation. Further assessment of community health resources by the community health nurse revealed that the Sunvalley Clinic, as part of the Hampton Health Department, had access to various audiovisual aids and printed materials on the subjects; however, all materials were in English.

R E V I S E D   P L A N

One Spanish–English–speaking staff member from the Third Street Clinic and one Vietnamese–English–speaking staff member from the YMCA would translate the materials into Spanish and Vietnamese free of charge with the provision that they be given copies of all the translated materials.

An additional constraint to each agency was that their staffs felt unprepared to do group instruction.

REVISED PLAN

The community health nurse would provide instruction in basic principles of group teaching, including methods of presenting information. In addition, the community health nurse would participate in the development and adaptation of materials and the teaching of classes.

For each constraint, a revised plan was proposed, discussed, and adopted. This is a period of intense collaboration between the community health nurse and community agencies, and only at the completion of this stage is the community ready for stage 5 of planned change—transformation of intentions into actual change behavior. This transformation of intentions is the actual program implementation (which is covered in the next chapter). However, before the plan is implemented, it must be recorded.

RECORDING

Community plans must be recorded in a standardized, systematic, and concise form that clearly communicates to others the purpose and actions of the plan as well as the rationale for revisions and deletions of actions. Discuss with each agency its present recording system and decide on a format and system for recording the plan. The format need not be elaborate, and a simple one such as that used at the Third Street Clinic would be adequate if agreed on by the agency.

SUMMARY

Before concluding, let's review the learning objectives for this chapter and their application to community health nursing. The planning process begins with validation of the community nursing diagnoses—a process that establishes the community's perception and value of community health needs. Next, using theories of planned change, the community health nurse and the community form a collaborative partnership to establish program goals and objectives. Last, based on resources and constraints, plans are proposed, recorded, and adopted. Although only one example is offered here, the process of community health planning was the same for all eight programs that were developed by the Rosemont Health Promotion Council.

REFERENCES

American Nurses Association. (1985). *Code for nurses with interpretive standards*. Kansas City, MO: Author.

Lewin, K. (1958). Group decision and social change. In E. Maccoby (Ed.), *Readings in social psychology* (3rd ed.). New York, NY: Holt, Rinehart and Winston.

Reinkemeyer, A. (1970). Nursing's need: Commitment to an ideology & change. *Nursing Forum, 9*(4), 340–355.

SUGGESTED READINGS

Bertera, R.L. (1990). Planning and implementing health promotion in the workplace: A case study of the DuPont Company experience. *Health Education Quarterly, 17*(3), 307–327.

deVries, H., Weijts, W., Dijkstra, M., & Kok, G. (1992). The utilization of qualitative and quantitative data for health education program planning, implementation, and evaluation: A spiral approach. *Health Education Quarterly, 19*(1), 101–115.

Dignan, M.B. & Carr, P.A. (1992). *Program planning for health education and promotion* (2nd ed.). Malvern, PA: Lea & Febiger.

Ervin, N.E. & Kuehnert, P.L. (1993). Application of a model for public health nursing program planning. *Public Health Nursing, 10*(1), 25–30.

Green, L.W., Kreuter, M.W., Deeds, S.G., & Partridge, K.B. (1980). *Health education planning: A diagnostic approach*. Palo Alto, CA: Mayfield.

Lippitt, G. (1973). *Visualizing change: Model building and the change process*. La Jolla, CA: University Associates.

Lippitt, R., Watson, J., & Westley, B. (1951). *The dynamics of planned change*. New York, NY: Harcourt, Brace and World.

Elizabeth T. Anderson **and** Judith McFarlane

IMPLEMENTING A COMMUNITY HEALTH PROGRAM

12

OBJECTIVES

Implementation is the action phase of the nursing process: it is carrying out the community-focused plan. Implementation is necessary to achieve goals and objectives, but, more importantly, the implementation of nursing interventions acts to promote, maintain, or restore health; to prevent illness; and to effect rehabilitation.

This chapter discusses the process of implementing a community-focused health program. Intervention strategies are presented, as well as resources that are helpful in program implementation.

After studying this chapter, you should be able to

- Suggest strategies to the community for implementation of health programs
- In partnership with the community
  - Implement planned programs
  - Review and revise interventions based on community responses
  - Use interventions to formulate and influence health and social policies that have an impact on the health of the community.

INTRODUCTION

Once goals and objectives have been agreed on and recorded during the planning stage, all that remains for implementation is to actually carry out the activities to meet those objectives. This probably seems straightforward and simple.

Indeed, at this point, you will have spent considerable time assessing, analyzing, and planning a program. You will be ready and eager to begin. But this very eagerness (and the associated impatience of the intervention stage) is a danger. You must take time to consider how you can promote community ownership, a unified program, and a clear health focus.

TAKE NOTE

This chapter focuses on the *process* of intervention and provides you with some general resources that may prove helpful in your community work. Many excellent examples of interventions in which community health nurses work as partners with the community are included in the following section, Part III.

COMMUNITY OWNERSHIP

Essential to achieving the desired outcomes of the interventions is the active participation of the community. The meaning of partnership and collaboration was discussed in the preceding chapter, but the present concern is ownership. The people of the community need to feel a sense of ownership of the program or event, which can only come with their full participation in the decisions regarding planning as well as their assuming some responsibility for implementation. Herein lies a potential conflict. The profession of nursing is one of nurturing, sustaining, and caring for others. It is part of our profession to do *for* others what they would do for themselves if they were able. Indeed, most nurses interact professionally with people during an altered health state that requires nurses to do for others; but this is not true in community health nursing. Stepping into the community requires an attitude of doing *with* the people, not doing things to them or for them. When things are done to us or for us, our emotional commitment remains limited.

How might you ensure community ownership for a proposed program and planned interventions? How can you facilitate involvement? In Rosemont, the Rosemont Health Promotion Council functioned to coordinate interagency planning for a community-focused health-promotion program. When the planning had been completed, the council directed its attention to the coordination of activities for the program's implementation. The important point in this example is that a coordination group was already in place. Usually the planning committee can coordinate implementation.

TAKE **NOTE**

When the Rosemont Health Promotion Council and designated staff in charge of program implementation reviewed the program objectives and needed resources, it was evident that before the program could proceed, resources had to be selected. (Resources means audiovisual aids, pamphlets, and other material for presentation of the program.) Council and staff members began to ask where such materials could be obtained. What was available in Rosemont? What could you have suggested at this point?

Examining the initial assessment of Rosemont, it was noted that the United Way listed 42 private and publicly supported social service agencies located in Hampton or Jefferson County. The United Way listing included identifying information for each agency as well as services and fees. Reviewing the list with the council and participating staff, the community health nurse suggested that selected agency representatives be invited to discuss programs and resources that they could make available, such as films and speakers. It was found that several could provide relevant material. The March of Dimes was sponsoring a campaign in Hampton to increase public awareness of the importance of a healthy pregnancy for the birth of a healthy child. The Mental Health Association had developed teaching modules on effective parenting, and the police department and the Woman's Center were offering programs on crime prevention. All of these programs had recently received a brief description, including the names of their contact persons, in the *Hampton Herald*. At this point, it was decided to complete program and learning objectives for each of the health-promotion goals established by the Rosemont Council. Therefore, as various agency personnel discussed their program with the council, decisions could be made on the appropriateness of the material for the Rosemont Community.

TAKE **NOTE**

Do not panic at this point and feel that you must be knowledgeable about all 42 agencies and their programs in the community that you have assessed. At the implementation stage, do refer back to your initial assessment and consider logically which service agencies may have resources helpful to the planned program(s). Then contact selected agencies, request information on their purpose and present programs, share with the agency your community-focused program plans, and solicit recommendations with regard to materials and resources. Table 12–1 includes a list of voluntary organizations that have professional staff at the national and local levels and an affiliated or community linkage structure. These voluntary organizations have ongoing programs for a wide variety of health issues, and most acknowledge health promotion as a vital part of their mission. The list is not inclusive and is meant to serve only as a guide.

TABLE 12–1 ■ Voluntary Organizations (a partial listing)

Voluntary Organizations

American Association of Retired Persons	March of Dimes
American Cancer Society	National Board of the YMCA of the USA
American Heart Association	National Coalition of Hispanic Mental Health and Human Services Organizations
American Lung Association	
American Red Cross	National Council of Alcoholism
Association of Junior Leagues, Inc.	National Health Council
Boy Scouts of America	National Kidney Foundation
Boys' Clubs of America, Inc.	National Recreation and Parks Association
Cooperative Extension Service	National Safety Council
Girl Scouts of America	National Urban League
Girls' Clubs of America, Inc.	United Way of America

In addition, the Office of Disease Prevention and Health Promotion (ODPHP), located within the Public Health Service (PHS) (which, in turn, is located within the US Department of Health and Human Services [DHHS]), publishes a tremendous amount of information that is designed to promote health and prevent disease among Americans. Special attention is given to facilitating the prevention activities of the five public health service agencies: the Alcohol, Drug Abuse, and Mental Health Administration; the Centers for Disease Control and Prevention (CDC); the Food and Drug Administration (FDA); the Health Resources and Services Administration (HRSA); and the National Institutes of Health (NIH). Several special programs, termed *initiatives,* are sponsored by ODPHP. A partial listing of the initiatives, services, and information available, as well as websites, is included in Table 12–2.

TAKE NOTE

Several libraries are designated as government depositories and, therefore, have many government publications. The government also has bookstores located throughout the United States. The Suggested Readings list for this chapter contains several government publications and websites that are focused on disease prevention and health promotion. You will find the websites easy to access and very informative.

Having discussed the importance of community participation and ownership of the program, the remaining issues to consider are a unified presentation of the program and an emphasis on health, not the program.

TABLE 12–2 ■ Office of Disease Prevention and Health Promotion: Selected Programs and Initiatives

Program	Description	Contact
Healthy People	Launched in 1979; guides efforts to identify objectives for nation	www.health.gov/healthypeople odphp.osophs.dhhs.gov/pubs/hp2000
healthfinder	A gateway website to link consumers and professionals to health and human services information from the federal government. Reliable information via the Internet	www.healthfinder.gov
National Health Information Center	Central health information referral service for consumers and professionals	1-800-336-4797 nhic-nt.health.org
Dietary Guidelines for Americans	Published with the US Department of Agriculture; federally mandated nutrition education activities	odphp.osophs.dhhs.gov/pubs/dietguid
Healthy Communities, Worksites, and Schools	With National Coalition for Healthier Cities and Communities, focuses on ways that communities can adapt the national Healthy People objectives for local use	odphp.osophs.dhhs.gov/pubs

Source: odphp.osophs.dhhs.gov/odphpfact.htm

UNIFIED PROGRAM

Because of limited resources, staff constraints, and other situations beyond the control of the planners, many good programs are implemented in a piecemeal fashion that minimizes their impact. A unified program requires collaboration and coordination between the agency personnel who will implement the program and the program's recipients (the target population). Allowing plenty of time for publicizing the program (and how you perform the mechanics of publicity–the how, where, and to whom) can make a crucial difference in whether people attend and what the subsequent impact will be.

After a time and place have been selected (based on initial input from the survey questionnaires), how might you publicize a program? Public service announcements, notification in the newspapers, bulletin inserts for civic and religious associations, flyers sent home with school-age children, and posters and notices in community service buildings and local shopping centers are some of the methods to consider. The Rosemont Health Promotion Council decided to publicize the first program on child health by sending home a flyer with each child at Temple Elementary. The flyer thanked the parents for their participation during the survey and invited them to programs at the Third Street Clinic and the YMCA Indo–Chinese Refugee Center. Public service announcements were made on the radio, and feature articles about the Rosemont Health Promotion Council and upcoming programs appeared in the Vietnamese and Spanish newspapers as well as in the *Hampton Herald* and Rosemont Civic Association's newsletter. Posters were placed in local grocery stores, churches, and gathering places. Because the parents on the Rosemont Health Promotion Council had expressed a concern that parents with young children might not be able to attend programs, arrangements were made for infant and toddler child care, and a separate health program for preschool and school-age children was planned during the adult programs. The program publicity was focused on health promotion for the whole family and not just on programs for selected family members.

HEALTHY PEOPLE

The idea of a health program based on unified goals and objectives is central to the Healthy People documents. In 1979, the first "health" initiative for the United States, *Healthy People: The Surgeon General's Report to the Nation* (US Office of the Assistant Secretary for Health and Surgeon General, 1979) promoted five goals. These broad goals were focused on reducing mortality among targeted age groups—infants, children, adolescents, young adults, and adults—and on increasing the independence of older adults. They were our first "health" goals for the nation, and their target date was 1990.

Healthy People 2000 (US Department of Health and Human Services, 1990) followed and was developed through broad collaborative efforts among government, voluntary organizations, professional organizations, businesses, and individuals. Three goals provided the framework:

1. Increase the span of healthy life for Americans
2. Reduce health disparities among Americans
3. Achieve access to preventive services for all Americans

In addition, and organized under the approaches of health promotion, health protection, and preventive services, more than 300 objectives were included under 22 priority areas.

A new report, *Healthy People 2010*, represents input from thousands of Americans. Additionally, this new set of objectives, according to the introduction, "will be distinguished from *Healthy People 2000* by the broadened prevention science base; improved surveillance and data systems; a heightened awareness and demand for preventive health services and quality health care; and changes in demographics, science, technology and disease spread that will affect the public's health in the 21st century" (US Department of Health and Human Services, 1998, Introduction 1).

Two broad goals (eliminate health disparities, and increase quality and years of healthy life) provide the framework and are incorporated into the model for *Healthy People 2010* (Figure 12–1).

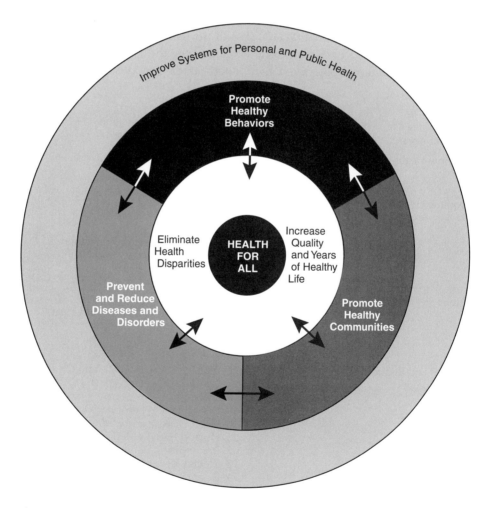

Figure 12–1. Healthy People 2010: Healthy People in Healthy Communities Model. Source: US Department of Health and Human Services. (1998). *Healthy People 2010 Objectives: Draft for Public Comment.* Washington, DC: Author.

Priorities for the specific objectives are listed in Table 12–3. For each area, there is a goal, a list of terminology, an overview, a description of progress toward year 2000 objectives, and the draft 2010 objectives. Numerous measurable objectives are included under each goal; for example, under Objective 22 (Immunization and Infectious Diseases) is "Achieve immunization coverage of at least 90 percent among children 19–35 months of age"(US Department of Health and Human Services, 1998). In that these objectives are based on national data, as well as rigorous criteria (Table 12–4), they can be used as standards against which we can compare local data.

As pointed out in the Healthy People 2010 draft document: "Healthy People 2010 is the United States' contribution to the World Health Organization's (WHO) 'Health for All' strategy. The US effort will be characterized by intersectoral collaboration and community participation. Through national objectives, the United States provides models for world policy and

TABLE 12–3 ■ Priority Areas for 2010 Objectives for the Nation	
General Area	**Specific Objectives**
Promote Healthy Behavior	1. Physical Activity and Fitness 2. Nutrition 3. Tobacco Use
Promote Health and Safety	4. Educational and Community-Based Programs 5. Environmental Health 6. Food Safety 7. Injury and Violence Prevention 8. Occupational Safety and Health 9. Oral Health
Improve Systems for Personal and Public Health	10. Access 11. Family Planning 12. Maternal, Infant, and Child Health 13. Medical Product Safety 14. Public Health Infrastructure 15. Health Communications
Prevent and Reduce Disease and Disorders	16. Arthritis, Osteoporosis, and Chronic Back Conditions 17. Cancer 18. Diabetes 19. Disability and Secondary Conditions 20. Heart Disease and Stroke 21. Human Immunodeficiency Virus 22. Immunization and Infectious Diseases 23. Mental Health and Mental Disorders 24. Respiratory Diseases 25. Sexually Transmitted Diseases 26. Substance Abuse

US Department of Health and Human Services. (1998). *Healthy People 2010 Objectives: Draft for Public Comment.* Washington, DC: Author.

TABLE 12–4 ■ Criteria for Objectives Development	
Objective Attribute	**Notes**
Important and understandable	Relate to 2010 framework and have broad audience
Prevention oriented	Should address health improvements that can be achieved through population-based and health-service intervention
Drive action	Including suggestion of steps that will achieve the proposed targets
Useful and relevant	Should be usable by states, localities, and private sector to target schools, communities, worksites, health practices, and other settings
Measurable	Should include a range of measures (health outcomes, behavioral and health-service interventions, and community capacity) directed toward improving health outcomes and quality of life
Build on *Healthy People 2000* goals	To provide continuity and comparability
Scientifically supported	Based on scientific evidence

US Department of Health and Human Services. (1998). *Healthy People 2010 Objectives: Draft for Public Comment.* Washington, DC: Author.

strategies for population health improvement" (US Department of Health and Human Services, 1998, Introduction 2).

TAKE NOTE

Are the goals and objectives for your community realistic in terms of the past and in relation to trends over time? Do the goals and objectives for your community-focused program further the national goals and objectives? When the Rosemont Health Promotion Council reviewed its goals and objectives, each was found to be congruent with the national plan as well as with Rosemont's state health department objectives for improved health.

HEALTH FOCUS

There is one remaining question to ask before initiating the program: Does it focus on health? This may seem to be a strange question. You might wonder, don't all community health programs focus on maintaining, restoring, or promoting health? Frequently, the answer is no.

In Rosemont, the council and designated staff had become very involved in planning specific activities and information modules associated with the community health program. Several programs had been enlarged to include screening and health fairs; additional activities were suggested at each council meeting. The initial goal of promoting the health of Rosemont residents had seemingly changed to providing Rosemont residents with lots of activities and information about health. What had happened? Remember, we discussed the impatience and eagerness that are often associated with new programs. This situation is normal. Committees tend to overemphasize activities and knowledge and forget the initial reason for the program—to improve health. But it should be remembered that it is the sustained day-to-day use of knowledge and lifestyle practices that improve health. Frequently, a program begins with enthusiastic momentum; media publicity attracts people to screening and information sessions—and then the program is over. Objectives are evaluated as having been achieved successfully, and another program is planned and implemented. But was there any real improvement in health? Did the participants change lifestyle practices? Will the changes be maintained and continued for a week? a month? a year? Most importantly, are the changed lifestyle or health practices supported by the surrounding environment and culture?

Environmental and Cultural Support

Many parents in Rosemont responded affirmatively to the survey questions about discipline. These parents believed that they or another person had hurt a child when the child was punished; the parents wanted to learn ways to keep from hurting children when adults were angry. The Rosemont Health Promotion Council responded with a series of programs on effective parenting that included information on various nonphysical strategies for disciplining youngsters as well as role-playing and open-discussion periods. However, as part of the community assessment, the community health nurse had recorded that the Hampton Independent School District (HISD) used physical punishment as a primary discipline method. Youngsters at Temple Elementary were hit on the buttocks with a wide board that frequently left large bruises. The conflict between the effective parenting programs and punishment methods at Temple Elementary was obvious. What could be done? What would you suggest?

In Rosemont, part of the planned effective-parenting classes included discussion sessions on the difference between discipline and punishment and the importance of inquiring as to disciplinary and punitive procedures when parents left their children for supervision, for example, at child care facilities and schools or with babysitters. Parents were asked to voice their feelings about the school district's policy on physical punishment. Although some parents were unaware of the school district's policy, most were aware of the punishment but believed the procedure could not be changed. After a discussion of parental rights and responsibilities, a group of parents made an appointment with the principal of Temple Elementary to discuss the situation. (After additional meetings with school board members, an open public hearing on public school discipline, and letters to state school board officials, the HISD changed the discipline policy to exclude physical punishment. The process took 2 years.)

Countless such incongruities exist between healthy lifestyles and environmental and cultural practices and policies. Here is one additional example: Recall that one community nursing diagnosis for youngsters at Temple Elementary was a high prevalence of dental caries. During the effective-parenting discussions, several parents commented that their children were given hard candy, usually suckers, as a reward for good behavior. When the nurse at Temple Elementary was contacted, it was verified that children exhibiting good behavior were given hard candy. This practice was done daily.

TAKE NOTE

Identify the environmental and cultural practices and policies that are in conflict with the proposed community-focused health program that resulted from your community assessment. What can be done to increase community awareness of these conflicts, and how can change begin? To focus on health and the maintenance of healthy lifestyles, all of the community must be involved.

The best way to maintain a focus on health and not on the activities of the program is to use your nursing practice model as a guide. The nursing practice model built and described in Chapter 8 (see Figure 8-2) defines intervention as primary, secondary, and tertiary levels of prevention. Do the programs proposed for Rosemont address these three levels of prevention?

Levels of Prevention

Recall that *primary prevention* improves the health and well-being of the community, making it less vulnerable to stressors. Health-promotion programs are primary prevention, as are programs that focus on protection from specific diseases. Usually health promotion is nonspecific and directed toward raising the general health of the total community (for example, teaching youngsters about nutritious foods or conducting adult exercise/fitness and stress-reduction sessions). Primary prevention can also be very specific, such as providing immunization against certain diseases. Additional primary prevention measures include the wearing of seat belts and the purification of public water supplies.

Secondary prevention begins after a disease or condition is present (although there may be no symptoms). Emphasis is on screening, early diagnosis, and treatment of possible stressors that may adversely affect the community's health. The tine test for tuberculosis, the Denver Developmental Screening Test for developmental delays, blood pressure assessments, and breast self-examinations are secondary prevention interventions.

Tertiary prevention focuses on restoration and rehabilitation. Tertiary prevention programs act to return the community to an optimum level of functioning. Adequate shelters for battered women and counseling and therapy programs for sexually abused youngsters are examples of tertiary prevention.

The distinction between prevention levels is not always clear. Is a program on the assessment of fever in children (and the prevention of febrile convulsions and dehydration through use of tepid baths and extra fluids) secondary or tertiary prevention? How would you classify an effective-parenting program? support groups for single parents? a crime prevention program? sessions on stress reduction and physical fitness? Can some programs be primary, secondary, and tertiary depending on the needs of the persons who attend? Certainly effective-parenting classes for the parent with a child who has a behavior problem will have a different purpose than classes designed for expectant parents of a first child. Likewise, the corporate executive who has been diagnosed with cardiovascular disease and placed on a low-cholesterol diet has very different nutritional learning needs from those of the senior citizen on a fixed income. Few programs are purely on one level of prevention.

The important point is to evaluate your programs (the implementation phase of the nursing process) and ask if the nursing interventions are consistent with the nursing practice model. If the focus is prevention, then are the programs directed toward prevention?

SUMMARY

Having considered the importance of community ownership of the program, the need to offer a unified program, and maintaining a focus on health, there remains one step in the process—evaluation. Before a program is implemented, the manner in which it is to be evaluated must be established. The following chapter explains why this final stage of the nursing process is essential before implementation.

REFERENCES

US Department of Health and Human Services. (1998). *Healthy people 2010 objectives: Draft for public comment.* Washington, DC: Author.

US Department of Health and Human Services. Public Health Service. (1990). *Healthy people 2000: National health promotion and disease prevention objectives.* Washington, DC: US Government Printing Office.

US Office of the Assistant Secretary for Health and Surgeon General. (1979). *Healthy people: The surgeon general's report on health promotion and disease prevention.* Washington, DC: US Government Printing Office.

SUGGESTED READINGS

Abraham, T. & Fallon, P.J. (1997). Caring for the community: Development of the advanced practice nurse role. *Clinical Nurse Specialist, 11*(5), 224–230.

American Public Health Association. (1991). *Healthy communities 2000: Model standards* (3rd ed.). Washington, DC: Author.

Anderson, E.T., Gottschalk, J., & Martin, D.A. (1993). Contemporary issues in the community. In D.J. Mason, S.W. Talbott, & J.K. Leavitt. *Policy and politics for nurses: Action and change in the workplace, government, organizations and community.* Philadelphia: WB Saunders.

Beddome, G., Clarke, H.F., & Whyte, N.B. (1993). Vision for the future of public health nursing: A case for primary health care. *Public Health Nursing, 1*(1), 13–18.

Chavis, D.M. & Florin, P. (1990). Nurturing grassroots initiatives for health and housing. *Bulletin of The New York Academy of Medicine, 66*(5), 558–572.

Courtney, R., Ballard, E., Fauver, S., Gariota, M., & Holland, L. (1996). The partnership model: Working with individuals, families, and communities toward a new vision of health. *Public Health Nursing, 13*(3), 177–186.

Dahl, S., Gustafson, C., & McCullagh, M. (1993). Collaborating to develop a community-based health service for rural homeless persons. *Journal of Nursing Administration, 23*(4), 41–45.

Durpa, K.C., Quick, M.M., Andrews, A., Engelke, M.K., & Vinvent, P. (1992). A collaborative health promotion effort: Nursing students and Wendy's team up. *Nurse Educator, 17*(6), 35–37.

El-Askari, G., Freestone, J., Irizarry, C., Mashiyama, S.T., Morgan, M.A., & Walton, S. (1998). The Healthy Neighborhoods Project: A local health department's role in catalyzing community development. *Health Education & Behavior, 25*(2), 146–159.

Farley, S. (1993). The community as partner in primary health care. *Nursing & Health Care, 14*(5), 244–249.

Flick, L.H., Reese, C., & Harris, A. (1996). Aggregate community-centered undergraduate community health nursing clinical experience. *Public Health Nursing, 13*(1), 36–41.

Flynn, B.C. (1997). Partnerships in healthy cities and communities: A social commitment for advanced practice nurses. *Advanced Practice Nursing Quarterly, 2*(4), 1–6.

Gamm, L.D. (1998). Advancing community health through community health partnerships. *Journal of Healthcare Management, 43*(1), 51–66.

Hawe, P., King, L., Noort, M., Gifford, S.M., & Lloyd, B. (1998). Working invisibly: Health workers talk about capacity-building in health promotion. *Health Promotion International, 13*(4), 285–295.

Hollinger-Smith, L. (1998). Partners in collaboration: The Homan Square Project. *Journal of Professional Nursing, 14*(6), 344–349.

Jenkins, S. (1991). Community wellness: A group empowerment model for rural America. *Journal of Health Care for the Poor and Underserved, 1*(4), 388–404.

Kinne, A., Thompson, B., Chrisman, N.J., & Hanley, J.R. (1989). Community organization to enhance the delivery of preventive health services. *American Journal of Preventive Medicine, 5*(4), 225–229.

Labonte, R. (1993). Community development and partnerships. *Canadian Journal of Public Health, 84*(4), 237–240.

Murashima, S., Hatono, Y., Whyte, N., & Asahara, K. (1999). Public health nursing in Japan: New opportunities for health promotion. *Public Health Nursing, 16*(2), 133–139.

Perino, S.S. (1992). Nike-footed health workers deal with the problems of adolescent pregnancy. *Public Health Reports, 107*(2), 208–212.

Primomo, J. (1990). Diapering decisions: A community education project. In *Notes from the field.* H. Tilson (Ed.), *American Journal of Public Health, 80*(6), 743–744.

Rutherford, G.S. & Campbell, D. (1993). Helping people help themselves. *Canadian Nurse, 89*(10), 25–28.

Scott, S. (1990). *Promoting healthy traditions workbook: A guide to the Healthy People Campaign.* St. Paul: American Indian Health Care Association.

Wardrop, K. (1993). A framework for health promotion. *Canadian Journal of Public Health, 84*(Suppl l), S9–S13.

Woodard, G.R. & Edouard, L. (1992). Reaching out: A community initiative for disadvantaged pregnant women. *Canadian Journal of Public Health, 83*(3), 188–190.

Elizabeth T. Anderson **and** Judith McFarlane

EVALUATING A COMMUNITY HEALTH PROGRAM

13

OBJECTIVES

Evaluation is determining the worth (or value) of something. During the evaluation process, information is collected and analyzed to determine its significance and worth. Changes are appraised, and progress is documented. This chapter discusses evaluation and the nursing practices that are necessary to plan and implement it.

After studying this chapter, you should be able to act in partnership with the community to

- Establish evaluation criteria that are timely and comprehensive.
- Use baseline and current data to measure progress toward goals and objectives.
- Validate observations, insights, and new data with colleagues and the community.
- Revise priorities, goals, and interventions based on evaluation data.
- Document and record evaluation results and revisions of the plan.
- Participate in evaluation research with appropriate consultation.
- Appreciate the complexity of program evaluation as well as the multiple paradigms that affect its implementation.

INTRODUCTION

The nurse evaluates the responses of the community to a health program in order to measure progress that is being made toward the program's goals and objectives. Evaluation data are also crucial for revision of the database and the community nursing diagnoses that were developed from analysis of the community assessment data.

Do you feel as if we are talking in circles? Evaluation is the "final" step of the nursing process, but it is linked to assessment, which is the first step. Nursing practice is cyclic as well as dynamic, and for community-focused interventions to be timely and relevant, the community database, nursing diagnoses, and health program plans must be evaluated routinely. The effectiveness of community nursing interventions depends on continuous reassessment of the community's health and on appropriate revisions of planned interventions.

Evaluation is important to nursing practice, but of equal importance is its crucial role in the functioning of health agencies. Staffing and funding are frequently based on evaluation findings, and existing programs are subject to termination unless evaluation evidence can be produced that answers this question: What has been the program's impact on the health status of the community? Recent years have witnessed a growing focus on program evaluation; training programs on evaluation have become commonplace, and evaluation has become big business. Unfortunately, evaluation is sometimes practiced separately from program planning. It may even be tacked onto the end of a program just to satisfy funding sources or agency administration. The problems of such an approach are evident. Effective community health nursing requires an integrative approach to evaluation; it is a unique aspect of the field.

EVALUATION PRINCIPLES

Congruent with the theoretical foundations of working with the community as partner, we base our program evaluation on principles explicated by the W.K. Kellogg Foundation (1998). These principles are summarized below.

1. *Strengthen programs.* Our goal is health promotion and improving self-reliance of the community. Evaluation assists in attaining this goal by providing an ongoing and systematic process for assessing the program, its impact, and its outcomes.

2. *Use multiple approaches.* In addition to multidisciplinary approaches, evaluation methods may be numerous and varied. No one, single approach is favored, but the method chosen must be congruent with the purposes of the program.

3. *Design evaluation to address real issues.* Community-based and community-focused programs, rooted in the "real" community and based

on an assessment of that community, must design an evaluation to measure those criteria of importance to the community.

4. *Create a participatory process.* Just as the community members were part of assessment, analysis, planning, and implementation, so too, they must be partners in evaluation.

5. *Allow for flexibility.* "Evaluation approaches must not be rigid and prescriptive, or it will be difficult to document the incremental, complex, and often subtle changes that occur..."(W.K. Kellogg Foundation, 1998, p 3).

6. *Build capacity.* The process of evaluation, in addition to measuring outcomes, should enhance the skills, knowledge, and attitudes of those engaged in it. This includes both professionals and nonprofessionals alike.

THE EVALUATION PROCESS

There is a burgeoning literature on evaluation (see References and Suggested Readings at the end of this chapter). Program or project evaluation has become a specialty with whole departments and consulting firms focused on measurement and evaluation.

For our purposes (that is, to provide an introduction to program evaluation), we will use a three-part model (Table 13–1). In this model, we look at the *process* of implementing the program, the program's *impact*, and the *outcome* of the program.

Our focus in this text is on health promotion, and health promotion programs are designed to "... influence target populations through planned activities (process) that may have immediate effects (impact) as well as more long-term effects (outcomes)" (Dignan & Carr, 1992, p 153).

Process or formative evaluation answers the question: Are we doing what we said we would do? That is, did we deliver the program, provide a place to meet, include handouts at our meeting, and so forth. For example, when the first effective-parenting training program was offered in Rosemont from 8 to 9 PM, only five parents attended. They stated that the time was too late for them to return home and complete bedtime activities for their school-age children. As a result of this formative evaluation, the time was changed to 7 to 8 PM, and attendance increased to 20 parents. Some authors (Green & Lewis, 1986) make a distinction between formative and process evaluation by using process to denote evaluation conducted during the program, whereas formative may be applied (as the name implies) at formative or preprogram stages.

TABLE 13–1 ■ A Model for Program Evaluation

	Process (formative)	Impact (summative; short-term outcome)	Outcome (longer-term)
Information to collect	Program implementation, including • Site response • Recipient response • Practitioner response • Competencies of personnel	Immediate effects of program on, for example: • Knowledge • Attitudes • Perceptions • Skills • Beliefs • Access to resources • Social support	Incidence and prevalence of risk factors, morbidity, and mortality
When to apply	Initial implementation of a program or when changes are made in a developed program (eg, moved to a new site, provided to a different population)	To determine if factors that affect health—both within the individual and in the environment—have changed. For example, did the person's behavior change? Was the new policy implemented?	To measure if incidence and prevalence have been altered. For example, has the immunization rate of 2 year olds increased? Did the rate of admissions for respiratory-related illnesses decrease? Did the industry filter its polluting smoke stack?

Adapted from Green & Lewis, 1986.

Impact (or summative) evaluation is concerned with the immediate impact of a program on a target group. If your program is aimed at changing a group's knowledge and behavior relating to sexually transmitted disease, for instance, you might build in a test to find out what they learned and what their *intent* is about modifying behavior. In the case of effective-parenting classes, summative evaluation criteria might include parental self-reports of changes in their attitudes toward physical punishment and disciplinary practices before and following the program, any alteration in discipline policies at Temple Elementary, and change in the number of reported incidences of child abuse.

It is in the long-term outcome evaluation, however, that you find out if the changes had a lasting and real effect. That is, did the incidence of sexually transmitted diseases drop in this group? Because we are getting closer to the cause–effect question, careful evaluative research is needed to determine the actual contribution of the program to the outcome being measured.

TAKE NOTE

An in-depth review of evaluation research is beyond the scope of this text. There are several excellent texts that focus on evaluation research, and two examples of evaluation research are included later in this chapter.

Before considering specific evaluation strategies, it is important to consider the "evaluability" of the program. To do this, review the program plan and ask yourself the following questions:

* Are program activities stated in precise words whose concepts can be measured?
* Has a time frame for attaining the change been included?
* Are the direction and magnitude of the change included?
* Has a method of measuring the change been included?
* Are the data that will be needed to measure the objectives available at a reasonable cost?
* Are the program activities that are designed to meet the objectives plausible?

If you find in your practice that any of these questions cannot be measured in one of your plans, review Chapter 11 and amend the plan to make it as concise and complete as possible.

TAKE NOTE

A positive response to each of the above questions would be an ideal state that few programs attain. Therefore, do not despair if your program is less than perfect but rather strive to increase your sensitivity to the issues that need to be considered in program planning in order to achieve optimum program evaluation.

COMPONENTS OF EVALUATION

Why collect evaluation data? To whom will the evaluation data be given, and for what purpose will it be used? What programs or activities will result from or be discontinued as a result of evaluation data? Before a strategy or method of evaluation can be selected, the reasons for and uses of the evaluation data must be established. An evaluation strategy appropriate for answering one type of evaluative question would not be useful for another. For example, if the Rosemont Health Promotion Council wanted to know the relevancy to community needs of a program on crime prevention, then questions would be asked of the participants concerning the usefulness and adequacy of the information that was given. Possible questions would cover a range of topics: Did the information make a difference as to how residents protect themselves from crime? What protection behaviors do the residents practice now that were not practiced before the program? Did the program answer the residents' questions? Did the program meet perceived needs? However, if the council wanted to know the outcome of the crime prevention program (such as if the program decreased the incidence of crime experienced by the participants), then self-reports and community crime statistics would be monitored. Usually questions of evaluation focus on the areas of relevancy, progress, cost-efficiency, effectiveness, and outcome.

Relevancy

Is there a need for the program? Relevancy determines the reasons for having a program or set of activities. Questions of relevancy may be more important for existing programs than for new programs. Frequently, a program is planned, such as a blood pressure screening, to meet an expressed community need. Then, it is continued for years without an evaluation of relevancy. The question should be asked routinely—is the program still needed? Clearly, evaluation is not necessary just for new programs but for all programs. A common constraint to beginning a new program is inadequate staff or budget. A remedy to that constraint can be a relevancy evaluation of existing programs. Staff and budgets from a program that is no longer needed can be redirected to the new program.

Progress

Are program activities following the intended plan? Are appropriate staff and materials available in the right quantity and at the right time to implement the program activities? Are expected numbers of clients participating in the scheduled program activities? Do the inputs and outputs meet some predetermined plan? Answers to these questions measure the progress of the program and are part of process or formative evaluation.

Cost-Efficiency

What are the costs of a program? What are its benefits? Are program benefits sufficient for the costs incurred? Cost-efficiency evaluation measures the relationship between the results (benefits) of a program and the costs of presenting the program (such as staff salary and materials). Cost-efficiency evaluates whether the results of a program could have been obtained less expensively through another approach. Cost–benefit analysis requires skills beyond the scope of this text, but references abound, particularly in economics and management literature.

Effectiveness (Impact)

Were program objectives met? Were the clients satisfied with the program? Were program providers satisfied with the activities and client involvement? Effectiveness focuses on formative evaluation as well as the immediate, short-term results.

Outcome

What are the long-term implications of the program? As a result of the program, what changes in behavior can be expected in 6 weeks, 6 months, or 6 years? Effectiveness measures the immediate results, whereas outcome evaluation measures whether the program activities changed the initial reason for the program. The fundamental question is this: Did the program meet its goal? (Was health improved?)

EVALUATION STRATEGIES

Program "... evaluation can be defined as the consistent, ongoing collection and analysis of information for use in decision making" (W.K. Kellogg Foundation, 1998, p 14). As such, the choice of approach or method to collect the information is an important decision in itself and needs to be agreed on by all involved from the beginning. Realize that there is no one best approach to evaluation, but whichever approach is chosen needs to "fit" the questions you wish to answer.

SELECTED METHODS OF DATA COLLECTION

Four key points need to be considered as you decide which method to use:

1. What resources are available for the evaluation tasks?
2. Is the method sensitive to the respondents/participants of the program?

3. How credible will your evaluation be as a result of this method?
4. What is the importance of the data to be collected? To the overall program? To participants? (W.K. Kellogg Foundation, 1998).

Consider, too, that there are several frameworks or paradigms that may inform your choices. A summary of five such paradigms is included as Table 13–2.

Taking the key points and paradigms into consideration, let's review the various methods of data collection.

Case Study

A case study looks inside a program to determine its adequacy to meet stated needs. The case-study method provides insight into an entire program and, unlike many forms of evaluation, can be started at any time during the program. The data collected during a case study include observation of program activity, reports prepared by the program, unstructured conversations with program personnel, statistical summaries of program activities, structured or unstructured interview data, and information collected through questionnaires. Subjective data and objective data can both be collected. Subjective data include information collected primarily through observations of participants or program staff. Objective data are collected from organization or program documents or structured questionnaires and interviews. The distinction between subjective and objective is not readily perceptible. All questionnaires, regardless of how carefully written, have a subjective component, and, likewise, "objective" records or documents are all written by people and, therefore, introduce a subjective factor. It is optimum to have a mix of both objective and subjective data.

Observation

Observation is one method of collecting data for a case study. Observation can be participatory or nonparticipatory. The participant observer assumes a working role in the agency or organization and collects data about the program while working within the group. The nonparticipant observer remains an "outsider," does not assume a working role within the agency, and reviews and examines the program for designated periods.

The types of observations that are made are determined by the questions that have been asked about the program. For example, if the question is one of relevancy, the observer would concentrate on the who, what, why, and when of

TABLE 13-2 ■ Paradigms for Evaluation

	Natural Science Research Model	Interpretivism/ Constructivism	Feminist Methods	Participatory Evaluation	Theory-Based
Roots	Western "science"; European, white, male	Anthropology	Feminist research, power analysis	Education, community organization, public health, anthropology	Application in comprehensive community programs
Key points	Control of variables	Study through ongoing and in-depth contact with those involved	Women, girls, and minorities historically left out; conventional methods are seriously flawed	Create a more egalitarian process, make process more relevant to all, democratizing	Every social program is based on a theory—the key to understanding what is important is through identifying the theory
Approach	Hypothetico-deductive methodology, statistics	In-depth observations, interviewing	Contextual, inclusive, experiential, involved, socially relevant	Practical, useful, empowering	Developing a program logic model—or picture—to describe what works
Purpose	To explain what happened and show causal relationships between outcomes and "treatments"	To understand the targets of the program and the program's meaning to them	To include the feminine voice in all aspects of evaluation, being open to all voices	Actively engage all in process, capacity building	Revealing what works in comprehensive, community-based programs

From W.K. Kellogg Foundation, 1998; Minkler, 1997.

the program. Who is using the services? Record the demographics of age, ethnicity, geographic location, educational level, and employment status. What services are the participants receiving? (For example, what services are offered in the well-child clinic? Immunizations? Physicals? Health teaching? Screening? How often are the services offered, and what are the ages of the children who use the services?) Why is the population using the offered services? (Availability? Affordability? No other options?) Lastly, when are the services accessed? (Do people come at appointed times or only when they are ill? Or do people tend to cluster at opening and closing times?)

Some data can be collected from agency records; other information can be collected by informal conversations with the participants—both the professional health care providers and the clients. When interviewing, always have a checklist of topics you want to consider, arranged in a logical sequence, along with the who, what, why, and when questions. Informal conversations, sometimes referred to as "unstructured interviews," afford the opportunity to explore with the participants their perceptions of the program. The results of unstructured interviews provide specific areas from which a "structured" interview can be developed. Recall from Chapter 11 that an interview is administered by an interviewer as opposed to a questionnaire, which is self-administered. Observations and interviews share the problem of selective perception.

SELECTIVE PERCEPTION

Selective perception is the natural tendency of everyone to consciously classify into categories the behaviors or statements of others. These categories have been established by our cultural values, learning, and life experiences. To a certain extent, this process is desirable because it limits the number of observations that need conscious consideration and permits the rapid and effective handling of information. For example, if it was observed that a client waited 1 hour for a scheduled appointment, most people, based on the common orientation to time, would classify that observation as a negative aspect of the clinic's functioning.

Herein lies the major problem of selective perception. Statements and behaviors are classified according to the selective perception of the observer, which may be completely different from the selective perception of the client or other health care providers. The most dangerous effect of selective perception in program evaluation is when the observer has a preconception that a program will be successful or unsuccessful. This can produce a self-fulfilling prophecy because the biased observer may unconsciously record only data that support the preconceived belief. Both selective perception and self-fulfilling prophecy are sources of subjective data. Perhaps the most important point is that you should be aware of the problem of selective perception and share your observation and interview data with a mixed group of clients and health care providers. Ask the group for categorization and summation implications.

INTERACTIVENESS

Interactiveness is an additional event to be aware of during all observations. When an observer, whether participant or nonparticipant, observes and records program activities, the person's presence affects and shapes the activities observed. Productivity may increase because staff members are aware of being observed or because they are concerned about client satisfaction or dissatisfaction. All evaluation strategies can have an interactive component, but perhaps the interactive consideration is strongest in case studies because of the presence of an observer.

Two additional techniques of the case study method are nominal group and Delphi technique. (References to both techniques and examples of their application are presented at the conclusion of this chapter in the Suggested Readings list.) Both techniques are based on the belief that the individuals in a program are the most knowledgeable sources on its relevancy.

Nominal Group

The nominal group technique uses a structured group meeting, during which all individuals are given a judgmental task, such as to list the functions of the program, problems of the program, or needed changes in the program. Each member is asked to write a response on paper and to not discuss it with other people. At the end of 5 to 10 minutes, all members present their ideas, and each idea is recorded (without discussion) so everyone can see all the suggestions. Once all ideas have been presented, a discussion is begun, during which ideas are clarified and evaluated. After the discussion, a vote is held to determine the order in which the group wants to address different areas. The nominal group technique allows all individuals to present their ideas before the entire group. Involving the entire group both decreases selective perception and promotes individual cooperation with the group's decisions because people believe they have been involved in the decision-making process.

Delphi Technique

The Delphi technique tends to be used in large survey studies but is also useful as a case-study method. It involves a series of questionnaires and feedback reports to a designated panel of respondents. An initial questionnaire is distributed by mail to a preselected group (this could be all nursing staff members, a group of clients, or program administrators). Independently, respondents express their thoughts through the questionnaire and return it. Based on the responses of the group, a feedback report and a revised version of the questionnaire are sent to the respondents. Using the feedback information, the respondents evaluate their first answers and complete the questionnaire again. The process continues for a predetermined number of feedback rounds.

Usefulness to Evaluation

The case-study method of program evaluation can help answer questions of *relevance*. Questioning clients and health care providers helps explore perceptions of how well the program is meeting its defined goals as well as ascertaining problem areas and possible solutions. The case-study method would not point to any one solution but rather would offer several possible choices.

Questions of *progress* can also be addressed through the case-study method. The extent to which a program is meeting predetermined standards of service indicates progress. Because the case study provides an examination of the program, much can be learned if program activities are already in place.

Cost-efficiency of the program is difficult to evaluate using a case-study method. First, to evaluate if the program could have been offered more economically, a comparable program must exist; and second, the case-study method is designed to look at only one program. The method is not formatted to look at two programs and compare them. However, judgments can be made as to the operating efficiency of the program. These must be based on the experience and knowledge of the evaluator and cannot be based on comparisons with other operating programs.

Effectiveness determines if the program has produced what it intended to produce immediately after the program, as opposed to outcome, which measures long-term consequences. Although the case-study method may determine aspects of effectiveness, such as whether the aims of the program have been met in the short run, it is very difficult to measure long-term consequences unless the case-study method is conducted over a long period that allows a retrospective view of the program.

Surveys

A *survey* is a method of collecting information and can be used to collect evaluation information. Surveys are usually completed by self-administered questionnaires (the process used in Rosemont to determine community perception of health information needs) or by personal interviews. Surveys are formulated to describe (*descriptive* surveys) or to analyze relationships (*analytic* surveys). (Actually, most surveys can be used to both describe and to analyze.)

Surveys can be used to describe the need for a program, the actual operations of a program, or a program's effects. Along with the descriptive information, questions of analysis can be answered through a survey. For example, a survey could be used to *describe* the composition of the groups that attend crime prevention or weight reduction classes as well as to *analyze* the relationship between descriptive data of sex and weight reduction success.

Surveys are usually performed for summative (impact) evaluation. Did the program accomplish what it was proposed to do? Was the program perceived as successful by clients? By personnel? If the program was considered successful, what parts were most helpful? Least helpful? What should be changed? Left unchanged? The questions asked by the survey are determined by the initial list of questions about program evaluation.

Like the case-study method, the answers on surveys come from the perceptions, values, and belief systems of the respondents. The response given to questions of program usefulness by the nurse who planned and implemented the program may be very different from the answers of the participants. Awareness of perception bias can direct evaluation efforts to consider the perceptions of all persons (providers, clients, and management) involved in program implementation.

Surveys that are used to measure program evaluation must be concerned with the *reliability* and *validity* of the information collected. Reliability deals with the repeatability, or reproducibility, of the data (that is, if the same questions were asked of the same people 1 week later, would the same responses be recorded?). Validity is the correctness of the information. If questions are written to evaluate knowledge, and the answers of the respondents reflect behaviors, then the questions are not valid because they do not measure what they claim to measure.

Usefulness to Evaluation

Surveys can be very valuable to answer questions of *relevance*, or the *need* for proposed or existing programs, especially if the perceptions of clients, providers, and management are solicited. In like fashion, *progress* can be measured. People critiquing surveys as an evaluation strategy may be concerned with the subjectivity of the survey—indeed, individual perception affects every response to every question. However, most decisions are based on subjective judgments, not objective reality. The important concern is to understand whose subjective impression is being used as a basis for judgment; it is imperative for community health nurses to ensure that clients' perceptions are represented alongside those of health care providers and management.

Cost-efficiency, effectiveness, and *outcome* are difficult to measure by using a survey. Although a survey can measure the perceived efficiency of the program or ideas on alternative ways of operating to make the program more cost-efficient, these perceptions are formed only in the context of the existing program. There is no other comparison program against which recorded perceptions can be measured. A survey can provide information on the characteristics of program activities that are perceived by the respondents to have caused changes in their health status, *but* these impressions are reported in the absence of any comparison group. A comparison group is especially important with regard to effectiveness and impact because it is impossible to tell if an alternative program (or no program at all) might have been more or less effective in accomplishing the same objectives.

TAKE NOTE

You may be wondering—if a comparison group is so important and if perceptions cloud the evaluation with subjective impressions, then why use surveys at all? Two pluses exist in surveys: a great deal of information for program evaluation can be obtained, especially about the activities of the program from the perception of several groups; and important evaluation data can be inferred if the instrument (questionnaire or interview schedule) is reliable and valid.

Experimental Design

Completed correctly, an experimental study can provide an answer to the crucial questions: Did the program make a difference? Are health behaviors, knowledge, and attitudes changed as a result of the program activities? Is the community healthier because of the programs offered by the Rosemont Health Promotion Council? However, the problem with experimental studies in program evaluation is that they require selective implementation, meaning that people who participate are selected through a process such as random assignment to a control group and an experimental group. For many ethical, political, and community health reasons, selective implementation is difficult to complete and is sometimes impossible. Despite these problems, the experimental study remains the best method to evaluate summative effects (outcomes) of a program and the only way to produce quantified information on whether the program made a difference.

Reviewing the steps of the research process at this point may be of help to you in understanding the examples to follow. Indeed, each issue—such as a theoretical framework, sampling, reliability, and validity—must be addressed if an experimental design is proposed for evaluation.

The following designs are the most feasible and appropriate to health care settings. Apply the research process to each design.

Pretest–Posttest One-Group Design

The pretest–posttest design applied to one group is illustrated in Table 13–3. Two observations are made, the first at Time 1 and the second at Time 2. The observation can be the prevalence of a health state (for example, the percentage of adults in Rosemont who exercise regularly, the teenage pregnancy rate, cases of child abuse, and so on), knowledge scores, or other important health facts in the community. Between Time 1 and Time 2, an experiment is introduced. The experiment may be a planned program aimed at a target group, such as teen sexuality classes, or with a community-wide focus, like a crime-prevention program. The evaluation of the program is measured by considering the difference between the health state at Time 1 and the health state after the program at Time 2.

If the experiment in Table 13–3 was teen sexuality classes for 10th-grade girls at Hampton High School, Time 1 was a teen pregnancy rate of 5 per 100, and Time 2 (1 year later) was a teen pregnancy rate of 3 per 100 among the girls taking the classes, then would you agree that the teen sexuality program was responsible for the decrease in teenage pregnancies? What other information do you need to know in order to decide? (Are there other factors that could account for the decrease in the teen pregnancy rate? Perhaps family-planning programs have been focused on teenagers, or maybe local churches and social service agencies have sponsored teen sexuality programs. Teen access and use of contraceptive methods may have increased, or laws regarding teen access to contraceptive methods may have changed.) None of these factors can be eliminated as unassociated with the decrease in the teen pregnancy rate. To eliminate other possible explanations for program effectiveness, a control group must be added.

TABLE 13–3 ■ Pretest–Posttest One-Group Design			
	Time 1		**Time 2**
Experimental group	Observation 1	Experiment	Observation 2

Pretest–Posttest Two-Group Design

A pretest–posttest with a control group design is illustrated in Table 13–4. The design has both an experimental group and a control group. At Time 1, an observation is made of both the experimental and control groups. Between Time 1 and Time 2, an experiment is introduced with the experimental group. At Time 2, second observations are made on both the experimental and control groups. Program evaluation is the difference between Observations 1 and 2 for the experimental group when compared to the comparison group (which has been selected to be as similar as possible to the experimental group). Will the pretest–posttest with a control group design eliminate the effect of outside factors that occurred simultaneously with the experiment and that might account for the change between Observation 1 and Observation 2, the very problem that plagued the pretest–posttest one-group design? The answer is yes, if the experimental and control groups are similar.

To explain, let's return to Rosemont and the idea of a teen sexuality class for 10th-grade students at Hampton High School. If a group of 10th-grade students, similar in social, economic, and geographic characteristics, were randomly selected and then randomly assigned to the experimental or control group, then it could be assumed that any other factors that influenced the experimental group would also affect the control group. However, frequently the decision is made that all students must be given the same program, thereby eliminating a comparison group. At the Rosemont Health Promotion Council, when the information was received that *all* 10th graders must be given a teen sexuality program that had been proposed by the school nurse as a response to an increasing number of teen pregnancies, the suggestion was made that perhaps another high school could be used as a control group. How would you respond to that suggestion? Perhaps another high school class of 10th graders could be used, *if* the students were similar in social, economic, and geographic characteristics to the students at Hampton High (an unlikely situation).

Another possibility mentioned by the Rosemont Health Promotion Council was to offer the program in one school year to one half of the Hampton High

TABLE 13–4 ■ Pretest–Posttest Two-Group Design			
	Time 1		**Time 2**
Experimental group	Observation 1	Experiment	Observation 2
Control group	Observation 1		Observation 2

10th graders (using the other half as a control) and then in the following year to offer the program to the remaining students. This method would ensure that all students would be given the program but would also allow for an experimental pretest–posttest design for evaluation.

A third method that was suggested to ensure an experimental design was to give the control group sexuality education and give the experimental group sexuality education plus assertiveness training. The assertiveness training would differentiate the groups and allow an experimental design. All the suggestions were discussed with school officials, and it was decided to offer a traditional sex education class to half the 10th-grade students (the control group); the remaining students (the experimental group) would get the traditional sex education material but would also receive classes on assertiveness training and values clarification. This design will not allow for evaluation of traditional sex education classes versus no information, but it will provide all students with the health information (an ethical compromise) and allow for evaluation of a traditional program on sexuality versus that traditional program plus assertiveness and values clarification information (an approach to reduce teenage pregnancies that is supported in the literature).

TAKE NOTE

Notice that the decision to offer information on assertiveness and values clarification as part of teen sexuality classes was based on documentation from the literature. Rosemont is not the first community to offer health-promotion programs. Many communities have assessed the health status and perceived health needs of the residents and have followed up with planned and implemented programs that have been evaluated, with the results reported in the literature. One contribution that the community health nurse can make is to review and synthesize the results of similar programs and present this information to the community for use in decision making. After the program topics have been decided, you should begin a literature review to study the ways in which other communities have addressed and evaluated similar programs.

Usefulness to Evaluation

An experimental design can yield data on whether a program has produced the desired outcomes when compared to the absence of such a program or, alternatively, whether one program strategy has produced better results with regard to the desired outcomes than some other strategy. However, the experimental design is not useful for evaluation of program progress or program cost-efficiency.

Monitoring (Process)

Monitoring measures the difference between the program plan and what has actually happened. Monitoring focuses on the sequence of activities of the program, specifically, *how* the program is to be implemented (the activities), *by whom* (the personnel and other resources), and *when* (the timing of activities). Monitoring is usually done with a chart, and, although there are several different styles of charts, all arrange activities in a sequence and specify the time allotted to complete each task. Figure 13–1 shows an example of a monitoring chart.

Monitoring Charts

To construct a monitoring chart for your program plan, information is needed on the *inputs* (resources necessary to carry out the program such as personnel, equipment, and finances), the *process* (the program activities, their sequencing, and timing) and *outputs* (the expected results of the program, including immediate and long-term health effects). It is helpful to make a list of inputs, processes, and outputs.

TAKE NOTE

You have already recorded this information as part of your program plan. Refer back to Chapter 11 and note that resources, program activities, and learning objectives were listed for the proposed class on common health problems of children. Resources are the same as inputs; program activities correspond to processes; and learning objectives designate expected outputs. So all that remains is to place the data into a chart for monitoring.

Figure 13–1 lists the inputs, processes, and outputs for the proposed program in Rosemont, along with a time sequence for beginning and completing each event.

It is difficult to decide on the amount of time that will be needed to complete any task. After assessing the organizational structure and management methods of the agency, you can determine the approximate amounts of time that will be needed to complete the activities of the program. Monitoring charts are easy to formulate and provide useful information for measuring program evaluation *if* the chart is realistic. The Suggested Readings list at the end of this chapter include references to several other types of monitoring charts, including the Gantt, Program Evaluation and Review Technique (PERT), and Critical Path Method (CPM). These provide a slightly different variation of the basic time-sequencing, activities-monitoring chart that appears in Figure 13–1.

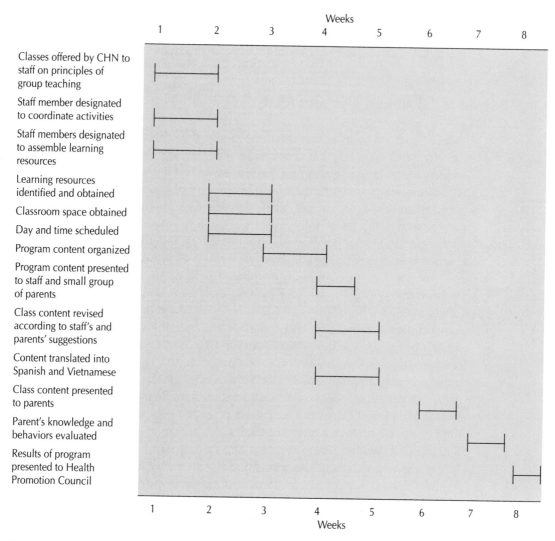

Figure 13–1. Sequence of events for program: Common health problems of children.

Usefulness to Evaluation

A monitoring chart measures progress and can be used to evaluate whether a program is on schedule and within budget. Perhaps no other evaluation method is as perfectly suited to *process evaluation* as the monitoring chart. In addition, monitoring can provide information on the *cost-efficiency* of the program by measuring the average cost of the resources required per client served.

The effectiveness of the program can be measured by monitoring the chart if the chart records outputs achieved. Monitoring charts cannot determine program relevance or the long-term impact of a program, however.

Cost–Benefit and Cost-Effectiveness Analyses

Much has been written and discussed about the escalating cost of health care services and on ways that cost can be reduced. The turmoil over health care reform in the United States and the intense debate regarding the pros and cons of various alternative approaches to health care delivery were testimony to the need to contain cost and yet increase access and maintain quality. Every program has a dollar price both in terms of the resources needed to offer the program (for example, personnel and equipment) and the dollar benefits to be gained from improved health (such as increased worker productivity).

Two of the most common methods of analyzing the economic costs and benefits of a program are cost–benefit analysis (CBA) and cost-effectiveness analysis (CEA). Both CBA and CEA are formal analytic techniques that list all costs (direct and indirect) and consequences (negative and positive) of a particular program. The distinction between CBA and CEA is based on the value that is placed on the consequences of a program. In CBA, consequences or benefits of a program are valued in dollar terms; this makes it possible to compare different projects, because all measurement is made in dollars. Therefore, the worth of a project can be judged by asking if dollar benefits exceed dollar costs and, if so, by how much. In contrast, CEA does not place a dollar value on either the consequences or the costs of a project. Another outcome is used for programs whose benefits or costs are difficult to measure. (For example, how could a dollar value be placed on each suicide prevented by a primary prevention program to decrease teenage suicide?) Therefore, CEA, unlike CBA, does not determine if total benefits exceed total costs.

However, CEA can be used to compare programs with similar goals and objectives. (For example, two different primary prevention approaches to decrease the incidence of teenage suicide share the same benefits, so only costs need be compared—a CEA.) A CEA can also be used if the costs of alternative programs are the same or if only a given amount of money exists and the objective is to select the program with the greatest benefits (not measured in dollar terms). The decision is obvious—select the program that produces the most effectiveness; that is, the most benefits per dollar spent or the least cost for each unit (individual, family, or community) benefited.

The choice between CBA and CEA depends on the type of questions and programs considered. Neither technique is superior to the other. Both techniques can be used in planning for future programs or as an evaluation strategy of present or past programs. The actual procedures for completing a CBA or CEA are beyond the scope of this book; however, several references that include the procedural steps are listed in the Suggested Readings list. Obviously, both CBA and CEA are strategies for measuring program cost-efficiency and do not address the issues of relevancy, progress, effectiveness, or impact.

SUMMARY

Several methods of evaluation have been presented and discussed. No one method will evaluate components of relevancy, progress, cost-efficiency, effectiveness, and outcome equally well. It is important to be knowledgeable about different methods of program evaluation and to discuss the benefits and limitations of each with the community as the program is being planned and before program implementation occurs. Table 13–5 presents a summary table of appropriate evaluation methods for program components. Once evaluation methods are selected, then the methods (case study, experimental design, or monitoring charts) become part of the program plan.

You may be wondering which evaluation methods were used to evaluate the health-promotion programs in Rosemont. A variety was used. To evaluate the relevancy of the health-promotion programs (crime prevention and effective-parenting classes), nominal group meetings were scheduled, and both health care providers and consumers attended. In addition, the use of rates and demographics of the participants using the health-promotion programs was assessed, as were the participants' perceptions of the value of the information.

TABLE 13–5 ■ Examination of the Appropriateness of Different Evaluation Methods for Program Components

Components	Method			
	Case Study	Survey	Experimental	Monitoring
Relevancy	Yes	Yes	No	No
Progress	Yes	Yes	No	Yes
Cost-efficiency	No	No	Yes	Yes
Cost-effectiveness	Some	No	Yes	Some
Impact	No	No	Yes	No

Program progress was evaluated with monitoring charts such as the one presented in Figure 13–1. The effectiveness and impact of individual programs were evaluated with knowledge, attitude, and behavioral intent surveys (that is, questionnaires, interviews, and tests) given to participants before the program, immediately after the program, and at predetermined follow-up times (6 weeks and 3 months following the program). As often as was feasible, an evaluation research design was followed, such as a one-group pretest–posttest. Additional measures of effectiveness and impact were community statistics on crime, child abuse, and teenage pregnancies before as compared to after the program as well as health policy changes that affected the residents of Rosemont (for example, access of minors to contraceptives, disciplinary practices in the public schools, and financial eligibility requirements for health services). Cost-effectiveness analysis was completed on several of the programs.

You are ready *now* for program implementation and the reinitiation of the nursing process; namely, assessment of the program's effects. As you implement the planned program, data will be added to the community assessment profile, which will demand addition, deletion, and revision of the community nursing diagnoses and the associated program plans and interventions. Let's take a final look at the community-as-partner model (see Figure 8–2) and ask: Will the planned programs assist the community to attain, regain, maintain, and promote health? strengthen the community's ability to resist stressors? enhance the community's competence and self-reliance?

TAKE NOTE

It is fitting that the final chapter of this section on the application of the nursing process in community health nursing ends with questions. Community health nursing is the constant questioning, prodding, probing, and pondering of the health status of a population. Although individual and family health are always important, the uniqueness of our field is the application of nursing techniques to the health of a community. Each community is unique and special. There is no other community quite like the one in which you are applying community health nursing. We have enjoyed sharing the uniqueness of Rosemont with you and the application of the nursing process to community health nursing.

REFERENCES

Dignan, M.B. & Carr, P.A. (1992). *Program planning for health education and promotion* (2nd ed.). Philadelphia, PA: Lea & Febiger.

Green, L.W. & Lewis, F.M. (1986). *Measurement and evaluation in health education and health promotion.* Palo Alto, CA: Mayfield.

Minkler, M. (Ed.). (1997). *Community organizing and community building for health.* New Brunswick, NJ: Rutgers University Press.

W.K. Kellogg Foundation. (1998). *Evaluation handbook.* Battle Creek, MI: Author.

SUGGESTED READINGS

Allen, J. (1993). Impact of the cholesterol education program for nurses: A pilot program evaluation. *Cardiovascular Nursing, 29*(1), 1–5.

Birch, S. (1990). The relative cost effectiveness of water fluoridation across communities: Analysis of variations according to underlying caries levels. *Community Dental Health, 7*(1), 3–10.

Fetterman, D.M., Kaftarian, S.J., & Wandersman, A. (Eds.). (1996). *Empowerment evaluation: Knowledge and tools for self-assessment and accountability.* Thousand Oaks, CA: Sage.

Finnegan, J.R., Murray, D.M., Kurth, C., & McCarthy, P. (1989). Measuring and tracking education program implementation: The Minnesota Heart Health Program experience. *Health Education Quarterly, 16*(1), 77–90.

Kohler, C.L., Dolce, J.J., Manzella, B.A., Higgins, D., & Brooks, C.M. (1993). Use of focus group methodology to develop an asthma self-management program useful for community-based medical practices. *Health Education Quarterly, 20*(3), 421–429.

Nas, T.F. (1996). *Cost-benefit analysis: Theory and application.* Thousand Oaks, CA: Sage.

O'Brien, K. (1993). Using focus groups to develop health surveys: An example from research on social relationships and AIDS-preventive behavior. *Health Education Quarterly, 20*(3), 361–372.

Rossi, P.H., Freeman, H.E., & Lipsey, M.W. (1998). *Evaluation: A systematic approach* (6th ed.). Thousand Oaks, CA: Sage.

Thompson, J.C. (1992). Program evaluation within a health promotion framework. *Canadian Journal of Public Health, 83*(Suppl 1), S67–S71.

Tonglet, R., Soron'gane, M., Lembo, M., WaMukalay, M., Dramaix, M., & Hennart, P. (1993). Evaluation of immunization coverage at local level. *World Health Forum, 14*(3), 275–281.

Wheeler, F.C., Lackland, D.T., Mace, M.L., Reddick, A., Hogelin, G., & Remington, P.L. (1991). Evaluating South Carolina's community cardiovascular disease prevention project. *Public Health Reports, 106*(5), 536–543.

STRATEGIES FOR HEALTH PROMOTION

Shirley Hutchinson **and** Judith McFarlane

DIVERSITY IN PRACTICE $\quad$ 14

OBJECTIVES

After studying this chapter, you should be able to

- Connect the historical development of community health nursing to present-day health issues.
- Elaborate on factors influencing community health nursing in the 21st century and the role of health promotion.

INTRODUCTION

The 21st century is finally here, bustling with phenomenal opportunities as well as troubling challenges for health care delivery and community health nursing. There is no better time to be a community health nurse than today. Yet nearly every professional, political, religious, and community group is trying to gaze into the future and determine what course of action seems most needed. It is important that community health nursing, and all of professional nursing, also try to anticipate the future. The discussion that follows represents some reflections on what is believed will characterize the practice of community health nursing in the 21st century. The term *community health nursing* is used to denote the practice of nursing by professional nurses who have been educated in processes of population-based nursing and whose principal client is the community or aggregate as a whole.

Traditionally, the role of population-based nursing was referred to as public health nursing. Public health nurses usually worked in health departments. This text uses the term *community health nurse*, which was adopted in recent years and intended to be more inclusive of population-based nursing practiced in a variety of community settings, including schools, worksites, shelters, health departments, and a multitude of other settings, some of which will be discussed in the following chapters. You will encounter both terms, *public health nursing* and *community health nursing*. Titles and practice setting are not as relevant as the nature of the practice itself. The essence and diversity of that practice are discussed in this chapter.

REFLECTIONS ON THE PAST

As we launch into the 21st century, it is both instructive and inspirational to reflect on the historic contributions of community health nurses. Examining our roots allows us to take the best from the past to shape the future. Community health nurses can gain motivation and direction from the work of Lillian Wald and her colleagues who, more than 100 years ago, faced the dawning of the 20th century. Observing rapid industrialization, large concentrations of people moving into cities, unsanitary environmental conditions, poor housing, poverty, misuse of child labor, infectious diseases, and a short life span, Lillian Wald and Mary Brewster were moved to action. Together, they founded the Henry Street Settlement House in New York City. There they lived and worked among the people, teaching hygiene practices, visiting the sick in homes, and crusading for better health care in all aspects of the community. Lillian Wald recognized the intertwining of health status, environmental sanitation, and societal and political forces. Her work targeted the root causes of ill health, which meant that she had to take on institutions, politics, and social policy to effect change for improvement of the community's health. Lillian Wald had an exceptional ability to inform and convince people of the need for social change (Backer, 1993). Wald first coined the term *public health nursing* and is regarded as the "mother of public health nursing" in the United States. Her contributions included establishing school nursing, advocating for better housing, working to change child labor laws, teaching preventive practices, advocating occupational health nursing, and improving the education of public health nurses, to name a few (Coss, 1989).

With the discovery of antibiotics in the 1940s and vaccines for mass immunizations in conjunction with tremendous improvements in environmental sanitation, the United States experienced a considerable decline in morbidity and mortality due to communicable diseases. Beginning in the 1960s, as communicable diseases declined, attention turned to prevention of chronic diseases and related risk factors such as cigarette smoking and dietary fat. Community health nurses, working in health departments, focused attention on screening, case finding, home visiting to individual clients, and health education activities related to disease prevention. This trend continued into the early 1980s when the focus of health shifted somewhat to health promotion, prompted by the Health for All era established by the World Health Organization (WHO, 1978). However, the 1990s were marked by considerable emphasis on clinical care and high-tech medicine as ways to increase life span in the United States. Health departments also began to emphasize clinical care, such as prenatal care, family planning, treatment of communicable diseases, and immunizations, particularly for citizens without access to basic preventive services. The 1990s can also be characterized as the era in which the high cost of health care in the United States became a major concern of policymakers.

In recent years, as official agencies have become more involved in direct clinical care, community health nursing has increasingly focused on clinical and illness-focused care or "clinic" roles and functions, assigning less importance to family- and community-focused roles and functions. This shift was primarily in response to the reimbursability of clinical services. To respond to the challenges facing community health nursing in the future, we must understand the changes occurring in health care delivery, including directions for population-based health embraced by the Essentials of Public Health Project (United States Department of Public Health Service [USDPHS], 1994).

COMMUNITY HEALTH IN THE UNITED STATES: THE EMERGING SCENE

Past debates about health care reform have largely ignored the contributions of population-focused community health, concentrating almost entirely on clinical care, with the exception of immunizations. Mechanisms to deliver and pay for illness care are driving the current health care system changes. The debate is really backward; we ought to talk about what can be done to make our population the healthiest rather than how we can best pay for illness. Elected officials have been reluctant to fund health promotion services at the level needed. This schism cannot continue. It takes excellent health promotion to minimize the cost of illness care. Health promotion results in wellness. Community health in the 21st century must offer integrated services and activities that focus on minimizing threats to health and promoting wellness and then focusing on illness management. This fact will become more apparent as managed care organizations develop more experience and realize that the key to their profits is investment in health promotion services. They are already turning more dollars toward health education and wellness activities of members. Clearly, to advance community health nursing, a focus on the core functions of public health (Institute of Medicine, 1988) and the ten essential public health services

(United States Department of Public Health Service, 1994) is essential. The three core functions include regular and systematic community assessment, policy development, and assurances that necessary services will be provided. The essential public health services can be used as a guide to ensure comprehensive community health nursing practice. The ten essential services are listed below.

1. Monitor health status to identify health problems (eg, community health assessment with vital statistics and risk profiles).

2. Diagnose and investigate health problems and health hazards in the community (eg, epidemiologic surveillance systems).

3. Inform, educate, and empower people about health issues.

4. Mobilize community partnerships and action to identify and solve health problems (eg, convening and facilitating community groups to promote health).

5. Develop policies and plans that support individual and community health problems (eg, leadership development).

6. Enforce laws and regulations that protect and ensure safety (eg, enforcement of sanitary codes).

7. Link people to needed personal health services and ensure the provision of health care when otherwise unavailable.

8. Ensure a competent public health and personal health care workforce.

9. Evaluate effectiveness, accessibility, and quality of personal and population-based health services.

10. Research for new insights and innovative solutions to health problems.

Granted, this is an impressive list, yet each essential service can be used to direct community health nursing practice in a diversity of settings. A term that is discussed frequently is *outcomes management*. Professionals are queried as to what measures they can offer to document improvements in health and well-being. Outcomes measures are being used to determine operating budgets.

OUTCOMES MANAGEMENT IN COMMUNITY HEALTH

Outcomes management is in the future of community health and, consequently, community health nursing. Community health nurses have acted to improve the health outcomes of Americans and will be part of outcomes evaluation of community health practice. The National Public Health Performance Standards Program is a partnership effort to develop structure, process, and outcome standards by which public health practice will be judged in the future. Measurement tools are being developed and tested at the local and state levels (Centers for Disease Control and Prevention, 1998). Quality improvement, accountability, and increased scientific basis for population health practice are among the goals of public health outcomes evaluation. The essential community health services (listed above) will serve as the basis for developing specific outcomes measures.

THE ESSENCE OF COMMUNITY HEALTH NURSING PRACTICE

To more clearly describe community health nursing, a group of four nursing organizations met. The four organizations were called The Quad Council and consisted of the American Nurses Association, Council of Community, Primary, and Long-Term Care; American Public Health Association—Public Health Nursing Section; Association of Community Health Nurse Educators; and Association of State and Territorial Directors of Nursing. The following components of community health nursing practice were identified (Quad Council of Public Health Nursing Organizations, 1997):

- Population-based assessment
- Partnerships with stakeholders
- Primary prevention
- Creating healthy environmental, social, and economic conditions
- Active outreach to those who might need service
- Dominant concern for group as a whole
- Wise stewardship and allocation of resources

We can use these tenets to guide our practice of community health nursing, regardless of the setting. Next, let's discuss some of the factors that will affect our practice in this century.

FACTORS INFLUENCING COMMUNITY HEALTH NURSING IN THE 21ST CENTURY

There is no disputing that the health care system is undergoing tremendous change. Much that seems familiar and comfortable will be altered, some for the worse and, we hope, most for the better. All health professions are being influenced by the changes going on in our health care system. The relevant factors shaping 21st century community health are summarized below.

- *Emerging health care delivery system.* All aspects of health care are becoming increasingly community based and population focused. The present goal of changes in health care delivery center around cost containment. Competition based on market forces is a major driver in the emerging health care system. Managed care has taken over nearly all aspects of individual and family care, including government-sponsored programs. Large, integrated health systems are rapidly developing with mergers of large hospitals, physician practice groups, nursing home care facilities, home health agencies, and other specialty groups. All of these factors create the challenge of balancing the needs of the individual within the broader social context. The increase in managed care organizations generally means fewer individual patients for health departments (and less revenue) in prenatal, well-child, and family planning clinics. This means that the Medicaid population will be cared for by managed care groups, causing less need for health department clinical services.
- *Demographics.* Two significant demographic factors shaping the future of public health nursing and all health care are age and increasing ethnic diversity. It is predicted that by 2040, one out of five Americans will 65 years of age or older. The graying of America will continue to shift the focus of medical care from acute to chronic illness and challenge the development of new and effective health promotion strategies for this population. Quality of life will become the priority, not merely a long life. There is no debate about the growing ethnic diversity of this country. Changes in immigration laws and differential fertility rates and age patterns among minority groups have dramatically altered the ethnic makeup of the United States. Nationwide, Asians and Pacific Islanders will constitute the fastest growing ethnic group, but Hispanics will contribute the largest number of people. There are many social and health implications of these changes for community health nursing.
- *Technology.* Technology will be both valued and scorned in the new millennium. With the openness and lack of control of what goes on the Internet, cyberspace community health nursing is a real possibility. Sexual abuse, violence, drugs, health misinformation, and other maladies are already being promoted by way of the Internet. Maximum use of technology will enhance the community health nurse's effectiveness in providing population-based health promotion. Telematics and informatics will expand to unforeseen levels in community health. Telematics includes the use of diagnostic software, record keeping, and communication of knowledge about health care and individuals to anywhere in the world. Telematics

has the potential of developing client profiles that include biochemical definitions of health, illness, and wellness for individuals. Such technology is in use in many aspects of health care, including health risk appraisals. Televideo nursing will expand, and self-care will be rampant with the use of this technology. Home telemedicine systems are also increasing in use as a home health variation.

- *Increasing globalization.* Viewing health care globally will bring challenges and opportunities for health care nurses worldwide. As free-trade agreements become more of a reality, international opportunities for freely exchanging expertise and ideas are more abundant. It also opens up the potential for rapid transfer of communicable diseases, terrorism, and other such undesirable health concerns. Preventing the spread of disease, protecting the environment, and reducing poverty will continue to be worldwide challenges. International public health surveillance systems will increase in priority in the coming century. There may even be another major war. No century, thus far, has escaped a major war. The tragedy of future wars is that the weapons (mass destruction and germ warfare) can be transported easily to any area in the world.

- *Increasing consumer involvement.* Increasing consumer involvement is in the future of community health and all of health care. Information dissemination, fueled by ready access to the Internet, television, and print media has created sophisticated consumers who seem to know what they want and who demand the best care that is available. Public health, in a reformed health care system, will forge partnerships between communities and all levels of government. As knowledgeable consumers become increasingly focused on health promotion, risk reduction, and quality-of-life issues, public health nurses will continue to play a major role in empowering the community to take responsibility for its health. Coalition building, collaboration, and partnership development will be essential skills needed by 21st century community health nurses.

- *Outcomes management.* As society continues to cope with the high costs of health care, policymakers want to invest resources in health services that seem to produce desired results in a cost-effective manner. Community health nurses must utilize evaluation research to show how they impact the health of communities.

- *Troubling signs.* Many of the community health skills needed in the 21st century will not be practiced exclusively by community health nurses. Although community health nurses have historically practiced in a generalist manner, demonstrating eclectic skills, other health professionals are marketing these specialized skills (eg, wellness specialists, health educators, and pharmacists who administer vaccines). Community health nurses must be willing to forge new partnerships and collaborative relationships in the emerging delivery system and yet maintain their tradition of going into the "field" where the people live.

COMMUNITY HEALTH NURSING: THE FUTURE AWAITS

The 21st century is bustling with opportunities for community health nursing. O'Neil (1998) has suggested that, in order to position nursing for the 21st century, nursing practice and education should focus on two core competencies that have always been a part of nursing: population-based approaches to health care and the incorporation of the psychosocial–behavioral perspective into the delivery of care. Salmon (1999) identifies five values of nursing that have sustained the profession in the past and that hold great promise for driving the future of nursing. These values are caring, courage, inclusion, reflective thinking, and social responsibility. As the 21st century unfolds, community health nurses must not forget these values.

The eight chapters ahead describe some of the diverse practice settings of community health nursing. Each chapter is riveted in the basic elements of practice—promoting healthy partnerships for community well-being. As you read through these chapters, our goal is for you to plan, implement, and evaluate wellness initiatives that promote health. We also hope you have fun and develop a life-long yearning to partner with populations for health. Here is to your future and the health promotion partnerships you forge.

REFERENCES

Backer, B.A. (1993). Lillian Wald: Connecting caring with action. *Nursing and Health Care, 14*(3), 122–129.

Centers for Disease Control and Prevention: Division of Public Health Systems Public Health Practice Program Office. (1998). *National Public Health Performance Standards Program.* Available at **www.phppo.cdc.gov/dphs/nphpsp/**.

Coss, C. (1989). *Lillian Wald: A progressive activist.* New York, NY: Feminist Press.

Institute of Medicine. (1988). *The future of public health.* Washington, DC: National Academy Press.

O'Neil, E. (1998). Nursing in the next century. In J. Coffman (Ed.), *Strategies for the future of nursing* (pp 211–224). San Francisco, CA: Jossey-Bass.

Quad Council of Public Health Nursing Organizations. (1997, July). *The tenants [sic] of public health nursing by the Quad Council of Public Health Nursing Organizations.* Draft white paper, unpublished.

Salmon, M. (1999). Thoughts on nursing: Where it has been and where it is going. *Nursing and Health Care Perspectives, 20*(1), 20–25.

United States Department of Public Health Service [USDPHS]. (1994). *Public health in America.* Available at **web.health.gov/phfunctions/public.htm**.

World Health Organization. (1978, September). *Report of the International Conference on Primary Health Care,* held in Alma Ata, USSR. Geneva, Switzerland: Author.

Charles Kemp

PROMOTING HEALTHY PARTNERSHIPS WITH REFUGEES AND IMMIGRANTS

15

OBJECTIVES

After studying this chapter, you should be able to

- Differentiate between the terms *refugees* and *immigrants*.
- Discuss the phases of health and adjustment for refugees and immigrants.
- Describe health promotion strategies that focus at the individual/family and community levels.

INTRODUCTION

Beginning in the 1970s and continuing into this century, the United States is experiencing the largest wave of immigration since the early 1900s. Refugees have come from Southeast Asia, Eastern Europe, Africa, and the Middle East; and immigrants (legal and illegal) have come from across the world, especially Latin America. Although some refugees and immigrants are at no population-specific risk for health problems, many are at very high risk for health problems in all spheres of being. To understand these populations, it is helpful to understand differences between refugees and immigrants.

- *Refugees* may be defined as people who are outside their own country and unwilling or unable to return because of persecution or a well-founded fear of persecution on account of race, religion, nationality, membership in a particular social group, or political opinion (Rasbridge, 1998).
- *Immigrants* are people who leave their homeland to seek economic or social benefit, and thus tend to be pulled to a new land by desire or need for benefit in contrast to refugees who are pushed from their homes.

Readers should understand that differences between refugees and immigrants may not be as clear-cut as presented above. For some immigrants, economic or social benefit may literally mean survival, whereas for others, the benefit may be a graduate degree or higher-paying job. For the purposes of this chapter, the focus is on refugee and immigrant communities that are at risk for acute and chronic health problems to a greater extent than the general population (ie, those who live in poverty, have little education, and exhibit other characteristics of vulnerable populations in general).

Refugees and, to a large extent, immigrants as described above go through a relatively predictable series of phases with respect to health and adjustment (Kemp, 1998; Rasbridge, 1998).

- The *acute phase* begins with arrival in the new country. Communicable diseases (eg, tuberculosis, parasitism, and hepatitis B) are of particular concern to health officials. The new arrivals themselves may be more concerned about chronic symptomatic health problems. Mental health problems are seldom identified by either the new arrivals or by health officials.

- The *transition phase* is characterized by the emergence of secondary or hidden chronic health needs once the initial and more acute health needs are met. Diabetes, hypertension, and goiter are examples of health needs viewed as secondary by many refugees and immigrants. Mental health problems, notably chronic posttraumatic stress disorder (PTSD) and depression, also emerge.

- The *chronic phase* is the negative outcome of the refugee or immigrant experience. Long-term sequelae of hypertension, diabetes, and other chronic illnesses begin to emerge with concomitant morbidity and mortality. People with untreated mental illnesses drift into individual or even community (underprivileged enclave) seclusion, often including alcoholism or other drug abuse. Family structure and roles deteriorate with marital breakup, family violence, and youth involvement in gangs common.

- The *resolution phase* is the positive outcome of the refugee or immigrant experience. When resolution occurs, individuals and families have access to health care and other essential resources. Physical, social, educational, mental, and spiritual needs are met to approximately the same extent they are met in other segments of the population. There is the essential characteristic of successful life: realistic hope for the future.

As with other theoretical or generalized stages applied to individuals, families, or populations, there are many exceptions or deviations from what is presented here. Nevertheless, these phases offer a structure to begin to understand refugees and immigrants and their health needs.

STRATEGIES FOR HEALTH PROMOTION: "COMMUNITY CARE"

"Community Care" had its roots in a community health nursing clinic in which students and faculty worked with Cambodian refugees in a large urban setting. Before beginning the health project, the class read Elizabeth Anderson's brilliant "A Call for Transformation" (1991), which discusses a district health model in which all people's health is addressed within the community. This would be a good time to stop, read, and discuss this short but very meaningful article. How does the article apply to the community you live in? work in? go to school in? or plan to do your clinical experience in?

As part of "Community Care," students and faculty took responsibility for providing health care to a culturally diverse (primarily Asian refugee and Hispanic) inner-city, low-income community with significant needs/problems. Rather than begin with a lengthy formal assessment process, students and faculty began working on one block of one street to assist people in the community to obtain health care and social services. Students went door to door, and every time a person was found with an unmet health or related need, the students stopped and, with the individual or family, figured out how to meet the need. In almost all cases, students later followed up on the solution.

Through the process of assisting people with the problems they believed were most pressing, students were able to develop a trusting and professional relationship with the community; identify needs and problems at all levels of care/prevention/promotion; and develop a meaningful understanding of available community services. Gradually, through this dynamic and continuing services-based community assessment, the program was expanded geographically from one block to more than 30 blocks and in terms of expanded individual, family, and community services as described below. Ultimately, the district health concept was realized.

District health is driven by individual, family, and community needs and encompasses individual- and family-oriented care such as outreach, primary care, case management, and home health care; and community-oriented care such as community assessment, disease prevention, and health promotion. Collaboration with a large number of providers and disciplines is necessary.

In addition to nursing students (from two universities), health promotion services are provided by seminary students, community health workers, lay health promoters, volunteers, and others. Services can be broadly classified as (1) individual- and family-oriented services and (2) community-oriented services. A differentiation of the two services follows.

INDIVIDUAL- AND FAMILY-ORIENTED SERVICES

Individual- and family-oriented services include outreach, primary care, case management, and home health care. These services are focused primarily on care for people who are sick and are the means by which the program is able to move toward disease prevention and health promotion. Outreach, for example, is focused on individuals and families, but, without these personal contacts, health screening would never reach the most isolated people in the community.

Outreach

As noted earlier, outreach is implemented door to door through the apartments in the district. Although students carry flyers on the program in Spanish, English, Vietnamese, Khmer (Cambodian), and Laotian, they seldom just leave flyers on doors. Instead, students knock and, if anyone is home, inquire about health problems and check blood pressures, vaccination records, medications, and address other issues that arise in the course of the visit. Always, as much as is possible, students stop to solve problems wherever they are found.

Language is an issue in outreach and other program components. The primary languages spoken in this district (in descending order) are Spanish, English, Vietnamese, Khmer, and Laotian. Everyone involved in this work is acutely aware that there often are breakdowns in communication! Although there are now caseworker/translators with capabilities in Spanish, Vietnamese, Khmer, and Laotian working with the program, it is important to note that had services been delayed to wait for these capabilities, thousands of opportunities to serve this community would have been missed.

Primary Care and Case Management

When people are found with health or related problems, nursing students or other persons involved with the program help find appropriate resources, help clients access the services, follow up on the care given to be sure that clients understand treatments and medications, and, finally, provide further follow-up to determine if treatments were effective and if any new problems develop. Common individual problems encountered in the community include clients having difficulty obtaining and understanding:

- Primary care for hypertension, infections, and similar problems
- Prenatal care and family planning
- Specialty care for cancer, diabetes, and other chronic illnesses
- Preventive care, such as childhood immunizations; or early disease detection

Many health and social problems are handled in a student-operated clinic in the community. The clinic is held at a police storefront with a church health program providing internist services on Thursday mornings and the county hospital community-oriented primary care clinic (COPC) providing pediatrician services on Friday mornings. Clinic services include medical care, teaching, vaccinations, refugee screening, social work, pregnancy testing and counseling, and volunteer services. The program takes pride in the fact that medical services came to the nursing education program rather than the far more common case of nursing education programs attaching themselves to medical services.

When patients require care beyond the level of this clinic, students help obtain appointments. Students often accompany patients to appointments and thus provide essential advocacy and/or teaching services. In all cases, a goal of care is increasing patient independence so that, ultimately, the patient is registered with a provider such as the COPC, knows how to make appointments, and is able to recognize the need to seek health care. This goal is not always reached. Access to care remains difficult for non-English or Spanish speakers, and current trends in health care have resulted in even public health providers demanding documentation that is impossible for some patients to provide.

Home Health Care

Home health care is provided independently of, or in cooperation with, home care agencies. Home care agencies have learned that, by cooperating with the program, the level of care exceeds that possible through funded sources. Some home care and hospice staff schedule visits on days when students are not available so coverage is doubled through cooperative care. In other cases, there is no coverage at all and students and faculty take on significant responsibilities for care.

For example, Mrs. C was a 58-year-old Cambodian woman who had undetected cervical cancer when students found her in door-to-door outreach. She had an 11-year-old son with Down's syndrome, a 13-year-old daughter who provided most of Mrs. C's care, and a 15-year-old son who was sent to prison midway through the course of care. Students and faculty were instrumental in the cancer being diagnosed, played a critical role in getting the patient through two courses of treatment (surgery and radiation), and took responsibility for her home care after crises related to very severe complications of disease and treatment (septicemia, stroke, seizures, bowel obstruction, malnutrition, and dehydration). For 2 years, Mrs. C received at least three home visits each week. She agreed to hospice care about 2 months before dying. A faculty member was with her when she died at home.

Care is continuous between students across semesters. In summers, the clinic is operated by volunteers, faculty, and church health and COPC staff.

COMMUNITY-ORIENTED SERVICES

Community services currently under way include community assessment, immunizations taken into the community, women's health services, church health, and community development. These are not one-time projects! They are ongoing community care activities that, over time and with reinforcement and repetition, will change lives. Each is summarized below.

Community Assessment

Assessment of the community is services based. In other words, the community (problems, needs, strengths, and resources) is assessed primarily through the process of delivering services. Biostatistical data are also used, but to a lesser degree than direct experience in the community.

Vulnerable communities have been extensively studied here and elsewhere. For example, it is known that, nationally, Asian women underutilize cancer screening. Is it ethical, then, to take time to determine the degree to which Asian women in this community also do or do not underutilize cancer screening? Or, is the community better served by developing cancer screening programs and, through the process of screening, determining the degree of utilization or underutilization? The answer is obvious.

Immunizations

In going door to door in the community, students assess the immunization status of every child encountered. Immunizations are provided free every

Wednesday by staff from a van from one of the nursing schools involved with the program and every Friday at the pediatric clinic by staff from the COPC or county health department. Influenza immunizations for adults are provided by the COPC and county health department at the community clinic site and at health fairs in the fall.

Women's Health

In addition to the already described outreach and assistance with family planning and prenatal care, each semester students plan and implement cancer screening events in which a portable mammogram unit is set up in the police storefront and women who otherwise would be highly unlikely to ever receive a mammogram come in for free screening. Along with mammograms, students teach breast self-exam one on one with the women, screen all participants (and others who come in the door) for other health problems (eg, diabetes, hypertension, colon cancer, HIV), and provide follow-up care for all problems. Except for operating the mammogram unit and HIV testing, students are responsible for all aspects of the screening.

Here is the ethnic breakdown of the 240 women screened for whom data are available in eight mammogram events: African American, 10%; white non-Hispanic, 5.5%; Hispanic, 0%; Khmer (Cambodian), 21%; Laotian, 14%; Native American, less than 1%, and Vietnamese, 23%.

An example of how screening helps to identify other family health needs is the story of Sarath. Sarath was a 15-year-old Khmer girl in a dangerously abusive relationship with an older man. After initial failures in intervening, students, police, and a child welfare agency were finally able to help her move back to her mother in California. Students first made contact with her when she was helping translate for an older woman at one of the mammogram events.

Church and Lay Volunteers

One of the underutilized resources identified in this community work were the churches. On the basis of a community assessment, students made contact with a clergy member and obtained his agreement to work with students 1 day per week in a small church health effort. This effort quickly led to a relationship with a group of volunteer Hispanic (mostly Mexican) women, named the "CoMadres," at one of the elementary schools in the community. With the CoMadres, students developed a lay health promoter curriculum and provided training to the CoMadres. This curriculum may be viewed at www.baylor.edu/~Charles_Kemp/welcome.html. Students work with the CoMadres on a weekly basis and have held one cooperative health fair at the CoMadres' school.

Student work with the CoMadres and the clergy led to a close relationship with the previously discussed church health program. The Community Care program became an integral part of the church health efforts, and faculty from the two involved nursing schools were among the first church nurses. As noted earlier, the church health program provides an internist for the Thursday clinic and is chiefly responsible for the presence of lay health promoters at the clinic and in the community on Thursdays and Fridays.

Community Development

In all aspects of working in this community, whether with individuals or as part of community care, students affirm and strengthen the community's ability to grow and care for itself. Many referrals to people in need come from others with whom students have worked in the past and who have learned basic health measures from students. There is a growing corps of volunteers and a strong network of concerned individuals whom students helped equip to reach out and more effectively help their neighbors. Rather than depend solely on caseworker/translator services, relatives, neighbors, and friends often assist with translation, transportation, and other such services. Existing community groups are used to assist and promote health as much as possible.

The program recently outgrew the police facility that students call "home base." A small Vietnamese church in the heart of the community offered part of its facility for the clinic. People from the community and from churches outside the community are giving countless hours cleaning, remodeling, painting, and in other work to prepare the facility.

Challenges and Problems

Follow-up and evaluation are a constant challenge. Through the alliance with the church health program, the program is able to track "preventable admissions" (diabetes, asthma, and so forth) to area hospitals from the district zip code. Data are encouraging, but direct cause and effect are difficult to show.

Compliance with treatment or health promotion is always an issue. Follow-up with patients with hypertension, diabetes, and other such diagnoses takes precedence over follow-up on compliance with health promotion measures such as breast self-exams after breast cancer screening. Efforts to utilize additional students to address the full spectrum of healthy behaviors are under way.

SUMMARY

This program was designed and has evolved for the specific purpose of addressing the health care needs and problems of a community that, despite the relatively near presence of several health and social service providers, remained significantly underserved. The program is driven and defined by human needs. Through meeting the needs and priorities of the community, students and their partners in this work are able to gradually introduce services directed to health promotion and disease prevention and early detection. Rather than students coming into the health care system as students (whose work would be done whether the students were there or not), they provide services that would not otherwise be available to the clients.

REFERENCES

Anderson, E.T. (1991). A call for transformation. *Public Health Nursing, 8*(1), 1.
Kemp, C.E. (1998). Mental health issues among refugees. In C.E. Kemp & L.A. Rasbridge (Eds.), *Refugee health & immigrant populations.* Online at **www.baylor.edu/ ~Charles_Kemp/refugee_health.htm**.
Rasbridge, L.A. (1998). Introduction: Background on refugees. In C.E. Kemp & L.A. Rasbridge (Eds.), *Refugee health & immigrant populations.* Online at **www.baylor.edu/ ~Charles_Kemp/refugee_health.htm**.

Nina Fredland   CHAPTER

PROMOTING HEALTHY PARTNERSHIPS WITH SCHOOLS

16

OBJECTIVES

After studying this chapter, you should be able to

- Design programs that are specific to the specialized school setting at the primary, secondary, and tertiary levels of prevention.
- Implement programs that teach healthy behavior to school-age children, their parents, and school faculty and staff.
- Involve the residents of the geographic community in which the school is located in program planning.
- Utilize community resources specific to school-age children and their parents.

INTRODUCTION

Most health care providers would agree that a major goal for this, the 21st century, would be to create a nation of children who are optimally well so that they can lead long, happy, productive lives. How do we as nurses achieve this goal? This chapter focuses on strategies and partnerships within the community setting of the school. The school nurse or the community health nurse, depending on the community, is ideally situated to provide health care to school-age children. Nurses with advanced preparation in child health, such as pediatric nurse practitioners and family nurse practitioners, are also well prepared to initiate partnerships with schools. An ideal model is one in which the school nurse or community health nurse collaborates with the advanced practice nurse. In this way, health promotion, disease prevention, and health maintenance are important components included within the delivery of health care. School-age children are a captive audience, and their parents are closely connected to the school community. This makes the school community an ideal center for health promotion activities for the entire family.

The health of our nation's children has been an area of concern for some time. Casual observations at any school note a high percentage of overweight children, youngsters easily fatigued while running around the playground, and children choosing non-nutritious snacks. Obviously, these children are at a disadvantage. Their health is compromised. One has only to observe adult role models to understand why children are making unhealthy choices. Therefore, health education approaches must be comprehensive and include the children as well as all groups of individuals involved in their care and nurturing. The school community encompasses:

- School-age children and adolescents
- Parents and guardians
- School personnel (faculty, staff, and administrators)
- Neighborhood residents, businesses, and service agencies

In addition to promoting the optimal health and preventing illness through the education of all members of the school community, school health programs must strive to identify and resolve existing health problems. Therefore, comprehensive school health programs should focus on delivering health services mandated by state laws and the individual school system as well as health education. Additionally, both internal and external environmental issues are critical areas of assessment and intervention for school nurses.

DELIVERING HEALTH SERVICES FOR HEALTH PROMOTION

Each state mandates certain requirements to maintain the health of school-age children. Programs for vision, hearing, and spinal screenings are required. Measurements of height, weight, and blood pressure are also usually part of these health services. Nutritional, dental, and developmental screening may also be required in the school setting. To find out about requirements in your state, contact your local state health department. The following list outlines some common state requirements.

Vision: Screen all new students within 120 days of enrollment. Screen students in kindergarten, 1st, 3rd, 5th, 7th, and 9th grades by May of each school year

Hearing: Screen all new students within 120 days of enrollment. Screen students in kindergarten, 1st, 3rd, 5th, 7th, and 9th grades by May of each school year

Spinal: Screen all 6th- and 9th-grade students

Certification is required to perform vision and hearing screening. Certification training is available through state health departments or through individuals the state has designated with this authority. To find out how to receive certification training, contact your state health department. Certification for registered nurses is not usually required for spinal screening; yet, ancillary personnel or volunteer assistants are required to have attended an approved educational program. Therefore, it is important that student nurses be taught a thorough procedure for assessing spinal deformities as part of their health assessment curriculum.

Immunizations are required by state law to be current and on file before or on the first day of school. A school district can establish a short grace period, usually 30 days. Immunization requirements must be strictly supported by the school administration. Each state sets a standard for immunizations. A school district can increase the requirements but must include the minimum standard. For example, tuberculosis screening for school-age children may not be required by state law; however, school districts can set a higher standard and require new students to have an approved skin test for tuberculosis screening within 1 year of initial enrollment. Furthermore, school districts can require school personnel to be tested biennially. The Centers for Disease Control and Prevention (CDC) is the best source for recommended immunization schedules for children and adults. The CDC web site is **www.cdc.gov**. This would be a good time to familiarize yourself with this web site and the current recommended immunization schedule for school-age children.

In addition to mass screening programs, a nurse in the school setting identifies and monitors existing health problems, both acute and chronic, such as common respiratory infections and asthma. The school nurse is a referral agent and case manager and offers education within his or her scope of nursing practice.

HEALTH EDUCATION FOR HEALTH PROMOTION

Major issues affecting American children can be categorized under headings of nutrition; interpersonal violence; substance abuse; mental health issues; safety; sexuality; and environmental hazards, such as lead, asbestos, and air pollution. Health promotion strategies should focus on these important areas. Some topics from which you might select for health education programs are listed here.

Some of these topics are more appropriate for children, parents, or teachers. As you are thinking of the topic, consider the audience you are targeting. For example, healthy food choices might be geared toward easy recipes that children can prepare. There are a number of cookbooks written with children in mind. My favorite is the American Heart Association's *Children's Help Your Heart Cookbook.* (To access this cookbook, contact your local chapter of the American Heart Association.) Eating disorders is a topic more suited for a parent session. The following health education list is not exhaustive. It is designed to promote your ideas. Consider how you might assess interest for any of the following programs.

Health Education Program Ideas

Nutrition
Healthy food choices
Healthy recipes for busy families
Healthy lunches children can prepare
Eating disorders (such as anorexia, bulimia, and compulsive eating)

Violence
Domestic violence—effects on children and sources of help for the
   whole family
Discipline versus child abuse
Anger management/Impulse control
Gang behavior
Date rape/Acquaintance rape
Signs of child abuse/Incest

Substance Use
Cigarettes and chewing tobacco
Underage drinking
Illicit drugs (marijuana, crack, cocaine, inhalants, speed, heroin, and
   so forth)

Mental Health Issues
Self-esteem
Attention deficit disorder/Hyperactive disorder
Depression
Suicide

Personal Safety
"Latchkey" kids
Problem-solving/Decision-making skills

Recreational Safety
Bicycles, in-line skates, sports
Vehicle safety (seat belts, booster seats, riding in open vehicles)
Water safety (swimming, boating, and skiing)

Sexuality
Personal hygiene
Sexually transmitted diseases

Teenage Pregnancy
Teen parenting

Environmental
Internal (air, water, space)
External (pollution, noise)
Psychological (grade stress, parent–child discord, parent–teacher and
teacher–teacher conflicts)

Societal Influences
Changing family structure
Peer pressure
Media Influences (video games, films, television)

HEALTH PROMOTION PROGRAMS FOR SCHOOL-AGE CHILDREN

Programs for children and adolescents in the school setting must be age appropriate. Obviously, breast self-examination and testicular self-examination are
not appropriate material for elementary school-age children. It is critical to
assess the developmental and maturity level of the children before deciding on
the educational content of a program or a strategy. Even if you think you know
how to relate to a certain age group, each class is different. The youngsters may
be a very young class for their grade level or they may be a very advanced
group. The students may or may not be well socialized. Several may have
attention deficit or exhibit hyperactivity.

Important information is gained from observing the student population
before planning programs. Always visit the classroom and observe how the
students and teacher interact. Classroom management skills are essential. It is
difficult to successfully manage the classroom if the nurse's contact with the
youngsters is only occasional. Relying on the regular classroom teacher for
assistance works best. It is helpful to include key people, such as the teacher,
counselor, school nurse, and parents in the planning phase of all health pro-

grams. Outlining individual expectations of the teacher counselor, school nurse, and parents will contribute to the overall success of the program. Another consideration is marketing your program. It may be the greatest idea; but, if no one comes or follows through, it is a waste of time and resources. Use flyers, bulletin boards, and public address announcements to reach your audiences.

Try various strategies to pique interest. For example, brightly colored signs and charts; guessing games; poster contests; door decorating competitions; age-appropriate, healthy food rewards (eg, juice bars, fruit) are a few suggestions. The following are examples of health promotion programs for school-age children:

- Red Ribbon Week
- D.A.R.E. Program
- Breast Self-Examination/Testicular Self-Examination (teens)
- Muscle Mover Club or Triathlon or Walk-A-Thon/Swim to Bermuda
- Monthly Health Bulletin Board
- Make a Cookbook
- Pet Responsibility

Red Ribbon Week

Red Ribbon Week occurs in October each year to celebrate being drug free. The Red Ribbon Campaign began in 1988 when the US Congress established Red Ribbon Week. The goal was to increase the awareness of the dangers associated with the use of tobacco, alcohol, and other drugs. Since then, Red Ribbon Week has become the standard in many schools. The Internet has many examples of how different schools across the nation celebrate the week. An agenda for a week's program focusing on drug abuse prevention, which can be incorporated into the curriculum of an elementary school, follows. Each student recites a promise to stay away from drugs and wears a red ribbon for the week. See the displayed material for a sample agenda.

The community should be involved in the program along with the students in various ways. Parents can be invited to some programs. The parents' organization can be asked to decorate the school with red ribbons. Community leaders (eg, church, civic, police) can judge contests. The police and fire departments can facilitate a parade route and provide security. Media coverage, such as local newspapers and radio and television stations, is an important strategy that schools should seek. (Often, worthwhile events are not covered by the media because media personnel have not been notified.) Older students and

Sample Agenda for Red Ribbon Week

MONDAY	Flag ceremony and recital of the drug-free pledge by student body.
PLEDGE:	

I SAY NO TO THE
UNLAWFUL USE
OF ALCOHOL
AND
OTHER DRUGS.

SIGNATURE

Designate a place for pledge signing for the students, faculty/staff.
Display the pledge cards in a central location.
Have a group of children, parents, and school staff deliver the signed pledge cards to an official person in city government (eg, the mayor).
Red ribbons are delivered to all classes by 5th graders (or oldest students in school). Each student wears a red ribbon.
Decorate school grounds with red ribbons.

TUESDAY	Wear red to school day
	Drug-free poster contest in art classes
WEDNESDAY	Classroom door decorating contest
	Display finished posters in halls
THURSDAY	Drug prevention programs per grade levels
FRIDAY	Judging posters and doors
	Assembly and drug-free pep rally
	Motivational speaker
	Drug-free songs and cheers
	Announce contest winners
SATURDAY/	
SUNDAY	Community parade

www.esc12.net/newsreleases/pre/.10.15.9br.html

campus leaders can influence younger students by positive peer pressure, such as wearing their ribbons, participating in all activities, and having a major role in organizing and implementing the activities.

It is very important to give clear messages to young people, particularly on the subject of drugs. The nurse should select speakers very carefully. Recovering drug abusers should not be used to speak to groups of students who are not users. It is also risky to choose high-profile role models, such as well-known sports or media individuals who may be positive non–drug users one day but in the news media at a later time for using drugs or violent behavior. Consider asking the students to give 1-minute talks on why they are not going to use drugs. Have a poem or smart saying contest. Get the speech club involved.

D.A.R.E. Program

The D.A.R.E. (Drug Abuse Resistance Education) Program is a substance abuse prevention program that originated with the Los Angeles Unified School District. The purpose is to teach students to resist peer pressure and say "no" to drugs. Decision making is emphasized, and alternative ideas for dealing with problems are explored. D.A.R.E. is sponsored by the local community police department in which a specially trained police officer is assigned to the 5th-grade class for a series of 17 weekly lessons. Other grade levels may be included in the educational process to a lesser degree than the targeted 5th grade. D.A.R.E. has also expanded to include high schools. The officer becomes an integral part of the classroom teaching team. This activity encourages positive relations between youth and law enforcement officers and provides children with accurate information about the hazards of drug use and useful strategies for staying drug free.

Muscle Mover Club or Triathlon or Walk-A-Thon

The Muscle Mover Club encourages physical activity by rewarding aerobic exercise, such as walking, running, swimming, and biking. Each child is given a badge and adds stickers for city blocks or track laps completed. Healthy competition can be encouraged by racing to a goal either individually or by a classroom. Another strategy is to include parent participation by having them sign off on triathlon or walk-a-thon mileage sheets. Encourage parents to do the activity with their child. A parent/teacher bulletin board recognizing athletic achievement, such as running a 5-mile race or marathon, highlights adults leading healthy lifestyles. Children are very proud to have their parents and teachers value their achievements.

HEALTH PROMOTION PROGRAMS FOR PARENTS

The following are ideas for healthy partnerships with parents:

- Parent information sessions
- Parent peer groups
- Late breakfast meetings; "Second cup of coffee meeting"
- Grandparents day
- Breast cancer awareness
- Parents' nutrition committee
- Parent information sessions

The most difficult part of planning health promotion activities that include parents is timing. Most parents are employed and have very little flexibility in their work schedules. Breakfast meetings that are short and occur as children are brought to school may be well attended. Issues must be appealing to parents, and it is always a good idea to conduct a "needs assessment" before deciding on topics. In this way, you can include important health information as well as meet parental expectations. Below is an example of an agenda for a parent information session on nutrition. This was a program held in the evening. Marketing strategies include credit for parent volunteer service hours, a cooking demonstration with samples, and prizes, such as a 1-year subscription to a parenting magazine or a healthy fruit or vegetable basket. Always try to involve the community merchants in the donation of prizes. Perhaps the local grocery store will donate a fruit or vegetable basket or the hair salon will donate a free hair styling. The more involved community businesses are in school activities the better the community health nurse can promote the health of all citizens.

Healthy Habits, Healthy Kids! (An Evening for Parents)
Registration, sign up for door prizes, complete survey related to nutritional knowledge
Welcome and panel introductions
Healthy Habits, Healthy Kids overview
Effects of cholesterol, sugar, and salt on our daily diet
Making sense of food labels
Making good choices in the grocery store
Making choices in the restaurant
Making your family recipes healthy
Healthy heart discussion
Door prizes awarded

Parent Peer Groups

Establishing a parent peer group in which parents agree to certain rules of behavior for the youngsters or teens, such as curfews and party rules, are helpful to parents and school personnel. Parents can agree not to allow drinking of alcohol, use of tobacco, or drugs at their house. Parents in the group can then feel comfortable when their children/teens are in the company of peers whose parents ascribe to the same rules. A consistent approach sets limits for youth while providing an atmosphere of positive peer pressure. Parents also feel comfortable consulting with each other and form a support system.

Grandparents Day

Grandparents Day is a day in which the school actively involves grandparents, many of whom may not have been in an educational setting for a long time. Activities of the day can include classroom visitation, a healthy lunch, and blood pressure screening. Seventh-grade (or higher grade) students can be taught to measure blood pressure in science, physical education, biology, math, or health class. You can work with the respective teacher and conduct the practice sessions together. Youths take the elders' blood pressure under the supervision of a health professional such as yourself and volunteer nurse parents or other trained adult. This activity provides a service for the elderly guests as well as increases the awareness of the young students regarding the importance of preventing heart disease and monitoring blood pressure. If elevated blood pressures are noted, have a referral plan complete with name and phone numbers of clinics, the local health department, or private medical care providers that the person with an elevated blood pressure can be referred to. Also follow up on elevated blood pressure measures and offer every participant written information on elevated blood pressure and the association with poor health.

Mother–Daughter Programs

Cancer prevention programs for mothers and daughters can promote breast self-examination and mammography. Culturally appropriate programs can be designed to attract women of various ethnic backgrounds. For example, if it is not culturally acceptable to discuss breast matters in public meetings, perhaps you can involve the local worship centers or other culturally acceptable agencies where the information could be hosted. (The worship center may also be able to provide a bilingual presenter for women not fluent in English.) Equally important is a cancer awareness for fathers and sons on testicular cancer and the correct technique for testicular self-examination. Perhaps mother–daughter talks can be scheduled at the same time with father–son talks. This can be fun for the whole family, regardless of age, and again involves the whole community. Girl Scout and Boy Scout troops or Future Farmers of America clubs might be interested in sponsoring a family awareness day because they are usually interested in hosting activities for the entire family.

Nutrition Awareness

If the school meal program is not healthy, form an ad hoc committee to study the problem. The committee should consist of parents, the community/school nurse, cafeteria personnel, representatives of the faculty and administration, and a dietitian, if available. (Hint: Seek consultation from parents. Frequently, a professional dietitian is among the parents.) Action steps would include:

1. Conduct a survey to assess parental interest and areas of concern. What would parents like to see happen? What are they willing to do to make change happen?

2. Conduct a survey to assess student opinion and food preferences.

3. Do a plate waste study to determine what children are actually eating (see below for how-to).

4. Form a committee, remembering to include the students.

5. Based on what you learned in steps 1, 2, and 3, identify other options to the present menu, such as hiring a nutritionist to study the present food service. You may also want to organize a committee to visit other schools to sample food, look at menus, and talk to those students about satisfaction.

6. Make recommendations to the school administration.

7. Make a presentation to the school board.

8. Pilot test alternatives.

Plate Waste Study

1. Recruit parent volunteers, cafeteria staff, and teachers to help you.

2. Choose at least 2 days of the week to conduct the study.

3. Place volunteers next to the tray return and trash containers.

4. Record types and amount of food put into the trash.

5. Look into lunch bags for type of discarded, uneaten food.

6. Record all information (perhaps onto form with different food types).

7. You now have important information, such as nutritious food waste and the amount of soft drinks and candy consumed (from the wrappers).

8. Write a one-page report.

9. Give the report to parents, staff, and students.

10. Present the results to school administration along with suggestions to decrease food waste.

HEALTH PROMOTION STRATEGIES FOR THE SCHOOL

The following are additional ideas for health promotion strategies that can be used with groups such as teachers or staff in the school setting. Again, this list is not exhaustive but meant to generate ideas for viable strategies.

- Blood pressure screening on the same day each month
- Cancer awareness programs
- Stuffing payroll envelopes with health promotion material
- Healthy heart lunches, such as salad day once a week
- Referral and resource information
- TB skin testing

HEALTH PROMOTION STRATEGIES FOR THE COMMUNITY

- Involve elderly in school activities, such as reading programs, mentoring, and monitoring lunch hour
- Collaborate with the local civic association
- Establish a drug-free zone
- Have a community parade celebrating being drug free
- Establish a safe traffic pattern
- Contact radio and television stations and newspapers and ask them to report health promotion events
- Immunization programs
- School-based family clinics

SUMMARY

This chapter has focused on health promotion strategies that can be implemented in the school setting to achieve the goal of optimum wellness for school-age children. We have reviewed the components of health services, health education, and environmental issues. Suggestions regarding ways to incorporate groups associated with the school children, such as parents, teachers, staff, and the neighboring community, in health promotion efforts have been outlined. Community resources specific to the school setting have been included in this chapter. Now, we hope you will have fun promoting healthy partnerships with schools.

INTERNET RESOURCES

The following list contains websites that are of interest to those health care providers working in the school setting. It is important to note that Internet sites change rapidly and the information included below may not be the latest version. It is provided as a resource, and the reader is encouraged to recognize the need for periodic updating.

www.aap.org
American Academy of Pediatrics
An organization of primary care pediatricians includes information promoting health, safety, and well-being of children.

www.cancer.org
American Cancer Society
Not-for-profit voluntary health organization provides information to consumers related to the prevention of cancer.

www.diabetes.org
American Diabetes Association
Not-for-profit voluntary health organization provides information and resources related to diabetes.

www.americanheart.org
American Heart Association
Not-for-profit voluntary health organization provides information to consumers related to prevention and treatment of cardiovascular diseases. School site programs are highlighted.

www.lungusa.org
American Lung Association
Fights lung disease through community education, service, and research, particularly related to issues of tobacco use and asthma.

www.ashaweb.org
American School Health Association
Promotes the health of the nation's youth by advocating for comprehensive school health programs.

www.cyfernet.mes.umn.edu
Children, Youth, and Families Education and Research Network
Website includes resources for youth, parents, and professionals to promote healthy,
 safe individuals, families, and communities. Links with national, state, and international agencies, foundations, and associations.

www.cdc.gov
Centers for Disease Control and Prevention
An agency of the Department of Health and Human Services, which promotes health by
 preventing or controlling disease, injury, and disability. Website includes data, statistics, and health information.

www.acf.dhhs.gov
Department of Health and Human Services, The Administration for Children and
 Families

www.nasbhc.org/
The National Assembly on School-Based Health Care
Nonprofit private association promoting school-based interdisciplinary, accessible,
 quality primary and mental health care.

www.nasn.org
National Association of School Nurses, Inc.
Nonprofit specialty nursing organization. Website includes conference announcements
 and publications related to school nursing practice.

150.216.8.8/schealth/
Partnership for School Health
Website contains school health resources, information, and many links to health organ-
 izations and agencies.

www.schoolnurse.com/
School Nurse Forum
Accessible resource to link school nurses with current information and with each other
 through the web for the purpose of sharing ideas.

SUGGESTED READINGS

Journals

Journal of School Health
 Monthly journal, except for July/August
School Nurse
 Health information publication; four issues per year
American Journal of School Nursing
 Four issues per year

Books and Articles

American Heart Association. (1993). *American Heart Association Kid's Cookbook*. New
 York, NY: Times Books. Random House, Inc. Healthful foods for ages 8 through 12.
 Available at local bookstores.
American Nurses Association. (1998). *Standards of clinical nursing practice* (2nd ed.).
 Kerneysville, WV: American Nurses Publishing.

Birch, D. & Hallock, B. (1998). School nurses' perceptions of parental involvement in school health. *Journal of School Nursing, 14*(3), 32–37.

Bryan, S. (1998). School nurses' perceptions of their interactions with nurse practitioners. *Journal of School Nursing, 14*(5), 17–23.

Cavendish, R., Lunney, M., Draynyak, B., & Richardson, K. (1999). National survey to identify the nursing interventions used in school settings. *Journal of School Nursing, 15*(2), 14–21.

Cowell, J., Warren, J., & Montgomery, A. (1999). Cardiovascular risk prevalence among diverse school-age children: Implications for schools. *Journal of School Nursing, 15*(2), 8–12.

Gaffrey, E. & Bergren, M. (1998). School health services and managed care: A unique partnership for child health. *Journal of School Nursing, 14*(4), 5–22.

Lunney, M., Cavendish, R., Luise, B., & Richardson, K. (1997). Relevance of NANDA and health promotion diagnoses to school nursing. *Journal of School Nursing, 13*(5), 16–22.

Newton, J., Adams, R., & Marcontell, M. (1997). *The new school health handbook: A ready reference for school nurses and educators.* Englewood Cliffs, N.J.: Prentice Hall.

Pavelka, L., McCarthy, A., & Denehy, J. (1999). Nursing intervention used in school nursing practice. *Journal of School Nursing, 15*(1), 29–37.

GREAT RESOURCES

D.A.R.E. (Drug Abuse Resistance Education). Contact your local police department

Guidelines/health manuals/continuing education programs for school nurses developed by local school districts

State and local health department guidelines and laws

State associations for school nurses. Websites: access through state associations

Volunteer agencies such as the American Heart Association, American Lung Association, American Cancer Society, and American Diabetes Association. Websites were given earlier.

Nina Fredland

PROMOTING HEALTHY PARTNERSHIPS WITH FAITH COMMUNITIES

17

OBJECTIVES

After studying this chapter, you should be able to

- Discuss the role of the community health nurse in promoting the health of faith communities.
- Design and implement health promotion programs for faith communities.

INTRODUCTION

In the face of the changing health care marketplace, congregations of worshipers are increasingly forming partnerships with nursing for health promotion programs. This movement of nursing in faith communities is based on the principles of holistic nursing that recognize the dynamic relationship of spirituality and health of mind and body throughout the life span (Solari-Twadell, 1999). Other influencing components are self-responsibility for health, increasing autonomous roles in nursing, and increasing lay ministry responsibilities in faith communities. *Congregational nursing* and *parish nursing* are descriptive terms found in the literature and apply equally to the concept of nursing in faith communities. For the purposes of this chapter, the term *faith communities* will be used. People of these communities will be addressed as *participants*.

INITIATING HEALTHY PARTNERSHIPS WITH FAITH COMMUNITIES

The roles of the nurse with faith communities are dictated as always by the needs of the people and include, but are not limited to, consultant, educator, counselor, referral-agent, advocate, and facilitator (Westberg, 1999). Frequently, nurses with faith communities are licensed professional nurses, with varied educational backgrounds and areas of expertise, who share their nursing skills as a means to give something back to their community of spiritual support. (However, in some settings, the nurses may be employed by the faith community.) Frequently, the professional nurses donate their time and expertise as well as their own equipment (eg, stethoscopes and/or sphygmomanometers). Some are advanced practice nurses in positions of clinical specialist in critical care, trauma, or ambulatory care, or are nurse practitioners with adult and family certification. Some are professional nurses in home health rehabilitation, nursing home, and acute care. Other volunteers are retired professional nurses. This is a rich group of nurses with varied experiences.

From the very beginning, nursing with faith communities has embodied the holistic approach to health care. This approach recognizes the dynamic relationship of all the needs (physical, psychological, spiritual emotional, social, and economic) to a person's health (Solari-Twadell, 1999). Nurses with faith communities are recognized members of the ministerial team. Home health care and invasive treatment procedures are usually not in this nursing practice; however, these procedures could be included should the faith community and the nurse so agree. Nursing with faith communities is not intended as a competitor to public or private health service organizations. Rather, a faith community-based program is simply another way to access the health care system. The holistic nursing approach is founded on the basic concepts of prevention, responsibility for one's own care, and partnership between clients and providers (Schank, Weis & Mateus, 1996).

If nursing with faith communities is based on a model such as the community nursing assessment, intervention, and evaluation model presented in Part II of this textbook, then the continuous growth and evaluation of programs are ensured. Assessments (monthly screenings), annual surveys, and analysis of the components of participants' needs tell us what intervention programs need to be implemented (eg, healthy eating classes, exercise classes, walking clubs, or diabetes management instruction). These programs are implemented in a timely fashion that is most supportive of the participants. Evaluations of the programs lead us to expand or to minimize programs depending on their effectiveness. Effectiveness is measured by the number of participants in the individual programs as well as individual goal accomplishment and overall satisfaction with the health outcomes (eg, weight loss, increased feelings of fitness, decreased fatigue, better perceived control of stress with lowered blood pressure, and actual control and direction of one's lifestyle choices).

Here are some strategies for identifying faith community needs.

* Distribute an educational needs survey to various parish groups, such as the women's organization, the young mothers' support group, the elder group, the men's organization, and the non-English–speaking community. The survey sample appears as displayed material.
* Attend meetings for the different groups.
* Form focus groups to discuss options to increase health or join an initiative already in progress, such as prayer groups or faith renewal focus groups.
* Provide a suggestion box.
* Form an ad hoc committee to study the health ministry and include key people such as clergy, lay ministers, school principal, social and health agency personnel, and so forth. Be sure that formal and informal leaders are included.
* Remember never to make decisions without input from the faith community.

Tool for Assessing Educational Needs of Faith Communities

Anonymous Demographic Data: Include age group, sex, language preference
Program Timing Preferences: Time of day, day of week, time of year
Topics faith community members are interested in:

■ CPR Skills	■ Navigating Managed Care
■ Cancer Prevention	■ Nutrition for Youngsters
■ Cardiovascular Risk Factors	■ Parenting and Child Care Issues
■ Community Safety	■ Retirement Issues
■ Diabetes Education	■ Screening Programs
■ Domestic Violence	■ Sexuality
■ End-of-Life Issues	■ Stress Management
■ Exercise	■ Warning Signs: Stroke/Heart Attack
■ First Aid	■ Weight Management
■ HIV+ Information	■ Other _____

The educational needs survey in the displayed material could be distributed at worship meetings to maximize the number of people reached. Of course, this should be available in all appropriate languages. It is helpful to have pencils available so surveys can be completed and collected at this time. After the information is gathered and synthesized, concerns and topics are prioritized. If an English version and non-English version are both used, respective priorities are noted.

HEALTH PROMOTION PROGRAMS FOR FAITH COMMUNITIES

After assessing the faith community's educational preferences, the nurse plans intervention programs based on the results. Here is a listing of classes that may be of interest to members of a faith community.

Exercise groups
Nutrition classes
CPR/Choking awareness/First aid
Positive parenting
AIDS/HIV information sessions
Planning for a healthy retirement
Immunization program
Health fair

If the community is interested in an exercise group, suggest a walking map. Walking maps are a self-directed exercise tool, which is popular particularly with the elderly. These maps have mileage-marked routes in each neighborhood. Many members may be trying to begin an exercise program but they do not know where to begin. Such maps can be helpful in starting and continuing a daily exercise program that contributes to the feeling of good health and, more importantly, can prevent or control high blood pressure.

To construct a walking map, here is what you do:

- Design a 1-mile map around the worship center.
- Extend the map to include shopping malls, a recreational park, or neighborhood school yards.
- Make sure the area is safe and accessible.
- Indicate ¼-mile markers, such as a retail store, a "no parking" sign, a mailbox, and so forth.
- Provide an opportunity for participants to learn how to do warm-up and cool-down exercises.

- Teach target heart rates and how to monitor pulses.
- Provide a mechanism for people to meet and become walking buddies, such as a kick-off party, convening at the worship center, or meeting at the mall if it is nearby.
- Provide for ongoing encouragement and follow-up.

The Healthy Heart Club combines nutrition and education in a monthly gathering at lunchtime. This nursing action can be geared to adults, teens, or children. It is designed to teach the basics of eating a balanced diet, to provide tips on how to shop wisely for healthy food, and how to make good choices in restaurants. Here is a plan for Healthy Heart Club activities.

Healthy Heart Club Activities
- Gather in the faith community center at a convenient time once a month.
- See if a faith community member who is a dietitian is available because it tends to attract people to the session.
- Identify content to be explored, such as healthy food recognition and preparation, economic purchases, eating out, and celebrating with healthy food choices.
- Include cooking demonstrations with healthy nonalcoholic drink or smoothie recipes that can be made in a blender and then sampled by participants.
- Recipe sharing that includes multicultural traditions is always popular for young and old alike.
- Offer tips on how to maintain favorite tastes in family recipes and still eat healthy, for example, substitution of 1% milk for full cream milk, egg beaters for eggs, or oil for lard.
- Field trips to ethnic restaurants and grocers can be scheduled.

This heart-healthy eating idea can be expanded to include children. Try starting a "Healthy Tots" or "Kid's Club" focusing on healthy food choices for healthy kids. How about serving chicken or tuna salad in an ice cream cone. Toss a banana, a peach (without the pit), some orange juice, and plain yogurt in a blender. Serve it over crushed ice. Challenge the children to come up with their own healthy, fruity concoction. Finally, celebrate with a heart-healthy party. Here is a healthy lifestyle program for youngsters that reinforces the notion that healthy choices can be incorporated into celebrations.

Pear and Apple Party Time Activity for Kids
- Pick a time when children are assembled. (Perhaps it is after the worship service.)
- Equipment you will need: pears, apples, toothpicks, little plates, napkins, a chalkboard (for tallying votes), cutting board, and knife.

- Have a variety of apples on hand (Red Delicious, Jonathan, McIntosh, Granny Smith, Golden Delicious).
- Have a variety of pears on hand (Anjou, Bosc, Comice).
- Cut the apples and pears into cubes.
- Have children taste each kind.
- Take a vote on what kind of apple and pear they liked most.
- Tally the votes on a scoreboard.
- Decorate the apple and pear with the most votes.
- Take a picture of everyone (and the pears and apples, of course).
- Celebrate and enjoy!

Cardiopulmonary resuscitation (CPR) training is another healthy lifestyle activity. This instruction is usually highly valued and can be an annual event. Because CPR for community groups is an awareness session instead of a certification, it is less difficult. However, it still provides people with valuable information and skill should they be faced with a life-threatening situation. Attendees gain confidence in their ability to recognize warning signs and initiate lifesaving measures that perhaps can save loved ones. This training can include children over age 10 and teens as well.

If a faith community undertakes the project of a health fair, timing is very important. One theory is that it should have its own special time of year. Another view is that it can coincide with an annual bazaar or fund-raiser. Personally, I always prefer as much fun as possible in everything I do. How about you? Because the community usually supports the annual fund-raiser, a captive audience is present. On the other hand, sometimes people would rather take health more seriously and not try to focus on fun and games and screening or health education activities at the same time. However, if immunizations are provided, sometimes this is an unpleasant association for children who set out for a fun time. Both situations can work with proper planning and marketing, depending on the commitment and support of the faith community. The following are steps to consider when setting up a health fair. This outline is not meant to be exhaustive but to provide ideas and some direction. Although the faith community is a church, synagogue, or temple, it is important to include the greater community in its health ministry. A health fair is a wonderful opportunity to open the boundaries of the faith community.

Organizing a Health Fair for a Faith Community
- Contact the clergy and lay council.
- Set the date (try to allow at least 6 to 8 weeks to arrange).
- Decide what health promotion areas to cover, depending on the audience (adults only, families, elders).
- Invite identified organizations to participate.

- Invite health care providers, health service vendors, and community resources from the geographic area.
- Solicit prizes from local merchants.
- Offer incentives for attendance, such as door prizes and coupons for free services (eg, mammograms, heart scans).
- Collaborate with other professionals, such as a dental school, pharmacy school, or optometrist.
- Offer free immunizations.
- Have a women's health booth, a men's health booth, a teen booth, and a children's health booth.
- Include screening stations such as vision, hearing, blood glucose, blood pressure, lead, tuberculosis skin testing, depression, HIV testing, and counseling.
- Have a plan for referral and follow-up.
- It may be a good idea to have an HIV-positive ministry booth providing information about HIV as well as providers from treatment centers.
- Have stations that focus on environmental health, including booths on mosquito control and water safety. People from rural areas can bring in water samples for testing.
- A home safety booth sponsored by the utility company and/or fire department can address ventilation, electrical hazards, and gas appliances.
- A Crime Watch booth sponsored by the police can address self-defense and home security.
- Set up computers for health risk appraisal programs.
- Assign booth areas considering flow pattern. Provide for privacy if breast self-examination is demonstrated or skin cancer checks are done.
- Invite the media.
- Include fun activities, such as craft booths for the children and adults.

Additional health promotion strategies for faith communities include:

- Blood pressure screening
- Glucose screening
- Vision and glaucoma
- Consultation and referral
- Bereavement program
- Weight management programs—how about "Weigh to go!" for a title?
- Smoking cessation programs
- Diabetic education classes
- Caregiver support groups
- Asthmatic support group
- Respite care programs

The nursing volunteers from the community ensure that the multicultural factor of the community can be mirrored in the nursing team. The problems of language are thereby mitigated by the volunteers who speak the same language as the clients. Cultural practices that contribute to healthy lifestyle (eg, Vietnamese and Chinese heavy use of vegetables in the diet) are emphasized at social and educational activities. Importance is placed on cultural recognition and adaptation of health-supporting behaviors.

Economic factors as well as cultural factors are essential concerns of problem identification and solution. The faith community is a microcosm of the larger economic pattern of the city. Services should be accessible to all members of the faith community as appropriate. The affluence of the community will affect the type of programs that can be implemented. It is an accepted fact that families that have more discretionary income are more able to engage in health promotion activities. This will impact the overall health of the community. Economics also influences how members of the community access health services. The faith community may be the only consistent health care they receive.

ESTABLISHING A LASTING PARTNERSHIP WITH FAITH COMMUNITIES

Now that background information and program strategies have been explored, let's focus on the essential elements of establishing a nursing partnership with a faith community. Here is one way to begin:

- Obtain support from clergy and administration.
- Identify a core of health professionals willing to participate. Ideally, they will be members of the faith community.
- Establish a marketing system.
- Find a college of nursing or a community college to assist you in developing the ministry.
- Identify sponsor support through parish members and neighborhood establishments. (Local businesses are usually supportive because they recognize that their clients are members of the faith community.)
- Acquire supplies, such as cotton swabs, rubber gloves, stethoscopes, blood pressure cuffs, glucose meters, and so forth, from various sources.
- Recruit additional volunteer health professionals to participate.
- Have a team meeting and plan nursing actions. Probably the first action would be to conduct a needs assessment. Be sure that it is conducted in languages that reflect the constituency.

It is acceptable to start small or to have volunteers who are only able to give a little time. The nature of the ministry is that it builds on itself as time and community needs dictate. A successful marketing strategy is critical to starting and maintaining an active program. Several approaches can be implemented. Depending on resources and community contacts, some may be more feasible than others. Local newspapers, radio and television spots, and civic association bulletins are possibilities. Posting on the church marquee or other community billboards is usually a very effective way of notifying the community of program activities. The most effective strategy is pulpit announcements during or immediately after regularly scheduled services. Surveys completed at this time usually yield excellent response. A nurse column in the faith community's bulletin announcing scheduled health-screening activities and health education programs can be a regular feature. Catchy names such as "Positively Healthy Choices," "Nurse's Notes," or "Here's to Healthy Choices" will focus attention on the health information, which should be published in all languages commonly spoken. Remember to partner with nearby or church-affiliated schools, community stores, and fast food restaurants. Ask to market the faith community "nursing news" and events in their flyers and newsletters and on their marquees.

Consulting with a community college or university school of nursing to assist with establishing the health promotion program really helps. Faculty members may be willing to assist with the writing of a needs assessment survey. Then, the church community can be assessed annually with a tool, an invaluable part of the process. Graduate student nurses can be lead players in the community assessment. They can work with lay members of the faith community and guide the actual assessment. This would be a tremendous asset to the nurse or nurses because most often they are volunteering and such needs assessments can be very time consuming. Reciprocally, the students would have an opportunity to participate in a valuable and realistic clinical experience. Another benefit to colleges is the opportunity for sharing research data.

Health care provider systems (hospitals, HMOs, PPOs) have come to realize the importance of collaborating with faith community health programs as a valuable model. Frequently, faith communities will sign agreements of support with health management systems such as hospitals, private clinics, or group medical practices. Depending on the type of agency, the sponsor provides continuing education for the volunteer nurses, screening services through a stationary or mobile health unit, and a speakers bureau for health education programs (Gillis, 1993). This sponsor, who may be a local public health department, may also provide low-cost immunizations at health promotion activities (King, Lakin & Striepe, 1993). Additionally, faith community nurses utilize the sponsor health care system, as well as other local health care providers, as referral options for faith community participants. Other types of non–health care sponsors include fast food restaurants, retail shops, businesses, colleges and universities, as well as civic and public service organizations (eg, Lions Clubs, women's organizations, League of Women Voters). Frequently, national foundations, such as the March of Dimes, or local foundations may be receptive to being a sponsor, thus providing needed money for supplies, brochures, and other essential items. Because space on church property is limited, the program is totally portable. Many volunteers bring their own equipment (eg, stethoscopes and sphygmomanometers). Representatives from drug companies and medical supply companies, who are members of the faith community, may supply the program with other needed equipment.

An example of how important this program is concerns a "healthy-feeling" parishioner who, because of his spouse's urging, had his blood pressure and glucose checked. The results were abnormal for age and gender. So, he was given the written test results, counseled, and referred to a health provider of his choice. A month later, the spouse reported that her husband was recuperating splendidly from coronary bypass surgery and learning to manage his newly diagnosed diabetes. Registered nurses, who are the diabetic management experts, and the nurse practitioners, with the support of the sponsor agent, can be the usual blood glucose screeners. Participants feel comforted and assured when their screening data are within normal range. The participants who regulate their type II diabetes without monitoring at home, usually because of limited income, can use the screening program for self-management evaluation and further education.

Classes that are age or content specific are popular and well attended. A nurse with a background in men's health issues can speak to the men's club. A male nurse can make a particular contribution speaking to the group about testicular self-examination, prostate and colon cancer, and penile erection issues. Nurses have an opportunity to discuss domestic violence and abuse. Presentations focus on defining abusive situations, identifying community resources available to victims and perpetrators of abuse, and especially skills for relationships without violence. A special meeting of teens by way of youth groups should address the subject of dating violence.

Nurses support other ministries of the faith community by assisting with emergencies at services. They promote the health of Boy Scouts and Girl Scouts as well as Boys and Girls Clubs through education and immunization programs. Nurses team with men's and women's groups for monthly celebration activities. All events have health literature displays with generous amounts of health materials in all appropriate languages. Through these efforts, the nurses are recognized as a visible ministry of the faith community. The visibility contributes to the ongoing success of the partnership between the nurses and the faith community (Miles, 1997).

In summary, nursing in faith communities is still in its early development phase. It has an enormous potential to grow and evolve into an enhanced health care delivery system. Nurses are singularly well equipped to use their multifaceted skills and their extensive body of knowledge to improve the health status of individuals, families, and communities in a changing health care arena. This nurse practice model is a relatively new and cost-effective way to help participants navigate the managed care environment. It is part of the solution to the problem of the ever-rising cost of health care. If programs such as this one can keep segments of society healthier through health promotion, disease-prevention activities, and, in some cases, home care options, the quality of health care will be improved (Rydholm, 1997).

Through expansion of the nurse role, more services can be brought to the faith community. The sponsor agent relationship can facilitate the addition of services. Faith community nursing can be expanded to include well-child care, adult health, and minor acute care. This can be addressed by employing nurse practitioners, who will actually practice in a clinic in the faith community setting (Souther, 1997). Eventually, a community-wide needs assessment can be conducted to expand the annual faith community survey. Nursing students can assist with this activity. Analyzing databases to identify community assets as well as problems will provide information for the program.

One of the most important steps will be acquiring physical space for the nurse ministry to provide services. Clergy and administrative personnel who are supportive of the program and eager for it to advance will see this as a necessity. If renovation plans are under way, space for the nurse ministry should be incorporated. Although the program can be entirely mobile, it is more practical to have a designated space for storage and to render services. To maintain focus, ensure quality, and preserve the volunteer and multicultural components of the congregation, both long- and short-term goals are required. Identify a variety of health promotion strategies and health education needs to be addressed in the future. Then set realistic short-term goals that focus on the specific areas identified, such as enhancing the diabetic education, restructuring the weight management classes, or offering stress-reduction methods (eg, aromatherapy, realistic relaxation techniques, caregiver support). Because members of the team are already often managing careers and professional commitments and family and personal responsibilities, limiting the focus at the beginning stage of development is the best strategy to ensure continued success of the program. The practice model of nursing partnerships with faith communities described in this chapter is in evolution. Nurses need to be proactive in this area of continuous health care reform. We must participate in and help shape future decision making for health care delivery. This nurse ministry, whether volunteer or reimbursed service, is a cost-effective enhancement of health care delivery systems. Nursing partnerships with faith communities are part of the solution.

REFERENCES

Gillis, V. (1993). Sponsorship networks. *Health Progress, 4,* 34–41.

King, J., Lakin, J., & Striepe, J. (1993). Coalition building between public health nurses and parish nurses. *Journal of Nursing Administration, 23*(2), 27–31.

Miles, L. (1997). Getting started: Parish nursing in a rural community. *Journal of Christian Nursing, 14*(1), 22–24.

Rydholm, L. (1997). Patient-focused care in parish nursing. *Holistic Nursing Practice, 4,* 47–60.

Schank, M., Weis, D., & Mateus, R. (1996). Parish nursing: Ministry of healing. *Geriatric Nursing, 17*(1), 11–13.

Solari-Twadell, P. (1999). The emerging practice of parish nursing. In P. Solari-Twadell & M. McDermott (Eds.), *Parish nursing: Promoting whole person health within faith communities* (pp 3–24). Thousand Oaks, CA: Sage.

Souther, B. (1997). Congregational nurse practitioner: An idea whose time has come. *Journal of Christian Nursing, 14*(1), 32–34.

Westberg, G. (1999). A personal historical perspective of whole person health and the congregation. In P. Solari-Twadell & M. McDermott (Eds.), *Parish nursing: Promoting whole person health within faith communities* (pp 35–41). Thousand Oaks, CA: Sage.

INTERNET RESOURCES

www.interaccess.com/ihpnet
International Network for Interfaith Health Practices
Includes practice models and resource links.

www.csbsju.edu/library/internet/parish.html
Parish nursing.
Ecumenical perspective on health care ministry including Internet resources for parish nursing.

SUGGESTED READINGS

Weis, D., Mateus, R., & Schank, M. (1997). Health care delivery in faith communities: The parish nurse model. *Public Health Nursing, 14*(6), 368–372.

Journals and Newsletters

Journal of Christian Nursing, published by the Nurses Christian Fellowship, Box 7895, Madison, WI 53707. Inquire about reprints of parish nursing articles and the availability of photocopies of selected articles.

Parish Nurse, a quarterly newsletter for practicing parish nurses. Issued by LCMS Health Ministries, The Lutheran Church—Missouri Synod.

Nina Fredland

CHAPTER

PROMOTING HEALTHY PARTNERSHIPS WITH HOMELESS POPULATIONS

18

OBJECTIVES

After studying this chapter, you should be able to

- Define *homelessness*.
- Describe problems unique to homeless people.
- Implement a program for a homeless population.

INTRODUCTION

Community health nurses focus on the needs of vulnerable populations. Those individuals who make up the nation's homeless are vulnerable to disease and disabilities. In the United States, up to 2 million people experience being homeless during a 1-year period. More than 700,000 people may be homeless nationwide on any given night. Some larger cities, especially in Southern regions where the climate is warmer, may have as many as 10,000 people who are homeless on any given night (National Coalition for the Homeless, 1999a; 1999b; 1999c). Demographics of the homeless have changed, especially in recent years. The alcoholic or illicit drug user is no longer the typical homeless person. Profiles of the homeless show that women with children comprise an exceedingly large portion of the homeless. A study by Shinn and Weitzman (1996) found that 40% of the people who became homeless were families with children. Certainly this percentage is higher in some cities. How can healthy partnerships with the homeless be initiated and sustained?

WHO ARE THE HOMELESS?

According to the Stewart B. McKinney Act, 42 USC 11301, et seq. (1994), the definition of a homeless person is one who "lacks a fixed, regular and adequate night-time residence." Those individuals whose primary night residence is a supervised temporary shelter, an institution that provides temporary shelter for those intended to be institutionalized, or a public place not intended for sleeping would be considered homeless under the McKinney Act, 42 USC 11302 (National Coalition for the Homeless, 1999d). The literature further defines the state of homeless people as literally homeless, marginally homeless, or at risk for homelessness. Homeless people who live in shelters, abandoned buildings, or other public areas are considered literally homeless. The McKinney definition is consistent with the literally homeless view including those people who face imminent eviction (ie, within 1 week). Marginally homeless people live doubled up in places they do not own or rent and consider their situation to be temporary. People at risk for homelessness live in a residence they own or rent but live with the threat of eviction (Steering Committee Report for the Coalition for the Homeless of Houston/Harris County, 1989). Estimates are that the number of people at risk for homelessness in the nation accounts for 250,000 people (Harris County Community Development Agency Report, 1995). These people may be an illness, an accident, or a paycheck away from eviction and usually depend on utility assistance. When these people are hospitalized, they often have no place to go after discharge.

Frequently, it is not one particular thing that causes homelessness. It is usually a multiplicity of factors such as low wages, inconsistent employment, inadequate social support, and/or health problems (National Coalition for the Homeless, 1999e). The inability to mobilize resources, such as transportation and child care, may prevent people from achieving gainful employment. A study by the Coalition for the Homeless of Houston/Harris County in conjunction with agency members of the Homeless Coordinating Council (National Coalition for the Homeless, 1996), in an interview of 483 people seeking public assistance, asked the individuals to identify the "last straw" that brought about their onset of homelessness. The responses were categorized as health-related illness (34%), domestic violence (31%), and loss of employment (23%). Some 12% stated the "last straw" was unknown. The same study found the following homeless characteristics to be true:

> 51% were women.
> 71% were over age 29.
> 44% were African American, 37% were white non-Hispanic, and 14% were Hispanic.

23% reported illicit drug abuse.
34% had a health problem, usually a chronic condition.
23% were unemployed.

HEALTH PROMOTION STRATEGIES FOR HOMELESS PEOPLE

Primary Prevention

Primary prevention measures to prevent people who are at risk for homelessness from becoming homeless are the first steps in health promotion for this population. The goal is to keep people in their homes. Some strategies are:

- *Emergency financial assistance*—Frequently, utility companies will have an emergency fund that can be used to prevent utilities, such as water and electricity, from being discontinued. To find out if such an emergency fund exists, call the local utilities and ask. Inform at-risk homeless people how to apply for this assistance, and advise them of the information they will need to have handy when they call.
- *Legal assistance*, such as consultation or mediation to prevent eviction— Is there a volunteer group of lawyers in the community? Find out where no-cost or sliding-scale legal assistance is available. Call the organization and learn about waiting time for an appointment, required documentation, and so forth.
- *Financial advisement*—Financial counseling programs are available free of cost in most communities. These programs can help inform people about money management. If instituted early enough, this strategy can effectively prevent homelessness.
- *Relocation programs*—Call community organizations, such as the United Way, churches, major social service agencies, to ask questions and find out details about temporary housing programs. Ask about employment opportunities. Are there opportunities for needed social support? It is very important that people at risk to homelessness not be disconnected from the social support that they currently have. Sometimes a small, one-time loan (ie, money that is paid back) or grant (ie, money that is not paid back) is all that is needed to pay the rent, thus preventing homelessness. Some state welfare programs have added a "one-time" emergency financial grant for housing and basic needs (water, electricity) in lieu of ongoing welfare assistance. Inquire about present assistance programs in your community. Such emergency financial aid for rent, security deposits, utility

bills, and moving expenses can maintain an at-risk person in his or her residence during a critical period until a paycheck is received.

Secondary Prevention

Secondary prevention focuses on the homeless people. Begin by listing all their perceived needs. It is helpful to categorize needs as housing needs, health care, or employment. Health care needs must be addressed first. Identify the barriers to homeless people receiving health care and how might these barriers be eliminated. Many times, homeless people cannot access the health care system because they do not have a permanent address or adequate identification forms, such as a valid driver's license. Perhaps the homeless person is a veteran of the military and is, therefore, entitled to health care and to other benefits such as financial support associated with a disability. Frequently, waiting at hospitals and clinics for health care can prevent homeless people from obtaining shelter for the night. This is because often there is a limited number of beds at homeless shelters, and, once the beds are reserved, no additional people are admitted to the shelter.

To promote the health of the homeless, assess and evaluate community resources for serving this population. How many shelter beds are available? Are there shelters for families? for teens? for pregnant women? for people with special dietary needs (eg, diabetics or those with lactose intolerance)? Are emergency shelters available on a "walk-in" basis? What is available in terms of social and psychological support for homeless people? Once in a shelter, rehabilitation may be necessary for medical or substantive problems such as alcohol or drug addictions. Is a counselor available to the shelter, a nurse or physician for emergency medical needs?

The primary goal for homeless populations is exiting homelessness and counteracting the effects of being homeless. To reverse homelessness, transitional housing is important. Transitional housing needs to be free or very low cost. Frequently, homeless people are allowed to live in such housing units for extended periods of time in order to save up to afford permanent housing. In addition to shelter, social support is usually available (and always essential) at transitional housing. We will discuss more about social support later in this chapter.

A common concern for homeless people is following medication and treatment regimens. The following is a list of common conditions that require your constant awareness as you promote healthy partnerships with homeless people.

- Frequently, medications cannot be easily refrigerated.
- It is difficult to follow special dietary restrictions when meals are eaten at a shelter. Food is often very salty, high in fat, with limited fruits and vegeta-

bles. It is important for nurses to learn about food served at shelters and day centers. Ask if you might stay for a meal.

* Food may not be allowed in the sleeping areas at the shelter, so taking medication along with food may not be possible.
* Swapping medicine among homeless people occurs. Sometimes, medicine is sold for cash or people are assaulted for the medicine. Counsel homeless people as to where medicines may be safely stored.
* Many homeless people request vitamins to compensate for nutritional deficits.
* Understand that homeless people are usually trying their best to follow treatment regimens. Acknowledge this fact.

Part of a healthy partnership with homeless populations is further assessment of health and social service resources. See the list below for additional community assessment information. (This is a good time to refer to your general community assessment and evaluate it in terms of information specific to the homeless.)

* Do shelters offer clinic services? Daily or weekly? What services are on site and what services are referred?
* Are local health departments and county hospitals within walking distance? Are bus tokens available for medical appointments? How long are the waits?
* Are mobile health vans operative in the area? Are they consistent in their delivery of health care, meaning do they come the same day of the week to the same street corner? What services do they offer? Some services are key to treating homeless people, for example, lab services including HIV testing and counseling, x-ray, and dental services.
* Are services linked to a religious group? There may be expectations associated with receiving services that may or may not be acceptable to the homeless person.

PROMOTING HEALTHY PARTNERSHIPS THROUGH EDUCATION

Being diabetic and homeless is especially difficult. Actually, having any chronic condition presents many challenges for the homeless person. The following is an educational program for diabetics. You may choose to make the necessary changes for another chronic condition such as hypertension.

- Arrange with shelter administration to have a diabetic teaching class in the main waiting area of the shelter.
- Emphasize the importance of foot care using posters written at the 3rd-grade level.
- Demonstrate proper foot care by having homeless people in attendance soak their feet in basins. Inspect feet with attention to any red, swollen, cracked, or infected areas. Be sure to discuss the importance of properly drying the feet.
- Discuss the importance of shoes that fit properly and dry, clean socks.
- Offer attendees socks perhaps donated from local merchants or collected by neighboring school children. A letter of solicitation to merchants for socks can be drafted from the educational institution with which student nurses are affiliated and/or with the shelter's name.
- Shoes can be gathered in advance by placing receptacles in city or suburban fitness clubs encouraging runners to donate slightly used athletic shoes. (Runners often replace shoes every 2 to 3 months. Although the shoes may no longer be suitable for running, there is usually a lot of wear left for day-to-day use.)
- It is important to distribute incentives in a fair, organized manner. This requires detailed advance planning. Distribution is best done at the end of the program.
- Referral for health needs (eg, foot infections, ingrown toenails, fungal conditions, circulatory concerns) and follow-up mechanisms must be in place.
- Blood pressure and blood glucose screening could be offered at the same time in conjunction with the educational program.

POSITIVE PARENTING SESSIONS

To assist women and men in shelters learn better strategies for coping with children, parenting classes can be offered. Suggested topics to include are:

- Normal behaviors for developmental ages
- Behaviors that indicate a child is ill
- Normal height and weight for age
- Nonviolent ways to discipline (eg, time-out, consistency, clear rules)
- Healthy, low-cost food choices (fruit, peanut butter, cheese, eggs)
- How to keep a positive outlook
- Assertive and empowerment training

ORGANIZING A HEALTH FAIR IN A HOMELESS SHELTER

A health fair is another way to cover a number of areas at once. Screening procedures such as dental, blood pressure, cholesterol, blood glucose, vision, hearing, lead poison, and scoliosis can be included in the agenda. Steps for organizing a health fair are listed below.

- Contact the shelter administrator.
- Set the date well in advance (6 months to 1 year, if possible).
- Decide what health promotion areas to cover, depending on the audience (eg, family shelter versus adult male).
- Invite identified organizations to participate.
- Solicit prizes from local merchants.
- Offer incentives for attendance, such as educational hours (most shelters require participation in self-help programs).
- Collaborate with other professionals, such as a dental school.
- Offer immunizations.
- Include screening stations, such as vision, hearing, blood glucose, blood pressure, lead, tuberculosis skin testing, depression, HIV testing and counseling.
- Assign booth areas considering flow pattern.
- Invite the media.
- Include fun activities, such as a magician for the children or massage therapy for the adults.
- Have a plan for referral and follow-up.

PROMOTING HEALTHY PARTNERSHIPS WITH PEOPLE EXITING HOMELESSNESS

Most people will exit their homeless state. To prevent recurrence of homelessness, it is imperative that a strong support system is in place. It is not enough to merely provide transitional housing. It requires a commitment to support those exiting homelessness for long periods of time (usually several years). Health promotion strategies to support people exiting homelessness include:

- Coordination of services, such as health, social, substance abuse, and mental health
- Continuity of care
- Case management services
- Transportation issues
- Job training

- Child care issues
- Sources for funding programs

Americans must realize that homelessness is a major health concern. The numbers of homeless people are growing although the demographics are changing. Multiple strategies are needed to combat this societal problem. To dispel the concept of a homeless underclass, concerted effort should target already successful programs for modeling. More research is needed to identify the composition of homeless aggregates according to location as well as their particular problems. Probably the most important strategies are politically based.

Community health nurses can lobby for changes in legislation that can prevent homelessness at the primary prevention level. Supporting legislation to raise the minimum wage is one example. The National Coalition for the Homeless (1999e) formulates a legislative agenda related to homeless populations, such as housing, benefits, income, protected class status, homeless veterans, and youth. (See Internet Resources at the end of the chapter for further information on the National Coalition for the Homeless.) Campaigns to raise the minimum wage and create adequate, affordable housing are top priorities. Lastly, one must recognize that some people choose to remain on the streets and continue their homeless existence. However, it is the opinion of this author that most homeless people do not want to remain homeless. They are caught in desperate situations. It is the profession of community health nursing to promote healthy partnership with homeless populations.

REFERENCES

National Coalition for the Homeless. (1999a). *Facts about homelessness.* Available at **nch.ari.net/facts.html**.

_____. (1999b). *Homeless families with children. NCH Fact Sheet #7.* Available at **nch.ari.net/families.html**.

_____. (1999c). *How many people experience homelessness? NCH Fact Sheet #2.* Available at **nch.ari.net/numbers.html**.

_____. (1999d). *Who is homeless? NCH Fact Sheet #3.* Available at **nch.ari.net/who.html**.

_____. (1999e). *Why are people homeless? NCH Fact Sheet #1.* Available at **nch.ari.net/causes.html**.

National Coalition for the Homeless (1996). *What was the last straw that brought about your homelessness?* Survey conducted by the Coalition of Houston/Harris County. Houston, TX: Author.

Report prepared for the Harris County Development Agency by the Coalition for the Homeless of Houston/Harris County. (1995). *Service demands in Harris County community development delivery area.*

Report on Hunger and Homelessness (1995). Washington, D.C.: United States Conference of Mayors, 1995.

Shinn, M., & Weitzman, B. (1996). Homeless families are different. In J. Baumohl (Ed.), *Homelessness in America.* Phoenix, AZ: Oryx Press.

Steering committee report prepared for the Coalition for the Homeless of Houston/Harris County. (1989). *Addressing the problem of homelessness in Houston and Harris County.*

INTERNET RESOURCES

The following references and websites are available to help you learn more about the plight of the homeless. Some offer practical, constructive ways to help with this societal issue.

nch.ari.net/wwwhome.html
National Coalition for the Homeless
A network of homeless people, activists, service providers, and others committed to ending homelessness through advocacy, education, technology, and grassroots organizing efforts.

nch.ari.net/advocate.html
NCH Advocacy Tips: Communicating With Congress
Information on ways to influence elected officials on behalf of homeless people.

www.hud.gov/hmless.html
Housing and Urban Development
A federal agency that funds programs to help the homeless.

www.census.gov
Census Bureau
Current population reports and poverty statistics.

SUGGESTED READINGS

Anderson, R. (1996). Homeless violence and the informal rules of street life. *Journal of Social Distress and the Homeless, 5*(4), 369–380.

Dillon, D. & Sternas, K. (1997). Designing a successful health fair to promote individual, family, and community health. *Journal of Community Health, 14*(1), 1–14.

Helvie, C. & Kunstmann, W. (1999). *Homeless in the United States, Europe and Russia.* Westport, CT: Greenwood Publishers.

Kroloff, C. (1993). *54 ways you can help the homeless.* West Orange, New Jersey: Behrman House Inc. This is out of print but available as a hyperbook at **http://earthsystems.org/ways/54.html.**

National Coalition for the Homeless. (1999). *The McKinney Act. NCH Fact Sheet #18.* Available at **nch.ari.net/mckinneyfacts.html.**

_____. (1999). *NCH's 1999 federal legislative agenda.* Available at **nch.ari.net/99agenda.html.**

Nyamathi, A., Flaskerud, J., & Leake, B. (1997). HIV-risk behaviors and mental health characteristics among homeless of drug-recovering women and their closest sources of social support. *Nursing Research, 46*(3), 133–137.

Tollett, J. & Thomas, S. (1995). A theory-based nursing intervention to instill hope in homeless veterans. *Advances in Nursing Science, 18*(2), 76–90.

Unger, J., Kipke, M., Simon, T., Johnson, C., Montgomery, S., & Iverson, E. (1998). Stress, coping, and social support among homeless youth. *Journal of Adolescent Research, 13*(2), 134–157.

US Conference of Mayors. (1998). *A status report on hunger and homelessness in America's cities: 1998.* Available for $15.00 from the US Conference of Mayors, 1620 Eye Street NW, 4th Floor, Washington DC, 20006-4005; 202/293-7330.

Zima, B., Wells, K., Benjamin, B., & Duan, N. (1996). Mental health problems among homeless mothers. *Archives of General Psychiatry, 53,* 332–338.

Pam Willson **and Ann Malecha**   C H A P T E R

PROMOTING HEALTHY PARTNERSHIPS IN THE WORKPLACE

19

O B J E C T I V E S

After studying this chapter, you should be able to

- Assess health promotion needs in the workplace.
- Discuss strategies for successful health promotion programs.
- Plan, implement, and evaluate programs that teach healthy behaviors to diverse groups of employees and their families.

INTRODUCTION

Health promotion, disease prevention and control, wellness, risk factor reduction, and *preventive health care* are some of the terms applied to workplace health programs. In this chapter, the term *health promotion* will be used to denote a process by which employees learn how they can improve their health and quality of life by developing new lifestyle behaviors. The process of promoting health in the workplace usually begins with the employee acquiring knowledge about a behavior, health risk, or disease process. It is followed by learning new skills, implementing them in one's daily life, and finding a means of sustaining the learned behaviors over the long term.

The occupational health nurse is often responsible for health promotion programs at the worksite and is an excellent resource person in establishing a community partnership. If the organization does not have an occupational nurse, health programs may be the responsibility of the safety officer or an employee in the company's human resources or benefits department. Ask who coordinates health activities. The nursing processes for promoting health at the workplace focus on the entire population of the company and may even extend to the employees' dependents (spouses and children).

Health promotion activities at the workplace begin with assessing the health needs of the entire workforce, including management. The next step is creating an awareness of the health issues through company-wide education, screening, and interventions that focus on lifestyle changes. This chapter discusses strategies for successful health promotion programs, describes the steps used in implementing various programs, and lists several available resources.

WORKPLACE HEALTH PROMOTION

More than 80% of American businesses employing 50 or more workers are involved in health promotion activities (Hunnicutt & Deming, 1999). Companies integrate health promotion into employee recruitment (eg, membership at a health club), job training (eg, back care), safety (eg, hearing conservation), health (eg, risk profiles and screenings), and recreation efforts (eg, fun runs and sport teams). Employers are interested in promoting the health and safety of their employees for multiple reasons including increasing productivity, reducing absenteeism, maintaining safety standard requirements, improving employee morale, and lowering workers' compensation and insurance claims.

TYPES OF HEALTH PROMOTION ACTIVITIES

Common workplace activities that promote health or prevent injury and disease are exercise, smoking cessation, back care, and stress management programs. Frequently, companies offer employee health newsletters, health risk appraisals, health fairs, and screenings, such as blood pressure checks and cholesterol levels. These examples fall within three types of health promotion.

- *Awareness programs* increase the employees' level of knowledge and interest (eg, flyers, seminars, and newsletters).
- *Behavior change* activities help participants develop healthier behaviors (eg, smoking cessation, regular exercise, and healthy nutrition).
- *Supportive environments* create work opportunities that encourage healthy lifestyles (eg, low-fat foods in the cafeteria, on-site aerobic classes, release time for health screenings, healthy snacks in vending machines).

When deciding on the type of health promotion program to offer, it is important to determine how consistent that program is with the company's mission and goals. Also consider the costs and benefits of the activity for both the employer and the employee. Whereas employers are aware of the potential for financial benefits, such as reducing absenteeism or improved work output, most employees participate in health promotion programs for personal reasons (weight reduction, increased physical fitness). The worker desires to look and feel better or to have an improved quality of life. Meeting the needs of both the organization and the employees will support wide employee participation and a highly successful health program.

PLANNING A HEALTH PROMOTION PROGRAM

Needs Assessment

Questionnaires and health risk appraisals are commonly used to identify employees' interest in educational topics and to describe present health and safety behaviors. Ideas for health and lifestyle survey topics to include on a questionnaire appear below. To include all these topics on one questionnaire would be overwhelming. However, if a plan for the year was developed with a different focus each month that began with a brief questionnaire to establish interest, then one could be ensured of success.

Exercise and fitness
Nutrition and eating well
Vitamins and natural remedies
Smoking cessation
Weight management
Vision care
Men's health
Women's health
Pregnancy and care of the newborn
Pediatric fever and pain management
Menopause, osteoporosis, and estrogen replacement therapy
Safety (bicycle, motorcycle helmets, safety belts, car air bags)
Safely traveling abroad
Violence (women, children, and the elderly)
Depression and anxiety
Stress management and relaxation
Adult pain management (back, neck, and wrists)
Heartburn and indigestion
Heart health (cholesterol and hypertension)
Diabetes

Cancer

Allergies and asthma

Employee health and insurance records can also be used to identify prevalence of chronic illnesses of the employees that need to be addressed. Safety records, workers' compensation forms, or employee and manager interviews are additional resources for determining employee and company health promotion needs.

Once the needs are identified, you may assist the occupational nurse or planning advisory committee in securing management support for a health promotion program. A proposal presentation or executive report is often one of the first steps in convincing management of the value of the project. A *business plan* approach to communicating your program is used to establish a common language and understanding of the project by everyone in the organization. A sample business plan might include the following:

- *Executive summary:* A short summary of the health promotion plan, which includes the *purpose* (eg, to decrease lower back strain), *methods* (eg, three 30-minute classes), *expected benefits* (eg, fewer work days missed, increased productivity), *costs* (eg, program costs, such as brochures, flyers, teaching time, and incentives, as well as avoidance costs, such as averted absenteeism and decreased insurance and workman's compensation claims)
- *Purpose:* Exactly what is to be accomplished and rationale. Include *Healthy People 2010 Objectives* for healthy adults.
- *Methods:* How, when, and where the plan will be put into action. List each task to be completed (eg, brochure and flyer design and dissemination) and who is the responsible person(s) along with a timeline for task completion. Outline the content of the program, including use of guest speakers, demonstrations, return demonstrations, and methods to increase employee participation and adaptation of the taught behaviors. Include program goal and objectives in this section of the proposal. A program goal might be: Eighty percent of employees completing the back care program will report a decrease in the number of sick days related to low back pain. A program objective could be: After lectures and demonstrations on correct lifting procedures, 90% of participating employees will demonstrate correct lifting procedures.
- *Expected Benefits:* List outcomes of program (eg, fewer work days missed due to low back pain). This is a good point in the proposal to note the number of days missed in the last year and by what percentage the proposed program will decrease that absenteeism. This is also a place in the report to cite other companies that you have found in the literature that implemented a similar program and the results the companies experienced.

- *Costs:* An accurate projection of program costs (materials, teachers' time, incentives) as well as profits expected due to decreased absenteeism and increased productivity. For further information on the business plan, consult the reference at the end of this chapter by Helmer and associates (1995).

RESOURCES FOR HEALTH PROMOTION PROGRAMS

Health Risk Appraisals

A health risk appraisal (HRA) is an easily administered, confidential instrument used to determine life expectancy based on current risk behaviors. The HRA can also calculate the amount of risk that could be avoided if lifestyle behaviors were changed. Some HRAs determine the person's readiness to change behavior. An HRA can be used as a teaching tool that gives positive feedback for healthy behaviors and encouragement and information for changing those unhealthy behaviors. An HRA is usually completed on an interactive computer program and provides an accurate individualized report to each employee in a timely manner (within 2 weeks). Anonymous aggregate data are provided to the company. The usefulness of the information to the employer depends on a significant proportion of the employee population participating (hopefully at least 70% to 80% of employees). Confidentiality of HRA information and publicizing highlights of the aggregate summary may boost future participation levels.

Specific HRAs exist to assess nutritional status, weight, and general fitness status. If you are ready for a study break (of sorts), stop and check out these HRAs on the Internet. (When you get the website, search for HRA). Consider how each may be used for a health promotion program at the worksite.

- Healthy Eating—**www.realtime.net/anr/10eattip.html**
- American Cancer Society—**www.cancer.org/index.html**
- National Cancer Institute—**www.nci.nih.gov**
- National Heart, Lung, and Blood Institute—**www.nhlbi.nih.gov**
- American Heart Association—**www.women.americanheart.org**

USING STAGES OF CHANGE IN HEALTH PROMOTION PROGRAMS

Because most health promotion programs involve lifestyle behavioral change, Prochaska's change process (Prochaska & DiClemente, 1983), Pender's Health

Belief Model (Pender, 1996), or your chosen model/theory can guide the process from planning through evaluation. A brief review of the stages of the change process follow.

Stages of the Change Process

- *Precontemplation:* In this stage, the employee is not even thinking about changing his or her behavior. The goal is to make the person aware of the benefits of change and to get him or her to start thinking about the possibility of change.
- *Contemplation:* In this stage, the employee is at least considering making an effort to change behavior. The employee is weighing the pros and the cons. The employee may not know how to change and may consider the change to be almost impossible. The attempt to change is not worth the effort if failure is to occur. The goal is to help the employee identify the benefits and to decide that putting forth an effort to change is worthwhile.
- *Preparation:* A person at this stage has decided to try and change a behavior(s). This employee desires help in making the change and is ready for information and skills to maintain the behavioral change.
- *Action:* At this stage, the employee is practicing the new behavior; however, it is not yet incorporated into his or her lifestyle. The new behavior requires lots of effort, which leaves the employee at risk for relapsing to the old behavior. The employee needs support, incentives, and sincere encouragement.
- *Maintenance:* The new behavior is ingrained in the lifestyle behaviors. A crisis or major stressor at work or personal life can become the impetus to revert to the previous behavior. The employee needs reinforcement, support, and opportunities to practice the new behavior. The employee benefits by sharing the newly learned behavior.

PROGRAM IMPLEMENTATION

Marketing is an essential part of successful program implementation. Some strategies for marketing include:

- *Posters.* Must be professional looking. Catchy words and titles are essential (eg, "Weigh To Go" for a weight reduction program). Change posters frequently to keep attention.

- *Electronic mail messages.* Count down to event; offer a related health quiz question and give the answer and rationale the following day.
- *Health newsletter.* Detail a success story, such as early detection of malignant melanoma, weight loss regimen using a walking program, not knowing a person had high blood pressure until participating in a screening program and how simple lifestyle changes helped control the disease (without medication).
- *Letter from the company's president or benefits manager.* Offering company time for health screening, announcement that company will pay for all or a portion of smoking cessation program/health screening test, or allowing a trade-in of 2 hours of sick time for wellness program attendance.
- *Offer incentive gifts* to participating employees, such as T-shirts, hats, sunscreen samples, a healthy fruit snack, water bottles.

PROGRAM EVALUATION

The evaluation process provides an opportunity to determine the outcomes derived by the health promotion program and directs improvement of employee health services. Evaluating the *structure* of the program, the *process* by which the program was delivered, as well as the *outcomes* of the program is a three-pronged approach common to quality assurance reviews.

Structural evaluation involves (1) reviewing the reporting mechanism to management and the support given to the health promotion program; (2) determining if the physical facilities were adequate for the program; (3) identifying equipment and supplies used; (4) identifying staffing requirements and their qualifications; (5) analyzing employee demographics and their health status needs; and (6) determining if the program mission, goals, and objectives were formulated to meet both the health needs of the employee and business needs of the employer.

Process evaluation addresses (1) whether the health promotion activity was appropriate for the setting, (2) whether the health promotion program was designed to meet workplace needs (this is where you can measure against the initial needs assessment), and (3) whether there was documentation and record keeping.

Outcome evaluation focuses on (1) were expected goals and objectives achieved; (2) did the program lead to positive outcomes; (3) did health outcomes demonstrate prevention of illness/injury, increase compliance, increase employees' self-care knowledge, restore function or relieve discomfort; (4) how did program benefits compare to program costs; and (5) satisfaction (of employees, employers, dependents) with the quality of health promotion services received.

Common methods for evaluation are postprogram rating scales, observation, and interviewing of employees about their opinions, attitudes, and satisfaction with the program. Chart and record reviews can be used to determine morbidity and mortality differences.

TIPS FOR MAINTAINING A HEALTH PROMOTION PROGRAM

To sustain a health promotion effort, always design the program according to the goals of the organization. Include from the beginning an identified, key workplace employee and/or manager. As part of the health promotion program, teach employees where, when, and how to utilize community resources. Include short- and middle-range evaluation of the program. If possible, give projections of long-range success, savings, health benefits (eg, morbidity and costs of finding early stage disease and averting possible surgery, pain, hospitalization, workman's compensation, and so forth). Always propose to incorporate health promotion into the employee benefits plan.

EXAMPLES OF HEALTH PROMOTION PROGRAMS

Skin Cancer Prevention

It is easy to incorporate skin cancer prevention and education into part of the activities planned for the company's annual fun run, summer picnic, or sport event. Here is a schedule.

- *Two weeks before event*—Add visual graphics to the event advertising that depict a runner with a hat on, a volleyball player putting on sunscreen, or other sun-appropriate activity.
- *Ten days before the event*—Give a brown bag lecture on or have a guest "expert" speaker from the American Cancer Society discuss skin cancer (incidence, prevalence, types of skin cancer, risk factors, warning signs, and prevention). Announce at the lecture that there will be skin cancer screening as part of the company event.
- *Seven days before the event*—Set up a table-top poster display on types of sun protection describing the amount of protection offered by each

product (broad-brimmed hat versus cap, white T-shirt versus tightly woven shirt, sun block versus sunscreen) or multiple types and forms of sunscreens (alcohol based, creams, waterproof, water resistant, gels, sprays) and have samples for testing.

- *Five days before the event*—Distribute an electronic mail announcement that a dermatologist and/or skin cancer specialist will be conducting skin cancer screenings at the picnic. Have them reserve a 5-minute time slot for each member of their family by phoning the "appointment hotline" number that you staff.

- *Four days before the event*—Distribute an electronic mail quiz regarding a fact about skin cancer prevention. Have the employees respond by electronic mail by the end of the workday. Place the prize and a flyer of congratulations on their desks or in their mailboxes the following morning. Continue the marketing by congratulating for several days. (Award ideas: lip balm with sunscreen, sun visors, sunglasses, sunscreens, and hats).

- *Event day*—Set up a booth and conduct skin cancer screenings and counseling. Distribute a list of dermatologists within the company's health benefits plan. Set up a station for demonstrating correct application of sunscreen. Dispense a medicine cup full of sunscreen to each passerby. Give the children red helium balloons imprinted with "Red balloons, NOT red children."

- *First day of work after the event*—Send short electronic mail evaluation to all employees regarding use of sun-protective products, number of family members sustaining sunburns, and value of the activities to the employee and their family.

- *Two and 4 weeks after the event*—Follow up on all written referrals given to employees and their families during the skin cancer screening. Determine outcomes and report to management concerning evaluation of the event.

Intimate Partner Violence Prevention

Each year in the United States about 1 million incidents of physical violence occur against women by an intimate partner, such as a current or former spouse or boyfriend. The effects of intimate partner violence spill into the workplace and can impact employment productivity. Working women who are being abused at home have reported being harassed by their abusive partners in person or by telephone while at work, being late, leaving work early, or missing work because of the abuse, and being reprimanded for problems associated with the abuse. Abused women have also reported losing a job because of the violence in their lives. More and more employers are recognizing that domestic violence is a major problem in the workplace and are willing to implement policies and procedures that address domestic violence prevention. The following are elements of a domestic violence prevention program that focuses on decreasing intimate partner violence against women.

- *A written domestic violence prevention policy statement.* Inquire if such a statement exists at the worksite. If not, you may want to initiate such an action. A clearly written company policy statement demonstrates concern and commitment to employees' safety and health. The policy should include nondiscrimination against victims in recruiting, hiring, and promoting, and sensitivity in performance evaluation.

- *Manager and employee education.* Educational opportunities, such as brown bag seminars, newsletters, posters, and brochures on domestic violence, will help create a work culture that recognizes and strives to prevent intimate partner violence. October is National Domestic Violence Awareness month, and many national organizations offer resources to raise workplace awareness about domestic violence. Consider having a panel of community experts, such as a police officer, counselor, and nurse, discuss different types of domestic violence, such as stalking, abuse during pregnancy, and sexual assault and offer available health, social, and legal services. Displaying a poster on the "safety bulletin board" about domestic violence prevention and changing to a different poster on domestic violence, such as child abuse or elder abuse, several times a year is an effective way to increase awareness. Organizing employees to collect food and clothing for a local battered women's shelter is another way to support prevention efforts.

- *Employee counseling and intervention.* Everyone at the worksite needs to be aware of the signs and symptoms of intimate partner violence. A flexible and empathic work environment allows abused employees to disclose the violence and seek help. Abused employees may need time off for criminal and/or civil court proceedings, health care and counseling, and safe housing relocation for themselves and their children. A current list of telephone numbers and addresses of community resources and social service agencies specializing in domestic violence should be available at all times. Posting hotline phone numbers and steps of a safety plan in the women's restrooms with a basket or box of business card size listing of community resources and telephone numbers (preferably available in individual toilet stalls) is a safe method for dissemination of resource information. Companies that offer an Employee Assistance Program (EAP) need to ensure that counselors are trained to provide appropriate assistance with domestic violence.

- *Provide adequate security to employees.* All employees need to be reassured of a safe worksite even if an abuser attempts to stalk and harass an employee at work. Procedures must be in place to deal with trespassing, violence in the workplace, harassment, and accessing law enforcement. Safety plans for victimized employees may include advising coworkers of the situation and possibly supplying a photograph of the abuser, temporary relocation of the victim to a secure area, reassignment of parking place, and escorting to and from the worksite.
- *Provide financial support to employees.* Examples of emergency financial assistance to abused employees include (1) making changes in benefits at any time during a calendar year to ensure adequate health coverage for the employee and dependents; (2) expediting requests for changing the process of electronic paychecks into different bank accounts; and (3) providing emergency funds for employees in crisis.
- *Implement domestic violence screening questions* on preemployment and annual health examinations. Information on domestic violence, safety measures, and community resources must be part of every health fair, screening, and health education event. Examples of domestic violence screening questions are available from the resources noted at the end of this chapter.

SUMMARY

This chapter has discussed many strategies for promoting healthy partnerships with people at the worksite. As you plan worksite health promotion programs, also consider programs discussed in other chapters, such as healthy partnerships with faith communities and schools (remember, many employees have children). Most adults spend about one third of each day at the worksite. This presents a excellent opportunity for promoting health lifestyles.

REFERENCES

Helmer, D.C., Dunn, L.M., Eaton, K., Macedonio, C., & Lubritz, L. (1995). Implementing corporate wellness programs: A business approach to program planning. *American Association Occupational Health Nursing Journal, 43*(11), 558–563.

Hunnicutt, D., & Deming, A. (1999). Building a well workplace. In Well Workplace University. Available at **welcoa.org/why_wellness_works/index.htm**.

Pender, N. (1996). *Health promotion in nursing practice* (3rd ed.). Los Altos, CA: Appleton & Lange.

Prochaska, J.O. & DiClemente, C.C. (1983). Protection motivation theory and preventive health: Beyond the health belief model. *Health Education Research: Theory and Practice, 1*(3), 153–161.

INTERNET RESOURCES

www.midwife.org
American College of Nurse-Midwives

www.eatright.org
American Dietetic Association

www.awhp.org
Association for Worksite Health Promotion

www.fvpf.org
Family Violence Prevention Fund

fido.nhlbi.nih.gov:70/1/nhlbi/about/othcomp/opec/ncep
National Cholesterol Education Program

www.cdc.gov/ncipc/ncipchm.htm
National Center for Injury Prevention and Control

www.ncadv.org
National Coalition Against Domestic Violence (NCADV)

www.dol.gov/dol/wb
US Department of Labor, Women's Bureau

www.osha.gov
US Department of Labor, Occupational Safety and Health Administration

Use a Search Engine and Request the Following:

American Association of Occupational Health Nurses, Inc.
American Industrial Hygiene Association
Bureau of Labor Statistics
Industrial Health Foundation
National Institute for Occupational Safety and Health
National Safety Council Public Health Foundation
Occupational Safety and Health Administration
Society for Occupational and Environmental Health

Shirley Hutchinson

CHAPTER

PROMOTING HEALTHY PARTNERSHIPS WITH COMMUNITY ELDERS

20

After studying this chapter, you should be able to

- Discuss selected health and social factors that impact health status and functional ability of the elderly.
- Differentiate between individual-focused and community-focused health promotion strategies.
- Design and implement a health promotion initiative for community elders.

INTRODUCTION

There is widespread agreement that a major challenge facing nursing and health care in this century is caring for the fast-growing elderly population. Most health care providers agree that a major concern is assisting the elderly live healthy and productive lives. The rapid aging of America can be attributed to a powerful combination of decreased birth rates and increased longevity, both a result of effective public health measures and advanced medical care. The needs of community elders are as diverse and multifaceted as the elders themselves. A thorough understanding of the issues facing community elders trying to maintain independence in their own communities is the basis for building communities in which elders can live satisfying lives. This chapter focuses on developing individual-focused as well as community-focused health promotion strategies and partnerships with noninstitutionalized elders.

The terms *elderly*, *older adults*, *aging*, and *senior citizens* are used interchangeably to denote people age 65 years and older.

DEMOGRAPHICS OF AGING IN THE UNITED STATES

Elderly growth has outpaced nonelderly growth each year since 1900. The percentage of Americans 65 years and older has more than tripled (4.1% in 1900 to 12.8% in 1996), and the number has increased nearly eleven times (from 3.1 million to 33.9 million). A child born in 1996 could expect to live 77.1 years compared to about 29 years in 1900. This phenomenal growth has occurred as a result of reduced mortality rates of children and young adults, an outcome largely attributable to public health measures such as immunizations and environmental sanitation (American Association of Retired Persons [AARP], 1996). The US Census Bureau predicts that by 2040, one of five Americans will be 65 years or older. Moreover, it is predicted that there will be as many people over age 65 years as there are people under 20 years of age. Of special note, the fastest-growing population of older Americans is the 85 years and older group. By 2025, it is projected that 7 million Americans will be age 85 and above. Growth of the elderly population is expected to rise even more rapidly as "baby boomers" (those born during America's post–World War II population explosion, beginning in 1946) begin to turn 65 years old (US Bureau of the Census, 1997).

HEALTH CHALLENGES, RISK FACTORS, AND CONCERNS OF ELDERS

Health Status

Morbidity and mortality patterns of the elderly generally follow patterns of the population as a whole, with cardiovascular disease and cancer as the top leading causes of death. Additionally, the elderly population has a high prevalence of chronic illness, with people over 65 years of age accounting for 33% of the chronic illness that causes many Americans some degree of dysfunction. In 1994, the top chronic physical disorders reported in the United States among the elderly included arthritis, high blood pressure, hearing impairment, heart disease, orthopedic impairment, chronic sinusitis, diabetes, and visual impairment. In 1994, 28% of the elderly assessed their health as fair or poor compared to 10% of the general population (AARP, 1996). As the percentage of elderly people 85 years and older grows, so will the severity and number of chronic ill-nesses. Because chronic illness is often related to frailty in the elderly, creative, multidisciplinary approaches to chronic illness management will be needed to optimize independence and functional ability.

Health Care

Accessibility and affordability of health care are challenges for the elderly, particularly for rural and poor elders. Many have not adequately planned for the medical expenses that often accompany chronic illnesses that older people incur. Access to preventive services is often limited for the elderly. Medicare, the primary health insurance for older adults, offers very little coverage for health promotion and preventive services. Medicare coverage is often poorly understood, sometimes leaving elders paying for services that are covered by Medicare. Additionally, Medicare has many necessary health-related costs, such as outpatient prescription drugs, that are not cov-ered by Parts A or B. It is generally known that the elderly are among the greatest consumers of prescription drugs, many times paying for them out of pocket. Moreover, many Medicare beneficiaries have no supplemental coverage for prescription drugs or other medical expenses. Some elders report going without food in order to pay for medicines. Although state Medicaid programs provide coverage for some low-income older people, stringent Medicaid eligibility requirements leave many without access to Medicaid health insurance. Some states have implemented pharmacy assis-tance programs to fill the void of prescription drug coverage for non-Medicaid low-income populations. Although older adults have health needs that require a range of services on a continuum, not all services on the continuum are available to older adults in a variety of settings, leading to potential fragmentation of care.

Preventive services for the elderly are often neglected, because many providers do not see any point in prevention during the last years on the age continuum. A related issue is the recruitment and training of health profes-sionals to provide medical and health care for seniors. Until the mid-1970s, there was little emphasis on geriatrics in medical schools (Gelfand, 1999). However, professional nursing has been at the forefront in educating advance practice nurses in gerontology and adult nursing as well as incorporating courses on aging in nursing curricula. Alternative forms of health care, such as acupuncture and herbal medicine, may not be covered by insurance plans. Medicare Managed Care is now available to older people as is Medicare sup-plemental insurance, which provides coverage for certain services that are not covered by Medicare. Elderly populations often need guidance in selecting Medicare supplement plans that can best meet their needs.

Transportation to health care is another issue that impacts access to health care by the elderly, and rural elderly are hit hardest by lack of transportation. Elderly people often rely on friends, family members, lay taxi drivers (people who use private cars and often charge high fees), church volunteers, public transportation, and other forms of community-sponsored transportation to access health services. Nurses can play a key role during debates on Medicare and Social Security reform by promoting health care coverage not only to prevent illness but to keep older Americans from losing their savings trying to pay for health care and, consequently, falling into poverty or sinking deeper, if already poor.

Elder Abuse

As functional status and sensory acuity begin to decline, the elderly become vulnerable to an assortment of abusive and neglectful situations. According to the National Aging Information Center (NAIC) (1998), there are three basic categories of abuse: domestic, institutional, and self-neglect. Domestic elder abuse refers to maltreatment of an older person residing in his or her own home or the home of a caregiver. Institutional abuse occurs in residential facilities whereas self-neglect refers to neglect inflicted by older people living alone which threatens his or her own safety or health.

The National Center on Elder Abuse reports an increase of 150% in state-reported elder abuse nationwide over a 10-year period, from 1986 to 1996 (NAIC, 1998). However, because abuse and neglect are largely hidden under the shroud of family secrecy, it is grossly underreported. Findings of the National Elder Abuse Incidence Study estimate that one half million older people in domestic settings were abused and/or neglected or experienced self-neglect during 1996 (NAIC, 1998).

Mistreated elders are often frail, dependent, over age 70, and women. Typically, family members, not strangers, are perpetrators of this abuse (Ham & Sloane, 1997). Elders who were abusive parents themselves are at higher risk of abuse. Elder abuse and neglect encompass a variety of events that harm older people, including trauma, swindling, fraud, unattended medical problems, poor hygiene, dehydration, malnourishment, battering, verbal abuse, forced confinement, and other types of mistreatment that come at the hands of family members, neighbors, and caregivers. Resolving abusive situations may require involvement of protective agencies as well as law enforcement. Community nurses need to be familiar with abuse reporting laws.

Community Safety and Fear of Violence

Many community-dwelling elders are virtually prisoners in their homes because they fear becoming victims of muggings, break-ins, rapes, and robberies. Elderly people often lack access to transportation and do not travel great distances; therefore, attacks are more likely to occur near where they live. The elderly are more vulnerable to crime. Due to declining physical strength to protect themselves, elderly people, especially women living alone, are easy prey for criminal victimization. Therefore, few venture outside and many take extraordinary measures to barricade themselves into their homes. This fear is compounded for the elderly poor who live in high-crime neighborhoods. The impact of criminal victimization is more devastating for the elderly than for younger adults. A low and/or fixed income makes it difficult for many older people to recoup from a robbery. They often live in aging neighborhoods that are undergoing change and economic decline (Gelfand, 1999, p 93). Fear for their safety can be a deterrent to elderly people engaging in walking as a form of exercise. This fear can also cause social isolation. Community health nurses can facilitate neighborhood safety campaigns, such as crime watch programs.

Mental Health and Mental Wellness Challenges

Mental health is an important aspect of healthy aging. Mental health issues faced by the elderly include social isolation and loneliness, depression, suicide, and alcohol addiction. Tremendous loss and role transition are associated with old age, including retirement, loss of friends and loved ones to death, loss of vitality and energy due to illness or disability, and, in many cases, less contact with children and grandchildren who may live in a different city or state. Social isolation is associated with the very old (age 85 and older), frail health, and the elderly living alone.

Depression is considered to be a significant problem for the elderly (Miller, 1995). The prevalence of depression varies by setting, affecting up to 20% of community-dwelling elders, 25% of hospitalized elders, and as much as 40% of nursing home residents (Ham & Sloane, 1997). Depression is one of the most common risk factors for suicide. Suicide is at least eight times greater in the elderly population than the general population (US Preventive Services Task Force, 1996). Community health nurses and other health care providers need to be aware of the signs and symptoms of elderly depression and suicidal tendencies. A number of depression scales are available for assessing levels of depression in elderly clients.

Accidents

Falls are the greatest cause of accidents in people over 70 years old. It is estimated that about two thirds of falls among the elderly are preventable. Whereas a fall in a younger person may not be problematic, a fall in an older person can have devastating results. Common risk factors for falls include use of medications or alcohol, poor physical condition, changes in visual acuity, inner ear disturbance, foot problems, gait and balance disorders, and hazards in home and community.

Several risk fall assessment tools have been developed and are widely available. Scores can be calculated and reviewed with elders to plan fall prevention strategies. Older adults are also at risk for accidental injury related to driving, fires, overmedication, and hypo-/hyperthermia. Decreased sensory acuity, impaired balance, decreased muscle strength, and decreased reaction time serve to diminish the ability of elderly people to interpret their environment. Community health nurses are in an excellent position to facilitate community-wide, as well as individual, injury prevention programs that target the elderly.

HEALTHY PEOPLE 2010 AND OLDER ADULTS

Healthy People 2010 has established a goal to increase quality and years of healthy life for all Americans (USDHHS, 1998). The document indicates that the most important aspect of health promotion for older adults is to maintain health and functional independence. Many of the *Healthy People 2000* health objectives (USDHHS, 1991) are included in *Healthy People 2010* objectives. When planning health promotion programs for community elders, community nurses should incorporate priority areas and specific objectives addressed in *Healthy People 2010*. One health promotion objective identified in *Healthy People 2010* that is directed at elders is: Increase to at least 90% the proportion of people aged 65 and older who have participated during the preceding year in at least one organized health promotion program.

Health Promotion and Health Protection Strategies for Community Elders

Health promotion and health protection are two elements of primary prevention. Health promotion denotes emphasis on helping people change their lifestyles and move toward a state of optimal health, whereas health protection focuses on protecting people from disease and injury by providing immunizations and reducing exposure to carcinogens, toxins, and environmental health hazards. The concept of health for the elderly must be revisited in planning health promotion interventions. Filner and Williams (1979) define health for the elderly as the ability to live and function effectively in society and to exercise self-reliance and autonomy to the maximum extent feasible, but not necessarily freedom from disease. More than any other age group, older Americans are actively seeking health information and are willing to make changes to maintain their health and independence. Health promotion efforts should be well focused on modifiable risk behaviors, matched to the leading health problems by age (USDHHS, 1998). Health care for the elderly, in general, has three common goals: (1) improved functional ability, (2) increased longevity, and (3) increased comfort and decreased suffering (O'Malley and Blakeney, 1994). To maximize health promotion for community elders, a multifaceted approach is needed. Interventions should target individuals and families as well as groups and communities.

Individual- or Family-Focused Interventions

Individual- or family-focused health promotion/health protection interventions are designed to increase the individual's or family's knowledge, skills, and competence to make health decisions that maximize health-promoting and health-protecting behaviors. The goal is empowerment of the elderly and their families to make rational health decisions. Some categories of health promotion and health protection intervention that target the individual and/or family are:

- Health screenings
- Lifestyle modification
- Health education (one-to-one or group)
- Counseling
- Support groups
- Primary health care
- Immunizations
- Home safety
- In-home care (home health, personal care, or household assistance)
- Home-delivered meals
- Social support (telephone reassurance and home visiting)
- Case management
- Home maintenance help

Community-Focused Interventions

Community-focused interventions are activities and programs that are directed toward community elders as a whole or various elderly subgroups in a community. The goal of community-focused interventions is to improve community capacity and availability of the appropriate mix of health and social services required to prolong independence and functional status of community elders. Interventions at the community level primarily involve advocacy, political action, and participation in policy making that affects community elders. Examples of community-focused interventions are:

- Community-wide health educational campaigns that emphasize older people
- Holding campaigns in May, which is designated as "Older American Month"
- Community coalitions to address specific elderly issues, such as development of local information centers, telephone hotlines, or Internet sites
- Political involvement to advocate for needs of the elderly, such as preserving or expanding Medicare coverage for in-home services
- Collaboration with universities, churches, senior centers, senior housing projects, and other established community organizations to provide comprehensive services to subgroups of elders
- Crime prevention activities
- Participation in community-focused health fairs

PARTNERSHIPS WITH COMMUNITY ELDERS

Elderly populations, in general, are open to new health practices and respond to a variety of approaches that have the potential to improve their health. To plan effective health programs, community health nurses should validate proposed goals and strategies with the targeted elderly group. Involving elders in planning health promotion and disease prevention activities is essential because older people are sensitive to potential loss of independence and involving them increases a sense of independence. Action steps for working with older adults in the community include:

- Take programs where elders usually congregate, such as churches, senior centers, and retirement centers.
- Incorporate outreach activities into all programs.
- Be prepared to offer transportation to group activities.

- Anticipate needs of those with poor sight and/or vision (eg, use large print, limit handouts, use quiet room and/or loudspeakers).
- Maintain slow pace for activities and allow adequate time for responses.
- Allow plenty of time for elders to share life experiences.
- Keep teaching sessions relatively short.
- Incorporate multiple repetitions and reinforcement of information.
- Structure health education activities so the elderly feel comfortable to ask questions and/or challenge information that is new or doubtful to them.
- Encourage involvement of families, friends, and significant others.
- Advocate for improvements in community resources and policies that affect the elderly.

Selected Health Promotion and Health Protection Needs of Community Elders

Health Services

People over 65 years of age need regular primary health care services to maintain health and prevent disabling chronic illness and life-threatening conditions. Health promotion services that can form the basis for a community nursing intervention include:

- Immunizations (influenza, diphtheria, tetanus, pneumococcal vaccine)
- Screening for chronic illnesses, such as cancers, cardiovascular disease, and diabetes
- Management and control of existing chronic illnesses (health education, case management, and medication management)
- Knowledge of coverage and reimbursement practices (including alternative medicine) of Medicare/Medicare Managed Care, Medicare supplemental insurance, and specific state health insurance programs
- Community outreach and advocacy efforts to ensure linkage of elderly people to needed resources, such as heath advocates, health coaches, and community gatekeepers. These may be trained employees of businesses, churches, and corporations that can refer elders to community resources (Florio et al., 1996).
- Referral to existing state pharmacy assistance programs and advocacy to establish such programs where they are needed
- Education on medication management (scheduling, adherence, calendars, and so forth)
- Continuous source of primary care

- One-stop shopping for health care
- Connection to chronic illness support groups

Nutrition

Adequate nutrition is important for older adults to maintain health, prevent disease, and slow down progression of existing chronic illnesses. To help the elderly improve or maintain nutritional status, it may be helpful to perform a nutritional assessment and build on existing strengths. An excellent tool that is readily available is the Nutrition Screening Checklist developed by the American Academy of Family Physicians, American Dietetic Association, and the National Council on Aging (Nutrition Screening Initiative, 1992). Consider the following nutritional health partnership program.

"Eating Healthy, Deliciously!"

Plan a class or a series of nutrition classes that focus on basic nutrition as well as risk management nutrition (less salt, less fat, less sugar, more fiber, and so on). If special diet needs are to be covered, consider a series of classes and stratify the group according to specific dietary needs. Nutrition classes are more effective if they are highly interactive with the audience—incorporate recipe tasting and recipe sharing, build on existing positive habits, and include ethnic food preferences. Use of colorful, large-print posters and videos is appropriate. Reinforcing handouts are also helpful. Remember, elderly people like to talk and share their experiences! Provide rewards for class attendance, such as canned goods, paper towels, macaroni, and other nonperishable food items. Enlist support of grocery stores for gifts. A major challenge is to get older people to attend these classes. Consider someone from the community or peer group to help with marketing and outreach.

Exercise and Fitness

The benefits of exercise are well established across the life span. Exercise activity for elders must be suitable to health and functional status. Here is a program idea for increasing exercise fitness.

"Sitting Down, but Kicking High: Exercise for Seniors"

While conducting a blood pressure screening clinic at a senior nutrition center, the nurse observed that the residents often arrive at site around 8 o'clock in the morning. Their time was spent sitting until lunch was served at 12 noon. A few played table games such as cards or dominoes, but there was little physical activity. While checking blood pressures, the nurse asked about physical activity and determined that most of them did not feel safe to walk in their neighborhood nor did they know of other forms of exercise. After validating the need for low-impact chair-type exercise, a program was developed and several of the participants were trained as exercise leaders. The program was titled "Sitting Down, but Kicking High: Exercise for Seniors." Under leadership of lay exercise leaders, the program was eventually incorporated into the daily activity schedule.

Fall Prevention

Falls among the elderly are a major concern. You may want to team up with occupational therapists and physical therapists to conduct a fall prevention class or classes at a location where elderly people normally congregate (yes, you probably won't impact the elderly needing this the most; they are at home because of fear of falling if they go out). Some can administer a fall assessment questionnaire, some can perform balance testing, some can demonstrate ways to prevent falls, and still others can provide individualized counseling regarding fall hazards. This collaborative multidisciplinary project can have tremendous impact on a problem that sometimes causes elderly their independence or even death. You will need to market the project and obtain space for all screening, balance testing, demonstrations, and counseling. Consider having waiver and consent forms for balance testing in the event of an accidental fall.

Community Safety

To reduce fear of violence that often haunts older people, community nurses need to work with local law enforcement agencies to develop community programs. Prototype programs include Neighborhood Crime Watch Programs, Citizens on Patrol, and other civic organization safety programs. Elders need education regarding physical and psychological self-defense programs. Population-focused media campaigns should concentrate on making elders aware of their vulnerability to specific types of crimes in the community, including frequency and time of day of occurrence. Additionally, direct deposit of monthly checks should be encouraged to decrease vulnerability to violence.

Driving Safety

As the percentage of older adults in America increases, so does the number of older drivers. It is recommended that older drivers relearn to drive to accommodate neuromuscular and sensory changes that occur with aging. Older drivers should be encouraged to periodically reevaluate driving ability, including vision/hearing checkups, and evaluation of other physical changes that might affect driving. Encourage elders to ask family and friends if there are concerns about their driving ability. AARP sponsors the 55 ALIVE/Mature Driving program to help older motorists improve driving skills, prevent car crashes, and avoid traffic violations (AARP, 1999a). AARP also publishes the *Older Driver Assessment and Resource Guide*, which is available free of charge. Older drivers should be referred to these resources or others that exist in the local community.

SIGNIFICANT LEGISLATION AND OLDER AMERICANS

Finally, some important pieces of legislation merit discussion. Two important pieces of legislation that impacted the lives of older Americans are the Social Security Act of 1935 and the Older Americans Act (OAA) of 1965. The Social Security Act mandated many programs to serve the elderly, including income assistance and health care. The main provisions included establishing a system of old age benefits and enabling states to make provisions for blind people, aged people, and dependent and crippled children. The act established a Social Security Board and mechanisms for raising money for retirement income and welfare benefits. One of the most significant amendments came in 1965, which established Medicare and Medicaid health insurance programs. The OAA gave national attention to the needs of the elderly and authorized the Administration on Aging within the Department of Health and Human Services. It funded research and training in gerontology and facilitated local, state, and national programs to improve quality of life of the elderly. Over the years, it has established many services for senior citizens, including area agencies on aging, multipurpose senior centers, nutrition services, volunteer programs, health education, transportation services, in-home health care, and preventive health activities. Other legislation that helped to improve the quality of life for the elderly includes the Age Discrimination Act of 1974, which prevented age discrimination in employment and prevented forced retirement; the Research on Aging Act of 1974, which created the National Institute of Aging in the National Institutes of Health; and the American Disabilities Act of 1990, which ensured the rights of Americans with disabilities.

SUMMARY

Promoting health partnerships with community elders is an exciting venture. A comprehensive paradigm of health for the elderly, including social and environmental health, is needed. For their own protection, the elderly of tomorrow will have to learn to stay well and become politically active (Alford and Futtrell, 1998). The focus of health care for this group will continue to shift from acute medical care to self-care and chronic illness management. Additionally, health promotion strategies will emphasize quality-of-life issues as more of the elderly are expected to experience a high level of functioning well into 80 to 90 years of age. Community health nurses have an opportunity to develop innovative approaches to improving quality of life for elders through advocacy and service delivery. Here are some questions to propel you forward toward health promotion for community elders.

- What impact does health promotion in younger years have on health status and functioning in older years?
- If frail elders residing in their homes are provided "lay case management" (such as a health advocate or health coach who calls or visits in-home periodically, supervised by professional nurses), will they experience longer independent living, better health functioning, fewer falls, and fewer hospitalizations than frail elderly who do not get such support?
- What is the appropriate mix of health and social services that can be provided through senior centers? Are such centers cost-effective?

REFERENCES

Alford, D.M. & Futtrell, M. (1998). Wellness and health promotion of the elderly. In J.A. Allender & C.L. Rector (Eds.), *Readings in gerontological nursing* (pp 77–79). Philadelphia, PA: Lippincott Williams & Wilkins.

American Association of Retired Persons (AARP). (1999a). *55 ALIVE/mature driving program.* Available at **www.aarp.org/55 alive**.

_____. (1996). *Profile of older Americans.* Available at **research.aarp.org**.

Filner, B. & Williams, T. (1979). Health promotion for the elderly: Reducing functional dependency. In *Healthy People 2000*. Washington, DC: US Government Printing Office.

Florio, E.R., Rockwood, T.H., Hendryx, M.S., Jensen, J.E., Raschko, R., & Dyck, D.G. (1996). A model gatekeeper program to find the at-risk elderly. *Journal of Case Management*, 5(3), 106–114.

Gelfand, D.E. (1999). *The aging network: Programs and services* (3rd ed.). (p 69). New York, NY: Springer.

Ham, R.J. & Sloane, P.D. (1997). *Primary care geriatrics: A case-based approach* (3rd ed). (p 262). St. Louis, MO: Mosby.

Miller, C.A. (1995). *Nursing care of older adults: Theory and practice* (2nd ed.). (p 504). Philadelphia: J.B. Lippincott.

National Aging Information Center (NAIC). (1998). *Elder abuse prevention.* Washington, DC: US Government Printing Office.

Nutrition Screening Initiative. (1992). *Nutrition screening checklist.* A cooperative effort of the American Dietetic Association, American Academy of Family Physicians, and the National Council on Aging. Washington, DC: Author.

O'Malley, T.A. & Blakeney, B.A. (1994). Physical health problems and treatment for the aged. In D.G. Satin (Ed.), *The clinical care of the aged person: An interdisciplinary perspective* (pp 27–61). New York, NY: Oxford University Press.

US Bureau of the Census. (1997). *Population projections.* Washington, DC: US Government Printing Office.

US Department of Health and Human Services (USDHHS). (1998). *Healthy people 2010 objectives: Draft for public comment.* Available at **odphp.osophs.dhhs.gov/pubs/hp2000/progrvw/olderprog.html**.

_____. (1991). *Healthy people 2000.* Washington, DC: US Government Printing Office.

US Preventive Services Task Force. (1996). *Guide to clinical preventive services: Report of the US Preventive Services Task Force* (2nd ed.). Baltimore, MD: Williams & Wilkins.

SUGGESTED READINGS

Clark, M.J. (1999). *Nursing in the community: Dimensions of community health nursing* (3rd ed.) (pp 551–588). Stamford, CT: Appleton & Lange.

Clemen-Stone, S., McGuire, S.L., & Eigsti, D.G. (1998). *Comprehensive community health nursing* (5th ed.). (pp 603–629). St. Louis, MO: Mosby.

Edleman, C.L. & Mandle, C.L. (1998). *Health promotion throughout the lifespan* (4th ed.). (pp 633-663). St. Louis, MO: Mosby.

Gorin, S.G. & Arnold, J. (1998). *Health promotion handbook.* St. Louis, MO: Mosby.

Hulse, J. (1998). Humor: A nursing intervention for the elderly. In J.A. Allender & C.L. Rector (Eds.), *Readings in gerontological nursing* (p 87). Philadelphia, PA: Lippincott Williams & Wilkins.

Pickering, S. & Thompson, J. (1998). *Promoting positive practice in nursing of older people.* London: Bailliere Tindall.

Swanson, E.A. & Trip-Reimer, T. (1996). *Advances in gerontological nursing: Issues for the 21st century* (Vol. 1). New York, NY: Springer.

AGENCY RESOURCES

Administration on Aging (National Aging Information Center)
USDHHS
330 Independence Avenue, SW
Washington, DC 20201
www.aoa.gov

Alzheimer's Association
919 North Michigan Avenue, Ste. 100
Chicago, IL 60611
www.alz.org

American Association of Retired Persons (AARP)
  601 East Street
  Washington, DC, 20049
  www.aarp.org

American Society on Aging
  833 Market Street, Ste. 512
  San Francisco, CA 94103-1824
  www.asaging.org

National Council on Aging
  409 Third Street SW
  Washington, DC 20024
  www.ncoa.org

Social Security Administration
  6401 Security Building
  Baltimore MD 21235
  www.ssa.org

Mary Wainwright   CHAPTER

PROMOTING HEALTHY PARTNERSHIPS WITH RURAL POPULATIONS

21

OBJECTIVES

After studying this chapter, you should be able to

- Discuss geographic and social factors that impact health status of rural populations.
- Describe health promotion issues that relate to rural populations.
- Design and implement a health promotion project with a rural population.

INTRODUCTION

What image comes to mind when you think of rural? Do you think of a farm at the end of a long dirt road where a large family is eating supper together? A place where neighbors know and care about each other? A place with close relationships and less hectic lifestyles? Most people have a favorable image of a rural lifestyle. Just like rural living, nursing in rural settings can be very rewarding and challenging. In this chapter, we describe some general characteristics of rural populations and discuss strategies for developing healthy partnerships with rural populations.

Although most people recognize rural when they see it, defining the term has been a persistent unsolved problem. There is no operational definition of a rural area that precisely differentiates rural from urban populations. A common distinction, especially for federal programs, is metropolitan areas and nonmetropolitan areas. These are designations made by the Office of Management and Budget (OMB) based on the integration of counties with big cities having a population of 50,000 or more (Baer, Johnson-Webb & Gesler, 1997). Obviously, a small rural town isolated in a county designated as a metropolitan area would be lost in the OMB definition. A more common definition of rural population is people living in a sparsely populated place usually somewhat distant from a large city. Rural has a difficult-to-quantify feeling of close ties and strong community identity. It is not necessary to adopt a single definition for the purposes of this discussion. However, nurses should be familiar with the OMB designation of metropolitan and nonmetropolitan areas.

Engelken (1997) articulates the concept that rural is a tangible asset. However, not all attributes of rural populations fit with an idyllic image. The negative features of rural life have implications for nursing in rural areas. There is a greater concentration of people who are uninsured and with low incomes in rural areas. Rural dwellers live longer, which contributes to the fact that rural populations have a greater percentage of the elderly than urban populations (18% vs 15%) (Dansky, Brannon, Shea, Vasey & Dirani, 1998). Geographic distance and inadequate transportation are typical barriers to health care access. Consequently, rural dwellers are more likely to have complex and chronic health care problems (Gariola, 1997). Access is also limited because of geographic maldistribution of health care providers. Whereas 20% of Americans live in nonmetropolitan counties, only 11% of patient care physicians practice in those counties (Crittenden & Myers, 1997).

Unfortunately, changes initiated by the Balanced Budget Act of 1997 have significant potential for altering the structure of the rural health delivery system (Mueller & McBride, 1999). These changes could result in increased rural hospital closings, reduction of home health services, and increased maldistribution of the health workforce. In most rural communities, nurses are the foundation and, in some cases, the sole source of health care.

RURAL NURSING THEORY

As a framework for building partnerships with rural populations, it is useful to consider the rural nursing theory development work of Long and Weinert (1989). They identified the following key characteristics of rural populations that affect nursing services:

1. Work beliefs and health
2. Isolation and distance
3. Self-reliance

4. Lack of anonymity
5. Insider/outsider and old-timer/newcomer designation

Work Beliefs and Health

Rural dwellers define health in terms of ability to work. A logger in a rural logging town probably considers himself in good health as long as he is able to work. He will try home remedies and neighborly advice before he seeks professional help. Only when the remedies and advice fail will the logger consult a clinician. Treatment that will get him back to work is his dominant medical care expectation. Nichols (1989) described rural residents' health care orientation as present-time and crisis oriented. As such, these work/health beliefs make rural dwellers only minimally interested in health maintenance and disease prevention activities (Muldoon, Schootman & Morton, 1996; Parrott, Steiner & Goldenhar, 1996). Infrequent participation in smoking-cessation programs, tobacco chewing, obesity, and disregard for regular exercise are common.

Isolation and Distance

Residents accept and adapt to isolation and distance. Distance is integrated into everyday life. Residents anticipate and even relish shopping trips that require a 1- to 3-hour drive each way. With little hesitation, a neighbor may devote a day to driving the distance required for a sick friend's specialty doctor appointment. However, even with significant adaptive strategies, distance is a barrier that increases the likelihood of deferring health care until one is very ill. Furthermore, recovery times and optimal rehabilitation are compromised by inadequate and untimely treatment.

Self-Reliance

For survival, isolation and distance require the development of strong, self-reliant attitudes. The high value placed on self-reliance is readily observed both in individuals and the community as a whole. For example, a rural community's aspiration to develop a regional medical center—and make the necessary financial commitment to support it—are consistent with the community's desire to take care of itself. Individual self-reliance is also typical. Take, for example, rural Rosebud resident Mr. Kane's response to his elderly wife's immobility. Rather than place his wife in a skilled-care setting, Mr. Kane fed her, bathed her, and changed her decubitus dressing as best he could. He maintained this exhausting care regimen until he developed pneumonia and had to be admitted to the hospital.

Lack of Anonymity

Rural communities are fishbowls. Everyone knows about everyone. It is all too true that "You know you are in rural America when you find out the results of your daughter-in-law's pregnancy test before she does." Each person is observed and judged equally on his or her personal life and professional ability. A health care provider is known throughout the community, and privacy is limited. In the grocery store, school, or church, the provider is expected to deal with health care issues. Because people with advanced education or leadership skills are so often away, lured to larger cities, the role of the health care provider in a rural community frequently includes expectations of leadership. This additional visibility magnifies the fact that a rural nurse's credibility, trust, and effectiveness as an agent of change in partnership building depend on the community's judgment of the person as a whole.

Insider/Outsider and Old-Timer/ Newcomer Designation

Rural community residents tend to be less mobile than their urban counterparts. Several generations live within close proximity, and friends grow up and remain together for a lifetime. People are identified in the context of their relationships: "You know her. She's Mr. Gray's daughter-in-law." If one's great-grandfather was the town drunk, one is always known as the grandchild of the town drunk. This is often expressed in comments such as "Jill has done well in spite of the fact she's old man Jones's granddaughter." In a similar vein, it's easy to learn who is an insider and who is an outsider by listening to comments like "Make sure you include Mr. Wallis on your invitation list. He's on every money-raising committee in town," or "Why are you inviting Mrs. Leroy? She's never been involved in this kind of meeting before." In fact, newcomers may not join the ranks of old-timers for as long as 15 to 20 years. Mrs. Taylor came to one rural community when she was first married and was referred to as "the lady from Missouri" until her grandchildren were born. Lenz and Edwards (1992) stated that these distinctions usually produce more favorable considerations for insiders and old-timers. However, the outsider position is sometimes advantageous when issues of confidentiality arise and emotional distance is preferred. Acceptance of a rural nurse and his or her community role is influenced by the insider/outsider, old-timer/newcomer mind-set.

BUILDING A PARTNERSHIP

With these five rural nursing theory concepts in mind, let us now consider how to develop a partnership with a rural community. We will include in the discussion examples from a rural community named Rosebud.

Assessment: Old-Timers and Insiders as Key Informants

In a rural community, nurses must pay special attention to personal contacts when implementing the community assessment strategies described earlier in this book. Before beginning the assessment process, or at least very early in the process, you should identify key informants in the community. If you are an outsider or a newcomer, an effective strategy is to have someone within the community "sponsor" you by introducing you to key informants, and you may want to refer to your "sponsor" when you make contact with others. Discuss with the key informants your assessment goals and their perception of community health assets and needs. Also, ask them to identify other important contacts. Rural communities are self-reliant and may resist activity they perceive as interference from outside. By engaging community old-timers and insiders early in the process, you can build a network that will help assess, plan, and implement strategies to meet community-identified health needs. This network of community informants can identify resources, overcome bar-riers, and help to find solutions to problems that reflect the community's perspective.

The most important concept to keep in mind is that the rural community's perception of their community health needs defines the reality of those needs. Many rural communities will accept help identifying their community needs. A reliable, comprehensive assessment is essential in securing resources for a rural community, but the resources to accomplish an assessment are frequently limited. Some communities may have strong public opinion regarding community health needs, with or without the benefits of a formal needs assessment. However, if a community places high priority on a health risk that you consider less critical than others, the community's perspective is the priority. To attempt to address the greater health risk without the community's support would be to invite failure from the beginning. By empowering the community and thereby contributing to "healthy community" behavior, you will offer a greater service. Often, when you help the community address the lesser risk, you build community awareness of the greater risk.

In rural Rosebud, several citizens were concerned about tobacco use by high school students. Our comprehensive community assessment revealed a high incidence of lung cancer in the community and no public activities to address the issue. We also identified as an asset the well-attended county fair, which contributes to Rosebud's economic health and civic pride. Utilizing both the community's identified need and the empirical evidence of an existing health risk, we make the community diagnosis: high prevalence of lung cancer related to long-term tobacco use.

Planning: Designing by the Community for the Community

The community needs information in a usable form about the results of the assessment process. An informed community can participate in effective planning. Key informants will again be excellent resources in suggesting a dissemination process for the assessment results. It takes time and energy to engage the community in the planning, but this "engagement" is the part of the process that builds the community's strength and ability to address its own needs. This empowerment is an important component of a community's "health."

Involving the community at every step is part of the partnership, whether you engage in a whole town meeting or an informal committee planning process with a few key informants. The plan should be achievable and appropriate for the rural culture. For instance, health promotion activities need to be threaded into the everyday activities of rural residents. A rural resident may not come to town just to participate in a free cholesterol screening session at the health clinic, but if the screening session was held at the grocery store on Saturday morning, he or she might take advantage of the opportunity. The action plan should include (1) clear objectives and action steps; (2) identification of resources needed, including people, budget, and materials; (3) identification of available sources such as grants, other funding, and volunteer time; (4) a timeline; and (5) an evaluation process.

In Rosebud, we posted the results of our community assessment, Rosebud's Top Ten Health Concerns, at the grocery store and the feed store as well as in the *Rambling Rose*, the weekly newspaper. Then, we convened five key Rosebud insiders to address the high prevalence of lung cancer related to long-term tobacco use. The informal group leader was a high school student's mom who was very concerned about smoking among her child's friends. By defining the goal, brainstorming, selecting interventions, and prioritizing the activities, we developed a project action plan. The plan included enlisting high school students to help us develop a "Health-Wise" booth at the county fair to promote anti-tobacco use behaviors and other health promotion activities.

Implementation: One Person Can Make the Difference

It is beneficial in the implementation process to enlist help from a community person who is energetic and enthusiastic about the project. Ideally, this person would have participated in the needs assessment and planning phases. Because of the "fishbowl" phenomenon in a rural community, a project's success may be linked to the person or people perceived as leading the project. That person may not be a "formal leader" of the community, but he or she must be able to influence others to participate in the intervention. One person does make a difference in rural settings. Furthermore, communities and community leaders need encouragement. Mark the milestones. Create opportunities to acknowledge publicly each incremental success. Develop effective relationships with news media. Signs in stores, newspaper articles, and radio and TV interviews are all effective strategies for maintaining the commitment and energy level of the community.

In Rosebud, when Ms. Carpenter, a local doctor's wife and community activist, learned of our "Health-Wise" booth project, she got excited and brought in all kinds of help. She was able to influence high school teachers to include research assignments about effective ways to prevent and change young people's tobacco-use habits. Students helped design materials and activities for the booth. Mrs. Carpenter's neighbor, the high school principal, allowed the students and other adults to use the wood shop to build the booth. Other project team members solicited donations for materials and coordinated work schedules. The newspaper editor wrote a small grant to the regional Lumber Industry Foundation to purchase sets of "Mr. Yuk Mouth," a bad-breathed, ugly-teethed model designed as a visual disincentive for tobacco use that targeted young people. We posted thank-you signs for every contribution. The local "investigative" reporter wrote a series of articles about youth and tobacco use and feature activities relating to the "Health-Wise" booth project.

Evaluation: Process and Outcomes

Rural community health needs rarely develop overnight. They are more often complex, chronic, and insidious problems. Evaluation strategies for community health interventions should include measures of anticipated long-term outcomes. In addition, assess the community's perception of the success of the project with respect to more short-range outcomes such as (1) partnership building and partnership strengthening, (2) numbers of individuals and groups involved, (3) quantity and quality of services provided, and (4) the impact of the project on the community diagnosis. Some of the outcomes may be new initiatives to address the problem or related problems. Acknowledgment of community assets is a healthy outcome. A community empowered to address its own needs is one of the most powerful outcomes possible. Finally, quantitative measures about behavioral changes and changes in health indicator trends should be reviewed in appropriate time frames. The results of the evaluation should be shared with the community.

In Rosebud, a feature article on the front page of the *Rambling Rose*, titled "Health-Wise Smoking Success," touted the community project's success. We received positive results from team members, including the high school students, who evaluated each action step and the overall project. The mayor acknowledged success of the project at the city council meeting. A new project was started in the elementary school, and the local merchants agreed to improve their strategies for preventing the sale of tobacco to minors. Another group began developing strategies to measure the actual tobacco use of children in their community. Although these outcomes were not anticipated in the original plan, they were legitimate and powerful project outcomes. Community empowerment was increased with this project, and Rosebud's self-image improved. It will be several years, if not decades, before the lung cancer rate health indicator may be affected, but Rosebud is proud of the changes that have already taken place.

SUMMARY

Rural communities are wonderful places to live and work. Understanding the rural dweller's work and health beliefs, the challenges of isolation and distance, the concepts of self-reliance, lack of anonymity, insider/outsider and old-timer/newcomer designations will increase our effectiveness in developing partnerships with rural populations. Throughout the nursing process, we can improve the strength of the partnership and healthy community behavior by engaging the rural community in each step of the process. One of the most rewarding aspects of developing partnerships with rural populations is the realization that "one person can make a difference" in the whole community. Perhaps you are the one nurse who has or will make the difference in your rural community.

REFERENCES

Baer, L., Johnson-Webb, K., & Gesler, W. (1997). What is rural? A focus on urban influence codes. *Journal of Rural Health, 13*(4), 329–333.

Crittenden, B. & Myers, W. (1997). Can Medicare medical education policies better address rural provider shortages? *Rural Policy Brief, 1*(3). Available at **www.rupri.org/brief/PB97-3/index.html**.

Dansky, K., Brannon, D., Shea, D., Vasey, J., & Dirani, R, (1998). Profiles of hospital, physician, and home health service use by older persons in rural areas. *The Gerontologist, 38,* 320–330.

Engelken, J. (1997). A wakeup call for rural health. *Rural Health FYI, 19*(1), 42.

Gariola, G. (1997). Developing rural interdisciplinary geriatrics teams in a changing health care environment. *Journal of Allied Health,* Winter, 27–29.

Lenz, C. & Edwards, J. (1992). Nurse-managed primary care: Tapping the rural community power base. *Journal of Nursing Administration, 22*(9), 57–61.

Long, K. & Weinert, C. (1989). Rural nursing: Developing the theory base. *Scholarly Inquiry for Nursing Practice: An International Journal, 3*(2), 113–127.

Mueller, K. & McBride, T. (1999). Taking Medicare into the 21st century: Realities of a post BBA world and implications for rural health care. Rural Policy Research Institute, Rural Health Panel Publication (pp 1–17), 2/10/99 P99-2.

Muldoon, J., Schootman, M., & Morton, R. (1996). Utilization of cancer early detection services among farm and rural nonfarm adults in Iowa. *Journal of Rural Health, 12*(4), 321–331.

Nichols, E. (1989). Response to rural nursing: Developing the theory base. *Scholarly Inquiry for Nursing Practice: An International Journal, 3*(2), 129–132.

Parrott, R., Steiner, C., & Goldenhar, L. (1996). Georgia's harvesting healthy habits: A formative evaluation. *Journal of Rural Health, 12*(4), 291–300.

INTERNET RESOURCES

www.nrharural.org/
The National Rural Health Association
A national membership organization whose mission is to improve the health and health care of rural Americans and to provide leadership on rural issues through advocacy, communications, education and research.

www.muskie.usm.maine.edu/rhsr/default.asp
National Rural Health Services Research Database
This site provides a database of funded rural health services research projects that are under way in the United States.

www.rural-health.org.au/
Rural Health WebRing
This is an Australian site dedicated to rural health issues. It includes government, educational, and hospital sites that contain information relevant to rural health.

Pamela Schultz

PROMOTING HEALTHY PARTNERSHIPS WITH THE CHRONICALLY ILL

22

OBJECTIVES

After studying this chapter, you should be able to

- Discuss the characteristics of chronic health conditions.
- Describe health promotion strategies for the chronically ill.
- Implement a health promotion plan for persons with a chronic health condition using strategies from other chapters.

INTRODUCTION

Typically, illness is viewed as a condition in which optimal health is not achieved. An acute illness is one in which the illness resolves as a result of an intervention or the lapsing of time. A chronic illness is one in which there is no resolution of the disease process. The implication is that the person will have this illness until his or her death; there is no cure. Because people frequently live long and productive lives with chronic illnesses, should they be labeled "ill"? Perhaps a more appropriate designation is chronic health condition. Many people in any community will be living with a chronic health condition.

On the surface, it seems that identifying those people with a chronic health condition is simple. But, upon reflection, this is a daunting task. How should "chronic health condition" be defined? What elements must be present to differentiate the acute health condition from the chronic condition? Can a health condition be both acute and chronic? Under what conditions?

The holistic approach to nursing care refrains from compartmentalizing the individual. The holistic approach emphasizes the interconnectedness of the person. When taken literally, this approach can be used to describe a person with a chronic health condition. The health of the person should not be compartmentalized, such as the diabetic, the person with cancer, the schizophrenic, or the person with HIV infection. However, the nurse is bombarded by the health care system's approach to label and categorize the person's health. So, in order to discuss the chronically ill, an attempt is made to describe this population in the broadest of terms.

CHARACTERISTICS OF CHRONIC HEALTH CONDITIONS

Progressive: The health condition worsens or becomes more severe over time. The time period may be over an entire life span or major portions of time. There may be periods of quiescence followed by periods of exacerbation or there is a slowly evolving deterioration. Examples of progressive health conditions are certain types of slow-growing cancers that are not curable and there is an inevitability of dying of the cancer. Chronic obstructive pulmonary disease characteristically is a slowly evolving deterioration of lung capacity. Congestive heart failure has periods of quiescence and control with patterns of acute bouts of heart failure. Diabetes mellitus, especially insulin-dependent types, becomes progressively more difficult to regulate.

Irreversible: The condition is not curable. The chronic health condition takes a toll on the individual. Damage that cannot be corrected occurs. Examples include some cancers such as those of the pancreas, which destroy the pancreas' ability to produce enzymes for digestion, which leads to nutritional deficits. There are several types of kidney diseases that eventually result in complete renal failure, which damages other major systems such as the central nervous system and the cardiovascular system. Chronic obstructive pulmonary disease causes a loss of pulmonary function, which is not reversible. Schizophrenia and bipolar disease are not curable but can be controlled; however, a long history of these conditions produces impairments in judgment, social skills, and activities of daily living.

Complex: The chronic condition may involve multiple systems. The impact of chronic health conditions reach beyond the arena in which they begin. People with asthma not only have physical manifestations of the process but they frequently restrict their activities in such a way as to cause isolation, which impacts their mental health and their recreation. Depression is a frequent sequelae of chronic health conditions (Davidson & Meltzer-Brody, 1999). The treatment of a chronic condition may have side effects, such as pain and nutritional deficits, that become a part of the condition. Diabetes mellitus can result in neuropathies; retinopathy leading to blindness; and circulatory problems leading to amputation, commonly of the feet and legs. Hypertension can lead to heart disease, stroke, and renal failure.

Treatment aimed at symptom control: The purpose of treatment is not to cure but to control symptoms. This implies an unknown cause and/or the lack of technology to enable a cure. In some cases, the condition is considered acute and treatment is aimed at cure, and, when this is unachievable, the condition becomes chronic. Some cancers follow this path.

A family affair and chronic sorrow: Chronic health conditions always have an impact on the significant others of the individual. Depending on the culture and the interfamily dynamics, this manifests itself with great diversity. Chronic sorrow is a condition that may be experienced by the individual and/or the family. This is a lasting phenomenon that can continue past the death of the individual with the chronic health condition. It is a sadness without end and comprises an accumulation of ongoing losses over time (Krafft & Krafft, 1998).

HEALTH PERCEPTION AND CHRONIC ILLNESS AND HEALTH PROMOTION

Every individual has a unique perception of the state of his or her health. This state fluctuates with various events, but usually a person has a static view of his or her health. People with terminal cancer may be heard to say that they are in good health if it wasn't for the cancer. People may maintain that they are in good health but be denied life insurance because of their medical history. People may perceive their health as being very poor but live well into their nineties. How is the perception of one's health important? If people perceive their health as good, then it is likely they will consider their quality of life as good. Studies have shown that the association between health status and quality of life is not clear (Covinsky et al., 1999). Covinsky and associates (1999) have shown that generally, one's health status is a reasonable indicator of perceived quality of life; however, incongruency is not uncommon. A person's perception of his or her health may sometimes lag behind actual health status. A 65-year-old woman is told she has severe osteoporosis and is at risk for hip fracture. She feels well and considers herself in good health. Within a few moments, she is given information about her health status that labels her as having a chronic health condition.

How a person perceives his or her health has a major impact on how he or she responds to health promotion strategies. If people see their health as good there may be resistance to health promotion strategies. If they view their health as not good, they may also be resistant to these strategies out of a sense of fatalism. Generalizations cannot be made. People with chronic health conditions typically are very informed about their chronic condition. They may have little patience with strategies aimed at areas of their health that are not perceived as part of that condition. Conversely, some people may choose to focus on an aspect of their health that can be improved.

IMPLEMENTATION OF HEALTH PROMOTION STRATEGIES

When planning to implement a health promotion program for people with chronic health conditions, there are several principles to consider.

Identification of specific health care priorities: People with chronic health conditions have special needs. Any health promotion activities must be tailored to those needs individually. The nurse must be knowledgeable about the person's health status as it pertains to his or her chronic condition. This requires a strong basic knowledge in the health care sciences. For instance, the nurse may want to emphasize the importance of drinking 8 to 10 glasses of water a day. For a patient on renal dialysis, this might not be appropriate.

Continuity of rapport: Stanley (1999) has described a program in which patients with chronic medical and psychiatric problems are placed in addictive treatment programs. Normally, these people would not be allowed to participate in the addictive treatment programs because of their conflicting chronic problems. But, because their program is designed to enable the health care professionals to respond to a variety of other health care needs, these patients can successfully complete programs aimed at addictive disease. This type of program allows for continuity of rapport. This partnership opens the nurse to intervene at all levels. It enables the psychiatric nurse to intervene in health promotion practices as well as the treatment for chronic conditions. In the milieu of managed care, continuity of care may become fragmented. Continuity of rapport is not only valuable in chronic health conditions but also in health promotion activities.

Social support: Social support has been linked to health and longevity in many studies (Lepore, 1998). It has been shown that social support enhances health. Many people with chronic health conditions develop a life pattern of isolation, which leads to difficulty in expressing themselves and relating to others (Jonsdottir, 1998). Many people with chronic health conditions have access to therapy and support groups focusing on particular chronic conditions. There are cancer support groups, AIDS support groups, sexual abuse support groups, and so forth. These types of groups provide comfort and camaraderie among the participants. Since 1960, group therapy has been shown to be a valuable tool of the helping professions (Bednar & Lawlis, 1971; Dies, 1986; Dies, 1979;

Kaul & Bednar, 1986; Orlinsky & Howard, 1986). These groups are fertile ground for health promotion by nurses. Many times, these groups are community sponsored. Support groups can be extended to family caregivers; this, too, increases the opportunities for health promotion, in some cases to the entire family (Ellgring, 1999).

Health professionals, particularly nurses, need to avail themselves of knowledge about the group process. This is not an unnecessary frill that exists on the periphery of medical and nursing practice or the private domain of a subspecialty (Sampson & Marthas, 1981). The skills required to work effectively with groups are not intuitive; they need to be learned.

Nurses state that providing support for their patients is a basic tenet of providing care. Support implies helping the patient make adjustments for the experience he or she lacks and problem solve in order to adapt to health care conditions (van Servellen, 1984). DeYoung and Dickey (1967) found that certain nursing behaviors expressed support defined by nurses. These included attention, presence, "thereness," acceptance, care, concern, interest, involvement, understanding, and empathy. van Servellen (1984) states that in the chronically disturbed family, the support provided by nurses takes many forms, such as restoration, facilitation of strengths, and resources that are present to maintain whatever level of wellness is possible.

Sampson and Marthas (1981) identify the roles of group process for health professionals. As we review the tasks of group process, it will become clear there is overlap in these group processes.

Human Growth and Development

Human beings learn how to be humans in groups. The early family is usually the most significant. As people grow, school and friends form other groups. As adults, these groups are changing and each person brings to each group situation a unique experience, which helps to further personal growth and development. People learn how to be human as children, teenagers, adults, the elderly, the disabled, the chronically ill, and the dying.

Behavior Maintenance and Change

Humans can learn and see modeled new or different attitudes or habits that need to be changed for certain health conditions. Smoking cessation, substance abuse, and obesity groups are examples of groups that use the group process to change health-related attitudes and habits.

Health Promotion and Maintenance

Physical fitness, cancer care, and stress reduction are examples of health promotion or health maintenance type tasks of groups. People learn through interaction with the group about the health condition common to all. Nurses uses this format to share their expertise and direct the group to share experiences concerning pertinent issues.

Team Practice

We are in an era of specialization, and groups of health professionals care for individuals as a team. This team functions as a group also. Each professional has different functions, and patient care is more effective when the team understands and uses good group process skills.

Family and Community Work

For example, cancer patients are not products of their disease alone. Interactions with their families and communities impact their disease process. Families are often caregivers; there are work and social concerns within the community that are critical for the care of that patient. The nurse can be instrumental, not only as a consultant, but may actually see a need and organize a specific group within the community.

Teaching, Training, and Supervision

Health promotion with a group is a vital role of community health nursing. Many examples are offered in other chapters on health promotion programs. As you work with groups that have a chronic illness, consider which of the health promotion strategies described in other chapters might be applicable. Here is an example of a support group for persons with cancer and their families.

Cancer Patient and Family Therapy Support Groups: A 6-Year Community Experience

This is the description of an ongoing support group that was begun in the community and is facilitated by two volunteer nurses with psychiatric and oncology experience. The basic purpose of the group was to provide support for cancer patients and their families. However, it became obvious that more than social support was needed as health promotion issues not related to cancer began to surface. The facilitators had to expand their knowledge base in the areas of exercise, nutrition, elder abuse, sexuality, heart disease, hypertension, postpolio syndrome, Parkinson's disease, hip and knee replacements, renal dialysis, and many other areas. Priorities in health concerns are in constant flux according to the individual. This experience highlighted the need for a comprehensive health education and promotion program. These people with a chronic disease sought information about how to be healthy. They also wanted new coping skills and new problem-solving techniques in living with their chronic disease.

Group Description

The group meets monthly for 90 minutes. The group is open, and there is no compulsory attendance. The group meets in a local church, and the one rule is confidentiality. There is no structured agenda, and the group members identify their immediate needs and the agenda for the group.

Group Demographics

The age range of the participants is 29 to 83 years of age. Sixty-seven percent are female. The length of time that members have attended the group is 1 week to 6 years. The majority are upper middle class; most are college graduates. The most common cancer diagnoses are breast and prostate cancer.

Evaluation

Evaluating a group process is problematic. The success of the program is best measured by its longevity. Some of these people have been attending these groups for 6 years. The social support they receive is apparent in their continued attendance. Some of these people know as much about their chronic health condition as can be known, but they continue to attend for the social support and other health information that they receive for themselves and their families. Families with chronic health conditions need to be able to talk with health care providers about quality-of-life issues. In today's health care environment, there is little opportunity for this. Community nurses with the appropriate education and expertise can use their unique knowledge to provide this service in the community.

The nurses have built a rapport with these people. They have formed a partnership with this community; they have become a part of it as well. They have brought to this experience their expertise, commitment, compassion, and, most importantly, themselves.

SUMMARY

Different from other chapters in this section of the textbook, there have been no specific health promotion programs offered in this chapter. This is because we hope you will review all the chapters and choose health promotion programs appropriate to the need of the chronically ill you encounter. Indeed, we hope you have enjoyed all the many strategies for promoting health partnerships. *Health to all.*

REFERENCES

Bednar, R.L. & Lawlis, G.F. (1971). Empirical research in group psychotherapy. In A. Bergin & S. Garfield (Eds.), *Handbook of psychotherapy and behavior change: An empirical analysis.* New York, NY: John Wiley.

Covinsky, K.E., Wu, A.W., Landefeld, C.S., Connors, A.F., Jr., Phillips, R.S., Tsevat, J., Dawson, N.V., Lynn, J., & Fortinsky, R.H. (1999). Health status versus quality of life in older patients; does the distinction matter? *American Journal of Medicine, 106,* 435–440.

Davidson, J.R. & Meltzer-Brody, S.E. (1999). The underrecognition and undertreatment of depression: What is the breadth and depth of the problem? *Journal of Clinical Psychiatry, 60*(Suppl 7), 4–9.

DeYoung, C. & Dickey, B. (1967). Support—Its meaning for psychiatric nurses. *Journal of Psychiatric Nursing, 5,* 46–58.

Dies, R.R. (1986). Practical, theoretical, and empirical foundations for group psychotherapy. In A.J. Frances & R. E. Hales (Eds.), *The American Psychiatric Association annual review, volume 5.* Washington, DC: American Psychiatric Press.

_____. (1979). Group psychotherapy: Reflections on three decades of research. *Journal of Applied Behavioral Science, 15,* 361–373.

Ellgring, J.H. (1999). Depression, psychosis, and dementia: Impact on the family. *Neurology, 52,* S17–S20.

Jonsdottir, H. (1998). Life patterns of people with chronic obstructive pulmonary disease: Isolation and being closed in. *Nursing Science Quarterly, 11,* 160–166.

Kaul, T.J. & Bednar, R.L. (1986). Experiential group research: Results, questions, and suggestions. In S.L. Garfield & A.E. Bergin (Eds.), *Handbook of psychotherapy and behavior change.* New York, NY: John Wiley.

Krafft, S.K. & Krafft, L.J. (1998). Chronic sorrow: Parents' lived experience. *Holistic Nursing Practice, 13,* 59–67.

Lepore, S.J. (1998). Problems and prospects for the social support-reactivity hypothesis. *Annals of Behavioral Medicine, 20,* 257–269.

Orlinsky, D.E. & Howard, K.I. (1986). Process and outcome in psychotherapy. In S.L. Garfield & A.E. Bergin (Eds.), *Handbook of psychotherapy and behavior change.* New York, NY: John Wiley.

Sampson, E.E. & Marthas, M. (1981). *Group process for the health professions.* New York, NY: John Wiley & Sons.

Stanley, A.H. (1999). Primary care and addiction treatment: Lessons learned from building bridges across traditions. *Journal of Addictive Diseases, 18,* 65–82.

van Servellen, G.M. (1984). *Group and family therapy: A model for psychotherapeutic nursing practice.* St. Louis, MO: Mosby.

POSTSCRIPT

It has been over 100 years since Lillian Wald coined the term *public health nurse*. It seems fitting that we "wrap up" this 3rd edition of *Community As Partner* with an editorial inspired by Ms. Wald's work in New York City at the turn of the last century.

We fervently hope that such an editorial will not need to be written (or recalled) at the conclusion of the next millennium.

▮ A CALL FOR TRANSFORMATION

Standing in the room where Lillian Wald once lived at Henry Street was an inspiring experience. More than 100 attendees at the American Public Health Association's annual meeting in New York came together to hear Clair Coss read her play about the woman who coined the term "public health nurse" and then visit the historic Henry Street Settlement. Each of us reflected on what public health nursing was in those early days: comprehensive health and illness care that embodied social reform and political involvement.

What happened to this once-glorious group that picketed against war, fought for the rights of women and children, aided the immigrant, initiated school health programs, and saw to it that the poor and disenfranchised received a fair wage and access to health care? In 1920 the public health nurse was described as ". . . one of the very greatest agents in the advancement of health, both individual and public, in this country".[1] These early professionals accomplished the goals of reducing mortality and morbidity so well that they became a threat to those in power. One of the strongest opponents of home visiting was the American Medical Association (AMA), which successfully fought against federally financed public health programs. In 1930 the AMA condemned such programs as ". . . unsound in policy, wasteful and extrav-

Continued

agant, unproductive of results and tending to promote communism. . . ."[2] In addition, health became a medical concern and, as a result, health problems were depoliticized. Those problems rooted in social disarray were reduced to individual, biologic, or situational factors, and the focus became the individual. Even the sacrosanct home visit became limited to the care of a medically diagnosed problem in order to carry out medically prescribed activities. Funding of programs outside the hospital was predicated on stamping out disease (always with medical prescription to back it up). Other funding was aimed at specific problems, so that we had (and still have) immunization clinics, Women, Infants, and Children programs, sexually transmitted disease clinics, and the like. But the community is not a series of fragmented risk groups. It is a collection of people who want and deserve comprehensive nursing care: primary health care given distributively whether the people are sick or well. The district nurses did that in the early part of this century. Where are they now?

Now is the time to end our focus on fragmented programs and to return to our raison d'etre, the improvement of health: not health as an end, but as a means to a full life. Health cannot occur when the means of achieving a living wage are controlled by a small minority; when agencies charged with maintaining and improving a safe environment are influenced by the polluters they are supposed to police; when the whole structure is predicated on health as a commodity to be doled out to the "deserving" (insured) by a group whose primary mission is to cure disease; when violence, from child abuse to war, is tolerated; when age defines usefulness and is given as a reason to withhold care and treatment; and when a majority of the population is relegated to second-class status because of gender, race, or ethnicity.

Public health nurses can transform our fragmented, disease-oriented "system," not by bemoaning the loss of our glorious past, but by looking to the future, by focusing on a goal and the strategies to achieve it. Health for all through primary health care means that the nurses first ask the people what they want to improve their health and then take the responsibility to work as partners with them to achieve it (empowerment). This means working with others, not just the health team, but community groups, business and education leaders, politicians, engineers, and others to overcome inequities.

Public health nurses in the model of Lillian Wald can make a difference. Let us begin immediately either to change our public health care system (now in "disarray"[3]) or forge out on our own as Ms. Wald did, get our own financing, and deliver district nursing as it should be. We know we can reduce mortality and morbidity as she did; our research has demonstrated this. What we need is a galvanizing force to do so. Our challenge is this: Join with the community to transform an unjust and failing health care system to one that reflects health for *all*, the legacy of Lillian Wald.

ELIZABETH T. ANDERSON, DR.P.H., R.N., F.A.A.N.
GALVESTON, TX

REFERENCES

1. Welch, W.H. (1920). *Papers and addresses*, Vol III (p. 165). Baltimore, Johns Hopkins University Press.

2. Donahue, M.P. (1985). *Nursing: the finest art* (p. 339). St. Louis: C.V. Mosby.
3. Committee for the Study of the Future of Public Health, Division of Health Care Services, Institute of Medicine. (1988). *The future of public health* (p. 19). Washington, DC: National Academy Press.

Source: Anderson, E.T. (1991). Editorial: A call for transformation. *Public Health Nursing, 8*(1), pp. 1–2.

A MODEL ASSESSMENT GUIDE FOR NURSING IN INDUSTRY

A

Components	Questions to Ask
The Company	
Historic development	How, why, and by whom was the company founded?
Organizational chart	What is the formal order of the system, and to whom are the health providers responsible?
Company policies	Is there a policy manual? Are the workers aware of existence of the manual?
Length of the work week	How many days a week does the industry operate?
Length of the work time	Are there several shifts? How many breaks? Is there paid vacation?
Sick leave	Is there a clear policy, and do the workers know it?
Safety and fire provisions	Is management aware of situations or substances in the plant that represent a potential danger? Are there organized fire drills? (The Federal Register is the source of information for federal standards and serves as a helpful guide.)
Support services (benefits)	
Insurance programs	Is there a system for health insurance and life insurance, and is it compulsory? Does the company pay all or part? Who fills out the necessary forms?
Retirement program	Are the benefits realistic?
Educational support	Can the workers further their education? Will the company help financially?
Safety committee	If there is no committee, do certain people routinely handle emergencies? The Red Cross First Aid Course through programmed instruction is excellent (for information consult your local Red Cross).
Recreation committee	Do the workers have any communication with or interest in each other outside the work setting?
Employee relations	Are there problems in employee relations? (This is difficult information to get, but it is important to get a sense of how employees feel generally about management and vice versa.)

Components	Questions to Ask
The Plant	
General physical setting	What is the overall appearance?
The construction	What is the size and general condition of buildings and grounds?
Parking facilities and public transportation stops	How far does the worker have to walk to get inside?
Entrances and exits	How many people must use them? How accessible are they?
Physical environment	What conditions exist in the physical environment? (Comment on heating, air-conditioning, lighting, glare, drafts, and so forth.)
Communication facilities	Are there bulletin boards and newsletters?
Housekeeping	Is the physical setting maintained adequately?
Interior decoration	Are the surrounding conducive to work? Are they pleasing?
Work areas	
Space	Are workers isolated or crowded?
Heights: workplace and supply areas	Is there a chance of workers falling or being injured by falling objects? (Falls and falling objects are dangerous and costly to industry.)
Stimulation	Is the worker too bored to pay attention?
Safety signs and markings	Are dangerous areas well marked?
Standing and sitting facilities	Are chairs safe and comfortable? Are there platforms to stand on, especially for wet processes?
Safety equipment	Do the workers make use of hard hats, safety glasses, face masks, radiation badges, and so forth? Do they know the safety devices that the OSHA regulations require?
Nonwork areas	
Lockers	If the work is dirty, workers should be able to change clothes. Are they accidentally carrying toxic substances home on their clothes?
Hand-washing facilities	If facilities and supplies are available, do workers know how and when to wash their hands?
Rest rooms	How accessible are they, and what condition are they in?
Drinking water	Can workers leave their jobs long enough to get a drink of water when they want to?
Recreation and rest facilities	Can a worker who is not feeling well lie down? Do workers feel free to use the facilities?
Telephones	Can a worker receive or make a call? Does a working mother have to stay home for a call because she can't be reached at work?
Ashtrays	Are people allowed to smoke in designated areas? Are they safe areas?
The Working Population: Include worker and management, but separate data for comparison.	
General characteristics	(Be as accurate as possible, but estimate when necessary.)
Total number of employees	(Usually, if an industry has 500 or more employees, full-time nursing services are necessary.)

Components	Questions to Ask
The Working Population: Include worker and management, but separate data for comparison.	
General appearance	Are there records of heights, weights, cleanliness, and so forth? Ask to see them.
Age and sex distribution	What are the proportions of the different groups? (Certain screening programs are specific for young adults, whereas others are more for the elderly. Some programs are more for women; others are more for men.) Is there any difference between day and evening shift populations? Are the problems of the minority sex unattended?
Race distribution	Does one race predominate? How does this compare with the general community?
Socioeconomic distribution	Are there great differences in worker salaries? (This can sometimes cause problems.)
Religious distribution	Does one religion predominate? Are religious holidays observed?
Ethnic distribution	Is there a language barrier?
Marital status	What proportion of the workers are widowed, singles, or divorced? (These groups often have different needs.)
Educational backgrounds	Can all teaching be done at approximately the same level?
Lifestyles practiced	Is there disapproval of certain lifestyles?
Types of employment offered	
Background necessary	What education level is required? Skilled versus unskilled?
Work demands on physical condition	What level of strength is needed? Is the work sedentary or active?
Work status	How many employees work full-time? Part-time? Is there overtime?
Absenteeism	Is there a record kept? By whom? Why?
Causes	What are the five most common reasons for absence?
Length	What are the patterns of absences? (Absenteeism is costly to the employer. There is some difference between one 10-day absence and 10 one-day absences by the same person.)
Physically handicapped	Does the company have a policy about hiring the handicapped?
Number employed	Where do they work? What do they do?
Extent of handicaps	Are they specially trained? Are they in a special program? Do they use prosthetic devices?
Personnel on medication	What medication does each of these employees take? Where does each person work?
Personnel with chronic illness	At what stage of illness is the employee? Where does the employee work? Will he or she be able to continue at this job?
The Industrial Process: What does the company produce and how?	
Equipment used	Is the equipment portable or fixed? light or heavy?
General description of placement	Ask to have each piece of large equipment marked on a scale map.
Type of equipment	Fans, blowers, fast moving, wet, or dry?
Nature of the operation	Ask for a brief description of each stage of the process so that you can compare the needs and abilities of the worker with the needs of the job.

Components	Questions to Ask

The Industrial Process: What does the company produce and how?

Nature of the operation

    Raw materials used — What are they and how dangerous are they? Are they properly stored? Check the *Federal Register* for guidelines on storage.

    Nature of the final product — Can the workers take pride in the final product or do they make parts?

    Description of the jobs — Who does what? Where? (Label the map.)

    Waste products produced — What is the system for waste disposal? Are the pollution-control devices in place and functioning?

Exposure to toxic substances — To which toxins are the workers exposed? What is the extent of exposure? (Include physical and emotional hazards. Remember that chronic effects of industrial exposure are subtle; a person often gets used to having mild symptoms and won't report them. The *Federal Register* contains specifications for exposure to toxins, and some states issue state standards.)

The Health Program: Outline what is actually in existence as well as what employees perceive to be in existence.

Existing policies — Are there informal, unwritten policies?

    Objectives of the program — Are they clear?

    Preemployment physicals — Are they required? Are they paid for by the company? Is the information used to select?

    First aid facilities — What is available? What is not available?

    Standing orders — Is there a company physician who is responsible for first aid or emergency policy? (If so, work closely with him or her in planning nursing services.)

    Job descriptions for health personnel — Are they in writing? (If there are no guidelines to be followed, write some.)

Existing facilities and resources — Sometimes an industry that denies having a healthy program has more of a system than it realizes.

    Trained personnel — Who responds in an emergency?

    Space — Where is the sick worker taken? Where is the emergency equipment kept?

    Supplies — What are they? Where are they kept? (Make a list and describe the condition of each item.)

    Records and reports — What exists? (The OSHA requires that employers keep three types of records: a log of occupational injuries and illnesses, a supplemental record of certain illnesses or injuries, and an annual summary (forms 100, 101, and 102 are provided under the act). Good records provide data for good planning.)

Services rendered in the past year — Describe as specifically as possible.

    Care needed — Chronic or acute? Why?

    Screening done — Where? By whom? Why?

Components	Questions to Ask
The Health Program: Outline what is actually in existence as well as what employees perceive to be in existence.	
Services rendered in the past year	
Referrals made	By whom? To whom? Why?
Counseling done	Formal or informal? (Often informal counseling goes unnoticed.)
Health education	What individual or group education was offered by the company?
Accidents in the past year	During working hours? After hours? (Include those that occur after work hours; some may be directly or indirectly work related.)
Reasons why employees sought health care	What are the five major reasons?
Stressors	
As identified by employees	What pressures are felt on the job?
As identified by health providers	What problems do they perceive?

Adapted from Serafini, P. (1976). Nursing assessment in industry: A model. *American Journal of Public Health, 66*(8), 755–760.

ASSESSMENT OF AN INDUSTRY

Components	Description
The Company	
	The AAB Chemical Company Hampton Industrial Complex Located west of State Highway 519 and Loop 177
Historical development	The AAB Chemical Company separated from the AAB Refinery in 1957, and the present plant was completed in 1961. The parent company is a major oil company with headquarters in Chicago. The plant is today the most complex and versatile in the AAB system.
Organizational chart	A formal organizational chart was not available. However, by observation and interview, a structure consisting of a plant manager, with a supervisor in charge of each production area, safety, and maintenance was noted. There are overseers for each area of operation for each shift. The medical staff, which consists of one doctor and one nurse, are not hired by the plant personnel department but by the parent company in Chicago.
Company policies	The plant operations are never shut down. There are shifts around the clock for operators and craftspeople. Employees such as clerical, administrative, and medical staff work 8-hours days, 40-hour weeks. Breaks are provided during the work period. Employees are eligible for 2 weeks of paid vacation per year after working 1 year. This increases in 5-year increments. A 20-year employee is eligible for 5 weeks of vacation. Employees are eligible for sick leave after 6 months of service. Benefits vary with length of service. All benefits are published in an employee handbook, distributed to all employees.
	Management is well aware of situations and substances that pose danger to the workers. The safety program, run by a safety supervisor and a safety engineer, is extensive. Organized fire drills are held frequently. Procedures for dealing with spills and other hazards are also

Components	Description
The Company	
Company policies	well organized. Fire-fighting equipment and an ambulance are available on the plant site at all times. Certain employees are trained as firefighters. There are EMTs available inside the plant in addition to the nurse. Fire extinguishers are placed throughout the plant in strategic locations.
Support services	A comprehensive medical expense plan is compulsory for all employees. In addition, disability up to 40 weeks owing to occupational illness or injury is provided to all employees regardless of length of service. Term life insurance under a group plan is available at a low rate. A long-term disability plan is available to employees covered under the basic life insurance plan. A retirement plan is provided at complete cost to the company. A savings plan in which employees may invest in company stock and US Savings Bonds is also available.
	Employees are offered an educational assistance program and are encouraged to advance their careers. On-line-job training is provided to help employees advance.
Employee relations	The workers are affiliated with the Oil, Chemical and Atomic Workers International Union, a part of the AFL-CIO. It was difficult to perceive how management and labor relate to each other. However, several workers mentioned the familylike atmosphere among employees, and hopefully, this bridges the gap between labor and management. The last strike occurred approximately 2 years ago.
The Plant	
General physical setting	The appearance of the plant is best described as an intimidating maze of pipes, towers, and vessels. The main building, in which the clinic is located, is modern and attractive, with well-tended grounds. Ample parking is available, with areas provided for the handicapped. The building is air conditioned, spacious, and clean, with a pleasing interior.
	The grounds and buildings inside the plant are also neat and will maintained. Scattered through the plant in strategic locations are eye-bubbling devices for flushing the eyes and showers for removing irritants from the skin. Danger areas are clearly marked with yellow paint and warning signs. Employees working in areas where hydrofluoric acid is used are provided with complete protective covering, and they shower immediately upon leaving the area. Earplugs and earmuffs are required in high-noise areas. Compliance in use of safety devices is good, and workers are aware of Occupational Safety and Health Administration (OSHA) regulations.
Work areas	Some work areas, especially where craftspeople are involved, are cramped and close, owing to the physical structure of the myriad pipes and lines. Some areas are also elevated in height. One problem noted by the plant nurse is occasional heat stress during summer months when employees are working in these areas on equipment that reflects heat. Another problem noted was the stress, manifested in muscle and joint discomfort, of working in cramped quarters, especially when employees work a lot of overtime. Occasionally employees are injured by falling objects, such as heavy wrenches. Burns are the most common

Components	Description
The Plant	
Work areas	type of injuries. Operators who work in the processing units and monitor the gauges and flow rates are in stressful jobs because a mistake could be costly and dangerous.
Nonwork areas	Each work area has a kitchen area, restrooms, and water fountains that are easily accessible. Lockers and showers are also available. Communication by phone is possible in all areas of the plant. Facilities are available in the clinic so that workers who are ill may lie down. However, in some areas, repeated visits to the clinic are discouraged. Employees are instructed regarding handwashing and prompt attention to small wounds by the nurse as part of new employee orientation. Smoking is permitted only in specifically designated parts of the fenced area of the plant, the docks, and warehouses.
The Working Population	
General characteristics	AAB Chemicals employs approximately 500 people. Age and sex distribution data were not available. However, the plant nurse stated that employees range in age from age 18 to retirement at age 65, and that male employees outnumber female employees. The nurse also stated that some women were moving into previously male-dominated jobs. Race distribution data were not available. By observation, the distribution appeared to be predominantly white, followed by black and then Hispanic employees, which is in line with the population distribution in the community. Data regarding religious and marital status were not available. Wages and salaries are commensurate with education, qualifications, and years of service. Educational backgrounds range from high school graduates to advanced degrees in engineering and the sciences. Therefore, health teaching must be geared to match the educational level of the group being instructed.
Type of employment offered	Types of employment include skilled craftspeople, operators, lab analysts, chemists, engineers, clerical and administrative personnel, and a nurse and a physician. The background required for each area varies with the complexity and nature of the job. Most employees are full-time and work overtime as required.
Absenteeism	Records of absences are kept in the employee's work unit. The nurse keeps records on illness- or injury-related absences. An employee who has been absent owing to an extended or serious illness, an injury, or surgery must report to the medical department before returning to work and must supply a statement from a doctor regarding the nature of his or her disability and the limitations, if any, on permissible work. The medical department then determines the physical condition of the employee and notifies his or her supervisor regarding the employee's return to work. Strict record keeping also is done for OSHA requirements. According to the nurse, the most common reasons for absence are not occupationally related. They are most often for upper-respiratory infections and other common health problems or for accidents that occurred away from the plant.
Physically handicapped	The AAB Company is an equal opportunity employer. Information regarding handicapped employees, the nature of their handicaps, and the jobs they fill was not available.

Components	Description
The Working Population Personnel on medication Personnel with chronic illness	The nurse keeps records of employees on medication. This information is confidential. The confidentiality of employees' medical records is strictly enforced.
The Industrial Process Equipment used Nature of the plant operation	The basic job of the plant is to produce specialty chemicals and petrochemical intermediates for manufacture of products that range from boats and surfboards to carpets and furniture. Production of these chemicals involves moving raw materials (called "feedstock") from AAB's Hampton Refinery and another chemical plant and mixing them with xylenes and benzenes. Some of the chemicals produced are propylene, styrene, paraxylene, metazylene, aromatic solvents, oil-recovering chemicals, oil-producing chemicals, and polybutenes. The equipment used involves miles of pipes and many towers and vessels. Process units are designed to be energy efficient, and in many instances, energy-producing hydrocarbons are a by-product of a process. These are then recovered and used as fuel in other operations.
	Flammability and danger of explosion are major concerns when dealing with the above-named chemicals. Proper storage is essential and is carried out with care in this plant.
	The final product of the production process is barrels of chemicals. Workers take pride in turning out a certain number of barrels in a time period and in keeping the plant operating efficiently.
	The treatment of wastewater is through an effluent water-control system that is one of the most sophisticated in the industry. the facility handles wastewater not only from AAB Chemical but also from the AAB Refinery and another chemical plant in the area. Air-pollution control is done in two steps: first by eliminating potential contaminants whenever possible and then through the use of devices such as scrubbers, filters, cyclone separators, and a flare system to burn up the waste hydrocarbons.
Exposure to toxic substances	The major substances of concern are benzene and xylene. Benzene is a colorless, flammable, volatile liquid. The major hazard with this chemical is chronic poisoning by inhalation of small amounts over a long time. It is one of the most dangerous organic solvents in common use. Benzene acts primarily on the blood-forming organs. Skin contact also is to be avoided. Benzene is suspected of being carcinogenic. Xylene resembles benzene in many chemical and physical properties but is not involved in causing chronic blood diseases. It has a narcotic effect and can cause dermatitis with repeated contact. Benzene screening is done on all employees on a yearly basis.
The Health Program Existing policies	The objectives of the program are to monitor the status of each employee's health in order to pinpoint problems at an early stage and to provide prompt attention to accidents or emergencies as they occur at the worksite. The employees perceive the second objective more readily than the first. Many of them perceive the yearly physicals as a low priority.

Components	Description
The Health Program	
Existing policies	Preemployment physicals are done by the nurse and company doctor at no charge to the client and are used as a baseline for future reference.
	The ambulance kept at the plant is equipped for all emergencies. Injured or ill employees requiring more than initial first aid are taken immediately to Jefferson Memorial Hospital.
	There is a set of comprehensive standing orders, written through collaborative effort by the nurse and doctor. Yearly physicals include chest roentgenogram, blood work that includes benzene screening, urinalysis, vision and hearing assessments, and physical exams by the physician. Pregnant women are seen each month by the doctor in addition to their own private doctors. No screening programs alone are done, but they are incorporated into the yearly physical. Health teaching and informal counseling are done on an individual basis by the nurse and doctor.
	CPR is taught to selected personnel throughout the plant by the nurse.
Existing facilities and resources	The medical department consists of one full-time nurse and a physician who cover this plant and AAB's larger plant near Avina, as well as a part-time secretary. The facilities include the nurse's office, where all medical records are kept and where employees check in when visiting the clinic; a treatment room; a small lab and dispensary; a roentgenogram room; an exam room; and the physician's office. First aid facilities are extensive and well supplied. ECG equipment also is available. The nurse sees between 12 and 15 clients per day in the clinic. The major reasons employees seek health care are nonoccupationally related sicknesses or accidents, stress-related complaints, and minor accidents on the job.
Stressors	
Employees	Job pressure, as with operators who control the process units
	Overtime hours, when worked frequently
	Knowledge of potential fire or explosion
	Shift work that may not be in sync with normal body rhythms
	Strikes or layoffs
Health care providers	Problems with role definition. Nurse wishes to do more health teaching but feels Safety Department has taken over many of her functions. Feels powerless to change the situation. Feels that physician also perceives her role as limited to specific, traditional areas.

Index

Page numbers followed by *f* refer to figures; page numbers followed by *t* refer to tables; page numbers followed by *b* refer to boxes.

A

B

C